SURVIVING THE AIDS PLAGUE

Taki N. Anagnoston, M.D.
Obstetrician - Gynecologist

Copyright © 1991 by Taki N. Anagnoston, M.D.

All rights reserved. Printed in the United States of America. No part of this book, either in part or in whole may be reproduced, transmitted or utilized in any form or by any means, electronic, photographic or mechanical, including photocopying, recording, or by any information storage and retrieval system without permission in writing from the Publisher, except for brief quotations embodied in literary articles and reviews.

For permissions, or serializations, condensations, adaptions, or for our catalog of other publications, write the Publisher at the address below.

Library of Congress Cataloging-in-Publication Data

Anagnoston, Taki N., 1931-
    Surviving the AIDS Plague / Taki N. Anagnoston.
      p.   cm.
    Includes index.
    ISBN 0-922356-44-0
    1. AIDS (Disease) – Popular Works. I. Title.
    [DNLM: 1. Acquired Immunodeficiency Syndrome.
    WD 308 A532s]
  RC607.A26A47 1991
  616.97'92 – dc20
  DNLM/DLC
  for Library of Congress   91-26126
                                                                      CIP

Published by
AMERICA WEST PUBLISHERS
P.O. Box 986
Tehachapi, CA 93581
1-805 822-9655

Printed in the United States of America
10 9 8 7 6 5 4 3 2 1

"In the following pages I offer nothing more than simple facts, plain arguments and common sense."

– Thomas Paine

DEDICATION

I would like to dedicate this book to my lovely wife,
Kathleen,
who provided much appreciated encouragement and support,
as well as endless hours of proofreading
and critique of the book.

ACKNOWLEDGMENT

Many people contributed their time and expertise to the completion of this manuscript. Pat Anderson, Joseph McCormack, M.D., Frank Orrell, and Joseph Barbara, M.D. read the manuscript and gave me invaluable input and suggestions. Dr. McCormack also provided the two pieces of artwork included in this book. I sincerely thank the above people for their time and interest.

My special thanks to John L. King, Ph.D., who guided me through much of the publication process and provided invaluable information as to the economics of AIDS. His suggestions and recommendations have been irreplaceable.

And finally, to the production staff, I would like to thank Janet Silva, who typed the manuscript, Carla Hewitt who edited and computer formatted the book for publication, Chris I. Stuker, who helped with the graphics and designed the cover of this book and Larry Isenhart who helped prepare the book for its second printing...

TABLE OF CONTENTS

PROLOGUE
"THE SECRET"

CHAPTER I
TRUISMS OF AIDS 1

CHAPTER II
AIDS TODAY 11

CHAPTER III
WHAT IS AIDS? 27

CHAPTER IV
MAN'S FUTURE: AIDS CURE OR EXTINCTION? 55

CHAPTER V
**RISK OF AIDS/
PRECAUTIONS TO TAKE TO PROTECT YOURSELF** 65

CHAPTER VI
POTPOURRI OF AIDS: Part I 73

CHAPTER VII
POTPOURRI OF AIDS: Part II 129

CHAPTER VIII
POTPOURRI OF AIDS: Part III 185

CHAPTER IX
**REFLECTIONS, COMMENTS AND OPINIONS
OF AN OBSTETRICIAN & GYNECOLOGIST** 223

CHAPTER X
RADIO QUESTIONS AND ANSWERS 241

CHAPTER XI
THE FINAL CHAPTER: AUTHOR'S CRITICS ANSWERED 293

"HAPPINESS USA REVISITED" 1995   317
DEFINITIONS   329
FOOTNOTES   333
AUTHOR'S MESSAGE TO THE READERS 1989   335
AUTHOR'S MESSAGE TO THE READERS 1991   337

THE BIBLICAL "END TIMES" JUST AHEAD?

The New Testament

There is growing evidence that the prophecies of Jesus the Christ of Troubled Times and the Millennium correspond to prophecies made by Tibetians, Egyptians, and others:

Then He said unto them, "Nation shall rise against nation,
and kingdom against kingdom
And great earthquakes shall be in diverse places,
and famines and pestilences; and fearful sights
and great signs shall there be from heaven.
For these be the days of vengeance.
For there shall be great distress in the land
and there shall be signs in the
sun, and in the moon, the sea and the waves roaring.
Men's hearts failing them for fear of those things coming
on the earth! For the powers of heaven shall be shaken.

Luke 21: 10-11, 22, 25-26

PROLOGUE
"THE SECRET"

Jack Well and Jill Healthy both lived in the little town of Happiness, U.S.A. and were deeply in love. Jack, a Harvard graduate, was 28 years old and had just started a private law practice. Jill was 22 years old, had also just graduated from college and was working as an elementary school teacher. After a short but romantic courtship, Jack and Jill agreed to marry.

After getting their mandatory blood tests for syphilis and German measles, they got their marriage license and were promptly married.

Their wedding was in a quaint, lovely church, filled with flowers and people. At the reception, Jack and Jill were hugging, kissing and dancing with each other and with as many well wishers as possible throughout the day. There was no shortage of food, spirits, music, laughing or toasting throughout the festivities. At the end of this long and memorable day, Jack and Jill excitedly departed for their honeymoon and the exhausted people, thankfully, to their homes. What a lovely, happy day for everybody!

Soon after the wedding, Mr. and Mrs. Well had settled into their new home and new routine of married life. After a few months, as luck would have it, Jill missed a menstrual period and shortly began having symptoms suggesting pregnancy (nausea, vomiting, breast tenderness and tiredness). A home pregnancy test was quickly done and, sure enough, it showed Jill was pregnant. Both Jack and Jill were delighted. Their happiness was magnified many times over: A new home, new careers, a marriage made in heaven, and now, a new baby – how could two people be so lucky?

After several weeks, Jill made an appointment with the town's most prestigious obstetrician, I. M. Smart, M.D. The Wells wanted nothing but the best for their baby. He thoroughly examined Jill, confirmed her pregnancy, and started her prenatal care. The routine prenatal laboratory work and medication was ordered. Jill was ecstatic. She announced this wonderful news to her husband, relatives, friends – anybody who would listen. She quickly and excitedly bought her maternity clothes and began preparing and planning for her baby. Jack was as proud as he could be; why not, he had fathered a child. He proved to himself and to the world, he was a MAN. Both could hardly wait until the baby was born.

For a few months, everything went just fine, but then Jill began to notice weight loss instead of weight gain and drenching night sweats. She felt exhausted most of the time and fatigued very easily. Dr. Smart told Jill, "Don't worry, these symptoms are all part of being pregnant. You'll be just fine." Instead, Jill's general condition worsened. She began having nausea and vomiting, diarrhea, loss of appetite and a host of other disturbing signs and symptoms. Finally Jack went to Dr. Smart and told him he was really worried about Jill. "Doctor," he said, "Jill doesn't act like, let alone look like, the woman I married. Something terrible is wrong and I want you to do everything you can to find out what it is!"

Dr. Smart then re-examined Jill very carefully. Now, he too noticed her sickly appearance and became alarmed. What was wrong? A battery of laboratory tests and chest X-rays followed, all essentially normal. After consultation with some of his colleagues, more tests followed. Again, all tests were normal. Jill's condition worsened and Dr Smart's concern for Jill increased. One night Dr. Smart happened to watch a TV documentary on the new disease, AIDS. He thought, "Could Jill have this disease? It sounds ridiculous, but Jill's signs and symptoms are much the same as reported in this program." So with nothing to lose and everything to gain, Dr. Smart obtained an AIDS test on Jill in the next few days.

When the results of the test came back positive, Dr. Smart was flabbergasted. He quickly called Jill in for a conference, where he told her she had AIDS. Jill became hysterical. She screamed, "This is impossible! It's a lie! It can't be! Jack is not a homosexual and I am not a lesbian. We have never used drugs nor have we ever had a blood transfusion. Both of us always used condoms in college with others and with each other. Doctor, you're crazy! I DO NOT HAVE AIDS! Jack and I did everything the AIDS experts said to do, not to get AIDS; so how is it possible for me to get infected by

Prologue

the AIDS virus? How can you be so cruel as to tell me this lie!"

Dr. Smart was upset, bewildered and apologetic. All he could say was, "I'm sorry, Jill, truly sorry, but the test is positive. I wish I could tell you how you got AIDS, even after you took all of the recommended precautions; but 6% of all AIDS cases are from unknown causes. I suggest you tell Jack as soon as possible – he has the right to know."

Jill hysterically grabbed her purse and coat and stormed out of the doctor's office. Sitting there quietly, Dr. Smart thought, "Oh my God, my staff and patients have all been exposed to the AIDS virus for months and they didn't even know it. Any of them, including me, could now be AIDS infected. What should I do? Who should or can I tell? I never thought I would ever see a person, let alone have a patient, with AIDS." Depressed and upset, Dr. Smart finally left his office.

That night, Jill told Jack the sad news. Jack was beside himself. He yelled, cussed, threw things, rationalized and cried. But nothing changed the situation – his wife was pregnant and AIDS infected. They agreed that night not to tell anybody the terrible news. Why should they? The government says they don't have to, because it would violate Jill's civil rights. In fact, it passed strict laws to help people keep such news confidential. Anyway, this would be their secret – a "personal secret" – that must never be revealed. If word got out that Jill, and maybe Jack, had AIDS, their lives would be changed forever. The most important thing to Jack and Jill now was to maintain their lifestyles, even if it meant accidentally infecting other people with the AIDS virus. The AIDS confidentiality and discriminatory laws the government had implemented will help them keep this horrible secret. Both Jill and Jack promptly and emphatically instructed Dr. Smart not to tell anybody Jill had AIDS. With mixed emotions, Dr. Smart reluctantly agreed to abide by their wishes – **what else could he do?**

Dr. Smart was eventually successful in convincing Jack to have an AIDS test. When it too came back positive, all of the problems for all the parties involved were multiplied. "What a terrible situation," thought Dr. Smart. "Both Jill and Jack have AIDS and I can't tell anybody, because if I do, I can be sued for everything I own for breach of confidentiality. How in the world and why did all this happen? AIDS is a problem for other people, not for people in Happiness, U.S.A." Anyway, Dr. Smart decided to make the best of a bad situation and tried to keep Jill from infecting as few people as possible, while he continued her obstetrical care.

As the months rolled by, life for the "happy" couple appeared as normal as could be, at least during the day. Jill continued to teach school and her pregnancy progressed without problems. Jack's law practice was growing better than expected, as was his reputation. Both met their social responsibilities and obligations without apparent difficulties.

At night, however, this facade of a happy, trouble-free life changed to one of misery, grief, terror and loneliness. Night after night, Jack and Jill tried to convince each other that their little secret wasn't hurting anybody and that the AIDS disease would somehow go away and would not change their plans for a long and good life. Why should it? Nobody they knew ever got infected by the AIDS virus and died, so why should they? The AIDS disease is for perverts, homosexuals and drug addicts – not for clean-cut, law-abiding, religious people like them.

One night, when Jill was seven months pregnant, Jack awoke to find her unconscious on the bathroom floor. She was in shock and lying in a large pool of her own blood. Frantically, Jack ran to the telephone and dialed 911 for an ambulance. Within minutes, the paramedics were on the scene and trying to save Jill's life. One paramedic was giving Jill mouth-to-mouth resuscitation while the other was giving her intravenous fluids. Once Jill's condition was stable for transport, the paramedics rushed her to the nearest hospital, State-Of-The-Art Community Hospital.

When the blood-covered paramedics delivered Jill to the emergency room, Dr. Smart was immediately called. Meanwhile, the doctors and nurses on duty continued Jill's emergency care. Emergency laboratory tests were immediately done (except one of the most important ones – the AIDS test), many blood transfusions were given, and ventilators and cardiac monitors were attached and activated – all in hopes of saving both Jill and her baby. In spite of all this care, however, Jill again began to hemorrhage and her general condition deteriorated. Now, both mother and baby were in great danger and near death.

Since Dr. Smart was still not on the scene, the doctors present decided not to wait and rushed Jill to surgery for an immediate Cesarean section. They felt that if there was any more delay, both Jill and the baby could be lost. So far, nobody knew or even suspected Jill had AIDS. Because the hospital had no AIDS policy and because the AIDS-uninformed emergency room staff minimized the AIDS danger, few AIDS precautions were followed during Jill's emergency care.

In any event, as the general anesthetic was given, Jill coughed and vomited all over the anesthesiologist's face and lap. The surgeon and assistant surgeon hurriedly entered Jill's abdomen and then opened her uterus. The limp, premature small baby boy was delivered and quickly handed to the pediatricians for resuscitation. The entire surgical team of doctors and nurses worked feverishly over both Jill and the baby until both were out of immediate danger.

The cause of Jill's hemorrhaging was bleeding from the placenta (afterbirth) of the baby, the official diagnosis being "hemorrhage from placenta previa." When the operation was completed, the doctors and nurses were exhausted and literally covered with Jill's blood, as were the surgical equipment, drapes and floor. Amniotic fluid from the gestational sac, as well as vernix from the baby, was also noted everywhere. During the operation, one of the surgeons accidently stuck his finger with a contaminated needle and several others tore their rubber gloves. After Jill and her baby were saved and out of danger, everybody felt good for a job well done.

When Dr. Smart finally arrived, Jill was in her semi-private postpartum room, resting quietly. Her roommate, who earlier delivered a beautiful set of identical twins, showered Jill with words of congratulations and encouragement. Baby Well was in the pediatric intensive care nursery with four other newborn babies. There, a team of pediatricians and nurses were successfully administering further medical care. Dr. Smart explained he was detained by a traffic accident and thanked everybody for their prompt and excellent medical care of Jill and baby during his absence. After satisfying himself that his two patients were out of danger, Dr. Smart went to the library to do some serious thinking.

"What should I do," he thought. "Nobody in the hospital knows that Jill, and probably Baby Well, have AIDS. Should I, or can I, inform everybody who came into contact with Jill or her baby about Jill's AIDS infection – the paramedics, the hospital emergency room staff, the surgical team, the postpartum ward patients and staff, or the newborn nursery babies and staff? Who else? Housekeepers? Engineers? Oh my God, everybody in the hospital should probably know, so they can take some kind of precautionary measures and get tested for the AIDS infection. But I dare not tell anyone, unless Jill and Jack authorize me to do so. I know they won't because they feel Jill's rights will be violated.

"But what about the rights of the people who worked so hard to help Jill and her baby live, and all the while were unknowingly being exposed to the 100% lethal AIDS virus? How unfair to all these poor innocent people! How can the government allow the rights of the many AIDS free people be trampled upon by the rights of the fewer AIDS infected people? How many other "Jack and Jill secrets" are out there – two, ten, one hundred, more? This "secrecy policy" is insane and inhuman. I never realized how ridiculous and unfair all this human or civil rights, confidentiality and discrimination talk is, when addressing the killer virus, AIDS. AIDS is a deadly medical disease, not a political issue. Something must be done to make everybody understand this!" Disgusted, frustrated and depressed, Dr. Smart left the hospital.

Six months later, Jill died of her AIDS disease. Both Baby Well and Jack were AIDS sick and dying. Dr. Smart eventually quit practicing medicine, because he feared becoming AIDS infected himself and because he was ashamed of both himself and his medical profession for allowing the politicians to interfere with the proper management of the AIDS virus and disease. "The medical profession should never have tolerated anybody to play with people's lives," including himself, he thought.

One of the paramedics, several of the doctors, several of the nurses and one laboratory technician (all who worked on Jill when she came to the hospital, hemorrhaging and in shock) became AIDS infected. One of the pediatricians and one of the nurses, who worked on Baby Well, also got AIDS infected. The many people, who had had contact with Jill, Jack or Baby Well, were terrified they might be or become AIDS infected. In short, Jack and Jill's horrible secret adversely affected the lives of many innocent people.

Within one year, the lawsuits started to surface. Jack sued Dr. Smart for breech of confidentiality, because the whole town knew Jill had died of AIDS and that both he and his baby were also AIDS infected. Most of the people who became AIDS infected from Jill's emergency care sued Jack and/or Dr. Smart for not informing them they were working on a patient who was AIDS infected. They felt their civil/human rights were violated, in order to protect Jill and Jack's same rights. The hospital was also named in these lawsuits, because it had no AIDS policy to protect its medical staff, employees, patients or visitors from the dreaded AIDS virus. Now, it was the lawyers' turn to jump into this saga of insanity, misery and death and complicate the situation further. Everyone involved will now have to relive these unfortunate events over and over, until everything is settled. Is there no end to this insanity and misery?

Several years after Jill's death, the AIDS infection had reached the plague stage in Happiness, U.S.A. As the days passed, more and more people became AIDS infected, AIDS sick or AIDS dead. The death toll from the AIDS disease reached and surpassed unbelievable levels. The graveyards were full and the crematory was working overtime. Terror, misery, fear, suspicion and horror filled the hearts of the people of Happiness, U.S.A.

Gone are the nonsensical cries of discrimination, unfairness or civil rights when it comes to the AIDS disease. Other "personal secrets" like Jack and Jill's were sooner or later revealed. Such "secrets" were finally made illegal, and when found, the parties involved were severely punished. Now the people wanted revenge and demanded punishment for the perpetrators of any AIDS deception and those minimizing the real AIDS dangers. The AIDS virus proved that it is a virulent killer, without vaccine or cure. Now, most people know it infects and kills anybody, anytime, anyplace. Life for the citizens of Happiness, U.S.A. had now changed forever. If a cure for AIDS is not found, life itself will surely cease to exist. **What a terrible price many innocent, unsuspecting people have** *paid and will pay for secrets like Jack and Jill's "personal secret."*

Author's Comment: This very real, fictional story could not only happen in any town or city in the United States, but in any country in the world. Because of the adverse influence of various self-interest groups, the inaction of the medical profession and the insane AIDS policies of our government, such stories will soon be both real (instead of fictional) and commonplace. Unfortunately, mankind will once again prove that he does not learn from his past mistakes.

The purpose of this book is to try and help people understand and survive the AIDS problem. Today, most people do not believe the world in general, and our country in particular, is threatened by the AIDS virus. As a result, most people are complacent, uninformed, and unconcerned about the present AIDS threat. As millions of Americans become AIDS-infected, AIDS-sick, and AIDS-dead, and as the plague continues to worsen worldwide, all people will come to fear AIDS for what it possibly is: **The Final Plague.**

I wrote this book as I see it, from the eyes of a practicing obstetrician/gynecologist. I strongly believe AIDS is now mankind's greatest and most immediate threat/enemy. Also, I feel few in the medical profession and government are leveling with the people and telling them the real seriousness and danger of the ever worsening AIDS plague. Since I am a full-time practicing physician and since both I and my patients are at great risk for the AIDS infection, I felt people would read a book I wrote on AIDS and, hopefully, evaluate and heed its information, warnings, and messages. Being on the battlefield or grass roots of medical care, I see the growing "fear of AIDS" people have, including patients, doctors, nurses, and dentists. People are scared, really scared, and this "fear of AIDS" has led most of them to not want to face the issue. Why should they? It's too frightening, too threatening, too horrible to even think about, let alone read about. Many people think if they ignore or minimize the AIDS disease, it will go away or, at least, it won't affect them or their loved ones. As the old saying goes, **"ignorance is bliss."** All this, I know is true, because I see and hear it every day – in the office, in the hospital, and in the community.

Since the topic of AIDS is too depressing and frightening for most people, I knew I had to approach this unpleasant subject from many directions. So, I have written this book in such a manner.

By using relevant historical information and present day articles, reports, and other information (as well as my own comments and opinions), I hope I have made this unpleasant subject informative, interesting, provocative, and controversial.

Hopefully, one of these many directions will entice readers to read part, if not all, of the book. Once read, I feel the reader will have a better understanding of the AIDS disease and its problems and, most important, a little better chance of surviving the AIDS threat. If these two goals are accomplished, I feel my reasons for writing the book have been met and the many hours of work to write it (between deliveries and operations) have not been in vain. After all, my work and purpose in life is not only to make people well, but to prevent them from getting sick in the first place. I know this book will help do both.

CHAPTER I
TRUISMS OF AIDS

*For in much wisdom is much grief:
and he that increases knowledge increases sorrow.*
                                    Ecclesiastes 1:18

My purpose for writing this book is to offer people hope, hope from what appears to be a hopeless disease – AIDS. Today, America's people have been lulled into a sense of complacency by misinformation, dysinformation and, often, no information at all about AIDS – both the virus and the disease. As a result, AIDS threatens the lives of all people, and the very existence of our country. I hope to repeatedly inform readers of all aspects of the AIDS virus and disease, at least enough to help them protect themselves and to hopefully survive.

The following are a few basic truisms about AIDS:

- AIDS (Acquired Immune Deficiency Syndrome) is a disease specific to man, very contagious and almost 100% lethal.
- Human beings appear to have *no immunity against the AIDS virus*.
- AIDS cases are doubling every 10 to 14 months.
- At this time, there is no known cure for AIDS or vaccine for the AIDS virus.
- The AIDS disease is now in the early plague stage, and is worldwide.
- The AIDS plague is threatening the survival of mankind and, in particular, the American people.
- The general public is *AIDS uninformed* and, therefore, more susceptible to the AIDS virus.
- By following recommended precautions, people can reduce their chances of becoming AIDS infected.

One of the most ominous and least understood characteristics of AIDS disease is the fact that the number of AIDS cases is doubling every 10 to 14 months. Why is this important fact so ominous? Economist Margaret Kennedy states:

> "We tend to believe there is only one type of growth, the growth pattern of nature which we, ourselves, experience and understand. However, there are three generically different patterns:

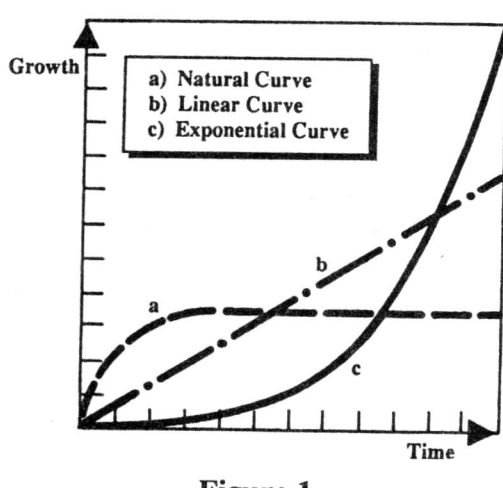

Figure 1

Curve a represents in an idealized form the normal physical growth pattern in nature which our bodies follow as well as that of plants and animals. We grow fairly quickly during the early stages of our lives, then begin to slow down in our teens, and usually stop growing physically when we are about twenty-one. This, however, does not preclude us from growing further – "qualitatively" instead of "quantitatively."

Curve b represents a mechanical or linear growth pattern, e.g. more machines produce more goods, more coal produces more energy, etc. It comes to an end where the machines are stopped or no more coal is added.

Curve c represents an exponential growth pattern which may be described as the exact opposite to **curve a** in that it grows very slowly in the beginning, then continually faster, and finally in an almost vertical fashion. In the physical realm, this growth pattern usually occurs where there is sickness or death. Cancer, for instance, follows an exponential growth pattern. It grows slowly first, although always accelerating, and often by the time it has been discovered, it has entered a growth phase where it cannot be stopped anymore. Exponential growth usually ends with the death of the guest and the organism on which it happens." (1)

Of the above three types of growth patterns, AIDS is following the exponential growth pattern (**curve c**) and this is the primary reason AIDS, if not controlled or eliminated, will prove to be the plague of plagues and the end of mankind. Margaret Kennedy continues:

"Through our bodies we have only experienced the physical growth pattern, of nature which stops at an optimal size (**curve a**). Therefore, it is difficult for human beings to understand the full impact of the exponential growth pattern in the material realm.

This phenomenon can best be demonstrated by the famous story of the Persian Emperor who was so enchanted with a new chess game that he wanted to fulfill any wish the inventor of the game had. This clever mathematician decided to ask for one seed of grain on the first square of the chess board, doubling the amounts on each of the following squares. The emperor, at first happy about such modesty, was soon to discover that the total yield of his entire empire would not be sufficient to fulfill the 'modest' wish. Recently, somebody calculated the amount needed on the 64th square of the chess board: in 1982 it would have been equal to 440 times the yield of grain of the entire planet.

A similar analogy, directly related to our topic, is that one penny invested at the birth of Jesus Christ at 4% interest would have bought in 1750 one ball of gold of the weight of the earth.

In 1990, however, it would buy 8,190 balls of gold. At 5% interest it would have bought one ball of gold already in 1403 and by 1990, it would buy 2,200 billion balls of gold the weight of the earth. The example shows the difference 1% makes over a longer period of time. *It also proves that the continual payment of interest and compound interest is arithmetically, as well as practically, impossible.*" (2)

The alarming point here is that AIDS is not infecting arithmetically (1,2,3,4, etc.), but exponentially (2,4,8,16,32, etc.). This is most important to understand. With this type of growth pattern, AIDS will literally *devastate earth's human population in just a few years*. Some AIDS experts question this rate of growth (100% per year), and state other lesser rates, like 25% or 50% or 75% a year. But even if the growth (infection) rate of AIDS is only 25%, it would take just 2.9 years to double instead of 4 years. In any event, the AIDS growth rate is not 25%, but approximately 100% per year, and it has the growth rate of **curve c** (exponential curve) on Figure 1. It is this elusive compounding growth rate of AIDS that should be understood and feared.

I have heard it said that there are more people alive today than have ever died. "From the beginning of the Christian era, the size of the human population grew gradually for about 16 centuries and then with increasing speed through the nineteenth century. This gradual but progressive acceleration was followed by a sudden steep rise in the twentieth century – a consequence of the scientific-technologic-industrial revolution – which has had the effect of making it possible to sustain a human population far larger than ever before." (See Figure 2) (3)

Whenever a species of life on earth is out of kilter with its environment, as the overpopulation of the human species now is, Mother Nature seems to correct the imbalance – one way or another. The mysterious AIDS virus may be just the vehicle by which mankind's numbers are decreased and controlled, if not eliminated.

The following Gallop Poll was reported by the *San Jose Mercury News,* November 27, 1988, page 15A):

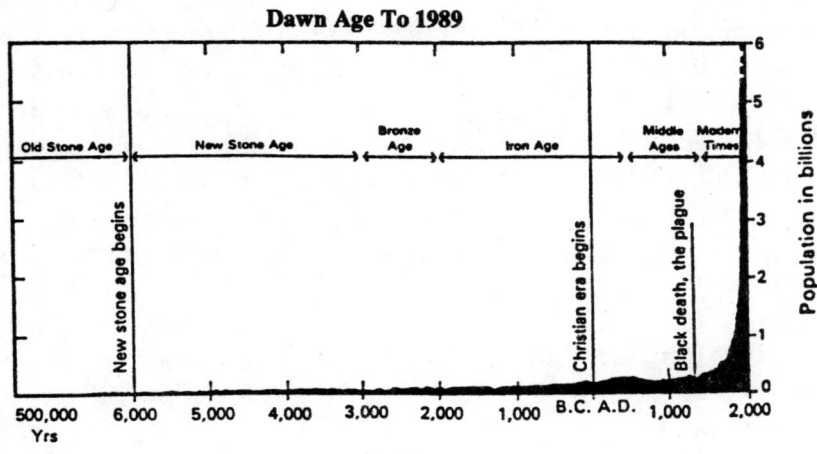

Figure 2

(1) "How concerned are you that you, yourself, will get AIDS – very concerned, a little concerned, not very concerned, or not at all concerned?"

Fear of contracting AIDS	1988	1987
Very concerned	19%	20%
A little concerned	19%	22%
Not very concerned	26%	21%
Not at all concerned	36%	37%

(2) "Do you think it is likely or is not likely that AIDS will eventually become an epidemic for the population at large?"

Epidemic for total population	1988	1987
Likely	69%	51%
Not likely	23%	42%
No opinion	8%	7%

It is interesting and upsetting that the majority (69%) of the polled people think AIDS will become an epidemic for the total population, but only a minority of them (38%) are a little or very concerned about becoming infected by the AIDS virus themselves. In other words, most people polled are assuming AIDS will infect *someone else,* not them. What a false and dangerous assumption this is. The AIDS virus can infect anybody, anytime; it doesn't respect age, sex, race, religion, or anything else. To assume anything about it is sheer folly and could result in many unnecessary deaths.

People must begin educating themselves on how to protect themselves from the AIDS virus. The goals at this time are:

(a) To not get infected by the AIDS virus.
(b) If infected, to stay alive until a cure is found.
(c) To survive financially and socially, in spite of the AIDS plague.

I feel certain (at least I hope) that some people will have a natural resistance to the AIDS virus and will therefore never get infected; it was probably this natural resistance by some people that saved them from the Black Death a few centuries ago. However, I'm afraid this number might be very small. Don't assume you are one of these lucky people!

If one wants to decrease their chances of becoming infected by the AIDS virus, the following precautions are presently recommended:

- Do not have sexual contact with AIDS-sick patients, with members of the high risk groups (sexually active homosexual or bisexual men, present or past abusers of intravenous drugs, prostitutes, or heterosexuals who have had sexual contact with an AIDS infected person), or with people who test positive for the AIDS virus. If you do, use a condom and avoid sexual practices such as anal intercourse, which may injure tissue.
- Do not use intravenous (IV) drugs. If you do, do not share needles.
- Do not have sex with people who use IV drugs.

- Women who are sex partners of AIDS-infected or AIDS-high risk people should consider the risk to their babies before pregnancy. These women should have an HTLV-III (AIDS) antibody test before they get pregnant. If they become pregnant, they should have a test during pregnancy.
- Do not have sex with multiple partners, including prostitutes (who may also be IV drug abusers). The more partners you have, the greater your chances of contracting AIDS.
- Know your sex partners and talk to them about AIDS. Ask the things you need to know. Remember, people may carry the virus and not know they are infected.

The above precautions should help lessen the chances of AIDS infection, *but only help*. As we learn more about the characteristics of the AIDS virus and disease, the more we can do to help protect ourselves. Thus far, education about AIDS and the AIDS virus is the most effective weapon we have to fight with.

IMMUNE SYSTEM

What is the human immune system and what does it do? How does it protect us from disease? These questions are extremely important and complicated. Medicine knows much about man's immune system, but by no means does it know all of it. If all the answers were known, man could protect himself from all diseases and sickness, including AIDS.

Let me simplify all the complicated medical jargon and say our immune system protects us primarily in two ways: by producing antibodies (a protein in the blood produced by the body to neutralize an invading antigen [organism], thus preventing it from hurting our bodies), and by mobilizing white blood cells (specific cells in the blood which seek and destroy an invading organism).

An antigen is a substance to which the body reacts to by producing specific antibodies against it. Many antigens, such as some bacteria and viruses, are detrimental to the very survival of our bodies; therefore, when such antigens are present, our bodies' defense system, the immune system, is activated to protect us. If the body is successful in "neutralizing" (destroying) a particular invading antigen, the specific antibodies produced by the immune system (to destroy the "invader") remain in the blood forever, in case this same antigen re-invades.

If this antigen ever does re-invade the body, these ever-ready, on-guard antibodies quickly seek, attack, and effectively neutralize the antigen. When this situation exists, the person is said to be immune (not susceptible) to that particular antigen.

As an example, Rubella or German measles is a disease caused by a virus (a particular type of antigen). When this antigen invades a human body, the body becomes infected and the disease blossoms. In defense, the victim's immune system is activated and fights the disease by producing specific antibodies and by mobilizing its white blood cells against the antigen (Rubella virus). Once the Rubella virus (antigen) is neutralized and destroyed, the disease is "cured." Thereafter, and most important, the cured victim is immune to Rubella, because the specific Rubella virus fighting or neutralizing antibodies produced will remain and always be on guard. If this Rubella antigen ever re-invades the victim again, these antibodies will attack and neutralize it, thus preventing re-infection.

Knowing the above, then why is AIDS incurable, as it now is? *The reason is that the AIDS virus attacks the very system in man that attacks viruses, the immune system.* It's like a "head to head" battle within the victim's body. Further, the AIDS virus multiplies faster than it is destroyed; thus the AIDS virus becomes stronger as time goes on, because the immune system becomes weaker and less effective. Also complicating this battle within man's body is the fact that other antigens (bacteria, viruses, etc.) continue to invade the victim's body, causing further strain on the body's embattled immune system. Often, these other antigens are successful in causing additional serious diseases (such as pneumonia and cancer), which we call "opportunistic diseases." People who are infected with both the AIDS virus and an opportunistic organism are in the ARC (AIDS Related Complex) stage of the AIDS disease.

Even further complicating this war is the AIDS virus' ability to, almost at will, change its form or mutate into another virulent type or form, which is resistant or safe from any anti-AIDS antibodies already produced by the victim's beleaguered immune system.

This characteristic of the AIDS virus is why a vaccine against it is so highly improbable. Unfortunately, thus far there are no known cases where an AIDS-infected person has survived. The human immune system is proving to be no match for the virulent AIDS virus.

Considering the above, the future looks pretty bleak. However, I don't feel the situation is as hopeless as it sounds for several reasons. As stated previously, I suspect (but of course can't prove) that there are people who are "naturally resistant" to the AIDS virus. Throughout history, people have survived all kinds of life-threatening situations, including plagues. Why did 60% of the people survive the Bubonic plagues years ago? No one really knows, but I suspect it was in part this inherent strength of man – "natural resistance."

In addition, I feel the human body will eventually somehow adapt itself to effectively overcome the AIDS threat. The human body is a complicated and wonderful machine and, thus far, has been able to adjust itself to anything. No doubt about it, the AIDS virus is a formidable foe, but *I'm betting on the former instead of the latter*.

Having stated and expanded on the above truisms, I believe the readers can now proceed with the following material and, hopefully, understand my message and warning – *the AIDS virus is very contagious, almost 100% lethal, and a mystery to mankind*. If we continue to underestimate its ability to spread, infect, and kill; if we continue not to recognize it for what it is, a devastating and worldwide plague; if we continue to protect the AIDS-infected people at the expense of the uninfected people; and if we continue fighting the AIDS virus with our minds closed and our hands tied – *man's very existence on earth is threatened*.

On the other hand, if people recognize the dangers of the AIDS virus and follow what are considered appropriate precautions, the chances of becoming AIDS-infected decrease significantly. Our final goal is to *survive the AIDS threat!*

CHAPTER II
AIDS TODAY

One generation passeth away, and another generation cometh: but the earth abideth forever.
Ecclesiastes 1:4

I recently attended a very good medical meeting on the subject of "Critical Care in OB-GYN" put on by the American College of Obstetrics and Gynecology in San Francisco, California (June 1988). This meeting was very informative and helpful, and attended by well over 200 physicians from many different parts of the world.

But as good as this meeting was, I left appalled! Not once during this three-day conference was AIDS mentioned or addressed by the lecturing physicians. Further distressing was the apparent lack of knowledge or concern by my fellow colleagues.

During several of the brunches and discussion groups, I brought up the topic of "AIDS," hoping to generate some interesting and informative conversations. The only thing I learned was that 99% of the physicians present didn't know much, if anything, about AIDS and their fear of it prevented them from even wanting to discuss or address it. There we were, well-trained OB-GYN specialists, spending three days learning how to save patients from occasional/infrequent critical OB-GYN conditions and completely ignoring AIDS, a highly contagious disease which is infecting and killing thousands of women (pregnant or not) and babies all around us. How ironic! How NEGLIGENT!

I think that the AIDS disease is a horrid plague. It will probably prove itself to be the worst plague ever to afflict mankind. I'm convinced it will kill more human beings than all the people killed by previous plagues *combined!*

Some knowledgeable people believe that AIDS will destroy the entire human race in just a few short decades if a cure and/or vaccine isn't eventually found. More than 5,000 San Franciscans have already died from AIDS thus far – more than all the San Franciscans who died in World War I, World War II, and the Korean/Vietnam wars *combined.*

Accurate worldwide statistics of this disease are unavailable and thus unknown, but the few numbers available are already mind boggling. The reasons why such statistics are unavailable are as follows:

(1) **Communist World.** No reliable statistics are being reported from this area. It is well known that alcoholism, drug abuse, and homosexuality are as high or higher there as they are in other parts of the world. To date, it is fair to assume that AIDS is as much of a problem there as it is elsewhere. To believe the communist countries have no AIDS problem is nonsensical.

(2) **Africa.** Only fragmented statistics are coming out of Africa, and these are questionable. We know the disease is running rampant, but because many African nations have no means of collecting reliable data and others fear damage to their economies, they cannot or do not reveal any HIV-infection statistics. In fact, some countries forbid or discourage their people to even talk or write about AIDS, for a variety of reasons. Also, no accepted accurate system to gather the correct numbers of AIDS cases/deaths has yet been developed. Piecemeal, terrifying information is coming out of Africa:

(a) 40% of the people of Zambia are now reported to be HIV positive (AIDS-infected) and many have the obvious, full-blown AIDS disease. Most of the Zambian army is feared HIV positive. Most of the Zambian copper/cobalt mines (the largest source for these metals in the world) are now closed because AIDS has decimated the work force. This is one of the main reasons why the price of copper and cobalt is now so high in the world markets.

(b) The South African government is now very concerned that AIDS may also force the gold mines, as well as many other types of mines, to reduce or even stop their operations. The resulting decrease of gold and strategic metal production would absolutely ruin the country's economy and force the worldwide market price of these metals to rise to unbelievable heights. Undocumented reports are coming out of this country that the fear of AIDS is so great that the government has made it a crime to openly talk about AIDS.

(c) Sources out of Africa have confirmed that the native population of many areas is now being decimated by AIDS. In some previously overpopulated areas, the forests, vegetation, and animals (crocodiles, fish, birds, etc.) are now coming back, because AIDS has virtually eliminated the people who were originally responsible for their destruction.

(d) Other undocumented sources from Africa, and some AIDS experts, fear the entire native population of Africa will eventually be destroyed by AIDS. The country will then be repopulated by other world peoples, much like what happened in the Western Hemisphere back in the 15th Century.

I disagree with this. New diseases (smallpox, measles, yellow fever, etc.) were brought to the New World by the explorers, which then literally destroyed the native population of the Western World. Thereafter, the New World was repopulated by Old World peoples *who were immune* to those same diseases and thus safe. In the case of AIDS, the people who will supposedly come and repopulate Africa after the natives are exterminated will either be HIV-infected already or will soon become HIV-infected because they too have no immunity to the AIDS virus at all. *The point here is, since AIDS is a new disease to man, all people worldwide are susceptible because they have no im-*

munity to it; therefore no people are safe from infection by the AIDS virus and the disease/problems it causes.

(3) **United States.** The statistics here are inaccurate, incomplete, and manipulated, and are thus confusing and incorrect. The manner by which the statistics are gathered and the criteria used for counting HIV-infection (AIDS) cases are certainly questionable. The main reason for this is that AIDS in America is considered a "political" disease instead of the "medical" disease it really is. Because of our leaders' complacency and ignorance of the AIDS virus and its effects, we are all now placed in great danger.

The responsible politicians, with the support of the gay community and other such self-serving special interest groups, are more concerned about the "rights" of their constituents than their lives. They are more afraid of losing votes at the polls than they are protecting the people from the AIDS virus. *How irresponsible.*

I predict that some day soon, when AIDS begins to decimate our population, the public will seek its revenge on all of the responsible people who delayed the real fight against AIDS. Fear and panic will then set in and then no one will feel safe anywhere.

(4) **Rest of the World.** Reliable statistics from other areas are not available for a variety of reasons – such as politics, economics, and fear.

The most important reasons for the inaccurate AIDS statistics is the fact that all the HIV-infected people in the first stage of AIDS and the second stage of AIDS (ARC), people with AIDS-dementia (CNS-AIDS), and people who die from any cause (and are also HIV-infected) are *not* counted or included (diagnosed or not) in American statistics. Here in the United States, *coroners are now admitting that unbelievable numbers of people who have died from various causes (such as suicide, accidents, heart attacks, and cancer) were also AIDS infected.* Unfortunately, only the AIDS-sick (people in the third stage of the AIDS disease) and AIDS-dead people are now counted and included in the AIDS statistics. These incorrect AIDS statistics are then reported by the media to the public. This policy is scientifically wrong and hides the true severity and extent of the AIDS disease in our country.

Since only a small percentage of our population is now being tested for AIDS and, by testing only some parts of the country and not others, many of the hot spots (areas where there are more AIDS cases than in others) are missed. This policy also leads to far less recognized numbers of AIDS cases than there really are. If the entire populace of our nation is ever *accurately* tested and counted, the true number of AIDS cases found would be *unbelievably high*.

To get the most accurate numbers of Americans infected with the AIDS virus, both living and dead people must be HIV tested. Everyone diagnosed as being HIV infected must be counted to get the true severity and extent of the AIDS disease. Without accurate information about AIDS, world leaders are unaware of the true extent of AIDS, and are thus underestimating the urgency and severity of the disease.

Today, AIDS is out of control. Our present "policy" for the control of AIDS is a disaster; in fact, there is no policy. It is estimated by some AIDS experts that more than 1% of all Americans, up to 1% of our college students, and up to 2% of our military are infected with the AIDS virus. A few AIDS experts estimate that up to 200 or more million people worldwide are now infected.

The number of new AIDS cases is said to be doubling every six to twelve months. The number of "unexplained" AIDS cases (AIDS-infected people not considered in "high risk" groups, such as homosexuals and IV drug users) continues to grow at alarming rates. Worldwide, the majority of cases fall into no identifiable "risk group" whatsoever.

No one is safe from contracting the AIDS virus. It has been found living in bodily fluids such as blood, saliva, respiratory fluids, sweat, and tears. The virus can survive from seven to 14 days outside of the body; thus some people are fearful the virus can be activated and infectious when coming into contact with human bodily fluids. (4)

Recent tests on normal, healthy human skin tissue have shown that skin cells react very positively to bringing the virus within the cell walls of the skin, eventually invading and infecting the entire body. There presently exists no cure and no vaccine for AIDS. This means that everyone infected today will most likely die.

Medical literature has documented cases of nonsexual, non-needle transmitted HIV infections. At least three health care workers and a mother caring for her AIDS infected child may pay with their lives for discovering that AIDS contaminacted needles or sexual intercourse are not needed to transmit the AIDS virus.

Research indicates that other infections in asymptomatic AIDS-infected people, like tuberculosis or herpes, can activate the AIDS virus and lead to full-blown AIDS. Also, other such infectious organisms can infect and kill HIV-infected people more readily. These HIV-infected people already have a weakened immune system and are thus unable to defend themselves against other invading organisms adequately.

On June 7, 1988, the people of California voted to turn down a proposition that would have extended the public health codes for communicable diseases to HIV-infected patients. This proposition would have required that the same public health codes that already protect Californians from other dangerous contagious diseases would apply to HIV-infected people, as well. This is only logical! But it failed by a wide margin. Why? Because the opponents misinformed the voters and accused the proponents of creating an atmosphere of fear, misunderstanding, poor health care, and panic.

In short, an uninformed and complacent electorate voted on this proposition. Worse, the President of the California Medical Association, the President of the California Nurses Association, and the President of the California Association of Hospitals and Health Systems all endorsed voting against the proposition. In my opinion, the opponents of this measure will someday regret their disservice to the citizens of California.

The American Medical Association (AMA) and the rest of the medical profession must face its responsibility to the people and properly address the entire issue of AIDS. *This they are not doing.* It is estimated that many millions of people in the world are already infected with the AIDS virus, most of whom (if not all) will eventually develop the full-blown disease and die. *Not to recognize AIDS as a plague and treat it as such, is irresponsible and insane.*

We need to convince our government (as well as ourselves) that AIDS is a lethal medical disease and not a political disease. We must begin immediate, appropriate preventive precautions for the protection of our people from the HIV and strive to minimize the cost factor for the medical care of AIDS patients. All world governments should cooperate to develop a cure and/or vaccine against this lethal disease, as soon as possible, because the survival of mankind depends on it.

Since the fact that the infectious AIDS virus is found in the bodily fluids of an infected person is generally accepted, then why isn't it also accepted that contact with such infected bodily fluids could infect an uninfected human being? Aren't physicians trained to respect bodily fluids from patients infected with contagious diseases (such as bacterium, septicemia, syphilis, gonorrhea, and tuberculosis)?

If so, why treat AIDS differently? Whatever the reason is, we need to stop our ridiculous rationalizing and face the reality and danger of the AIDS virus. The more we ignore the AIDS virus and the more we underestimate its contagiousness or lethalness, the faster it will spread and kill.

Anybody who believes AIDS is a disease of only homosexuals, drug addicts, hemophiliacs or prostitutes is either gullible or a fool. It is true that people in these high risk groups are more likely to become HIV infected, but the reality is that *all of us are in danger of contracting the AIDS virus.*

One of the most likely places to be exposed to the AIDS virus is in a hospital, especially in the Emergency, Obstetrical, and Surgical Departments. Physicians and other health care workers who have direct contact with patients are the most likely people to become infected by the AIDS virus. Of all the physicians, the obstetricians and gynecologists are the most likely to become infected.

Here in America, Organized Medicine must take the lead (which thus far it has failed to do) and wage an effective, all-out war against the AIDS virus. They could start by honestly and completely educating the physicians, politicians, and public about the AIDS virus and the disease it causes. Everybody must be as well informed as possible and begin to treat the AIDS virus with respect, caution, and a sense of great danger. If not, the HIV will literally destroy our population and country.

Organized Medicine and government together must set up and enforce stringent criteria/rules and regulations for everybody to follow, in hopes of stopping the spread of the AIDS virus. Medical societies (such as the AMA and the American College of Surgeons) must also assist in forming these guidelines. The government, in turn, should not only support but help enforce these guidelines. We must all forget about civil/human rights in this war with AIDS. What good are they if there aren't any people to enjoy them?

In California, it is considered a crime for a physician to order an AIDS test without the consent of the patient. Worse, if a physician knows he has an HIV-infected patient, he cannot tell anyone; otherwise he is considered as violating the patient's rights and thus, breaking the law. When such a patient is admitted to the hospital for treatment, the physician must keep their HIV-infectious condition "confidential," thereby unnecessarily exposing everybody in the hospital – health care workers, patients, and physicians alike – to the AIDS virus. In late 1988, the California Legislature passed a confusing law to correct this situation; instead (and predictably), this law worsened the problem.

For a physician to transfer care of an HIV-infected patient for any reason, he must first get the written permission from the patient and the accepting physician; otherwise he must continue his care. If he does not, he can be accused of patient abandonment.

Each state presently has its own rules and regulations concerning the management of this disease. This situation is literally insane. If any real progress is to be made in stopping the spread of AIDS, *all states must adopt and enforce the same rules and regulations as to how this disease will be managed.* In the past, governments usually protected their health care workers and providers at all costs during plagues. They did not place them in bureaucratic chains or unnecessarily expose them to great risks. No wonder California has had and is having increasing problems in the health care field – hospitals having difficulty filling their physician/intern/residency positions, a nursing shortage, a laboratory/X-ray technician shortage, physicians quitting medical practice or retiring early, etc.

In short, the increasing numbers of AIDS cases and the lack of proper precautions against the AIDS virus is now being adversely felt in the California health community, as well as in the general population.

The following are a few recommendations I believe will help contain the spread of HIV infection:

(1) Physicians should be free to order an HIV test on any patient they feel necessary, without fear of medico-legal liability.
(2) Mandatory HIV testing for all people at least once every twelve months, especially for health care personnel.
(3) Mandatory HIV testing on all patients entering the hospital.
(4) All people infected with the AIDS virus must be reported to the state health departments for contagious diseases. They then must be properly followed/educated/treated, so as to protect themselves and all HIV-uninfected people. Every attempt to find and HIV test all people who have had any contact with these HIV-infected people must be made.
(5) All hospital employees, allied health professionals, nurses, and physicians must be tested for the AIDS virus every six months. If HIV-infected, they must not be allowed to work/practice in hospitals.
(6) All physicians, allied health professionals, nurses, and employees in a medical office workplace must have HIV testing every six months. If such a person tests HIV positive and continues to work in the office, all patients coming to this office must be informed that one of the medical personnel is HIV infected.
(7) All hospitals must be monitored very carefully by the state health departments to insure that:

   (a) All human bodily secretions are properly handled and disposed of.

(b) Protocols for admitted AIDS patients are properly set up and carefully followed and enforced, thus protecting other hospital patients, personnel and visitors.
(c) Appropriate precautions to protect hospital personnel and physicians from the AIDS virus are present and enforced.
(d) All apparel and equipment used in the hospital are approved for AIDS safety by the state health department, such as surgical gowns, rubber gloves, etc.
(e) Medical staffs of all hospitals be properly educated and regularly updated about the AIDS virus and disease, as well as the disease's course in the nation and the world.
(f) When possible, set up hospitals and facilities to medically treat only AIDS patients, thus separating those patients completely from other types of patients. Only HIV-infected health personnel and volunteers should be allowed to work in such AIDS-only medical facilities.

(8) All HIV-infected people purposely infecting an HIV-uninfected person be arrested and prosecuted as criminals (that is, consider such an act a felony, not a misdemeanor).
(9) Every effort be made by all nations to find a cure and/or vaccine for the AIDS virus and the disease it causes.
(10) All people handling food for the public have mandatory HIV testing every six months. People who are HIV infected must not be allowed to work in this line of work.
(11) All people working with the public be properly educated about the AIDS virus, emphasizing the precautions and encouraging their use against it at all times.
(12) All facilities for the public (such as hotels, restaurants, and restrooms) have stringent criteria, rules, and regulations for AIDS safety. *Cleanliness is a must.* These facilities must be carefully and frequently inspected for compliance by state health departments. For any infractions found, the responsible parties should be heavily fined and/or the establishment closed. The punishment must be severe and quick to be effective.

(13) The following are recommendations for legislative steps to halt the AIDS spread, made by Gene Antonio in his book, *The AIDS Cover-Up*:

   (a) Empower and support the Surgeon General to take practical measures to halt the spread of AIDS.
   (b) Federal order closing all known homosexual bath houses.
   (c) Federal bans on all high-risk group members from:
   - Donating blood or plasma
   - Contributing semen to sperm banks
   - Donating organs.
   (d) Hospital officials must allow medical personnel to take proper precautions when dealing with AIDS patients. Proper precautions must be taken to protect non-AIDS patients from those with AIDS.
   (e) Federal regulations for all persons diagnosed with full-blown AIDS, pre-AIDS (ARC), and those testing positive with the AIDS blood screening test.
   (f) There must be a federal crackdown on pornography soliciting persons for high-risk sexual activities. Computerized solicitations for high-risk sexual activities and the efforts of pedophiles to seek children must be stopped.
   (g) There must be a crackdown on massage parlors and vice rings promoting anonymous heterosexual promiscuity.
   (h) Federal authorization for public and private employers to utilize AIDS risk factor questionnaires and AIDS blood screening tests in hiring. Insurance companies must be permitted to utilize these means in screening applicants.
   (i) Sex education in the public schools must include instructions in sound healthful principles of sexual interaction.

These are but a few of the many things we can do to fight this horrid disease. The point here is to practice such effective preventative measures now – not wait until people are visibly AIDS-sick by the millions. Many of these recommendations may seem radical and even draconian, but we are dealing with one of the deadliest diseases ever known to mankind.

ECONOMICS OF AIDS

Manias, panics, and crashes are tragic enough by themselves, but never in the history of Industrial Capitalism, nor in the history of the United States, has our system been ravaged by a major plague. Now we have one: AIDS.

As an economic problem, AIDS has no parallel and, coming as it is when the economy by itself is probably plunging into another depression, the final consequences will stand our prevailing economic theories on their heads.

French writer Albert Camus called America "The country where everything is done to prove that life isn't tragic." Our habit is optimism, so it is difficult to believe that such chaos might actually happen to us.

C. Everett Koop, former United States Surgeon General, prepared a report for the U.S. public on AIDS which was distributed in December 1986. He wrote, "The number of people estimated to be infected with the AIDS virus in the U.S. is about 1.5 million ... of these, an estimated 100,000 to 200,000 will come down with ARC ... scientists predict that 20 to 30 percent of those infected with the AIDS virus will develop an illness that fits the accepted definition of AIDS within five years. The number of persons known to have AIDS in the U.S. to date (December 1986) is over 25,000; of these, half have died of the disease. Since there is no cure, the others are expected to also eventually die from their disease."

Senator H. L. Richardson, formerly the Senior Senator in the California State Senate, wrote his constituents in his *Weekly Richardson Report* of June 25, 1987, "We live in a time of madness, a time when public and private foolishness reigns. We have among us a plague, a disease so deadly that anyone who is contaminated will most likely die. The official estimate is that *one to two million*

Americans are carriers of this plague; some estimates run as high as four million. We can observe two hundred Americans and know that, mathematically, one is a deadly transmitter of AIDS virus and poses a threat to us all. But the 'one' who is contaminated is unidentified. Why? Because the law protects AIDS carriers from disclosing their identity, thereby concealing the magnitude of the problem. Imagine that! A deadly disease with "civil rights."

Let's proceed with a simple mathematical exercise, always keeping in mind we are using estimated figures. If there are now three million carriers of AIDS, and since the disease doubles every year, there will be:

6 million carriers in 1989
12 million carriers in 1990
24 million carriers in 1991
48 million carriers in 1992
96 million carriers in 1993
192 million carriers in 1994 (75% of the population)

Remember, these are carriers ONLY. But, nonetheless, official estimates state that as many as 30 % of those will become AIDS-sick or, looking at 1994, 57 million people (about 20 % of the total U.S. population).

If, by 1994, there are 57 million sick with AIDS, and the most conservative current estimates of cost-per-treatment-to-death is $100,000 a year, then medical bills in 1994 could be as high as $5.7 trillion!

If you think this is too grim an assessment, reduce the numbers by 50 percent. The total cost in 1994 is then $2.85 trillion – still an impossible amount of money. Obviously, other ways of treating AIDS will have to be implemented.

We, as a nation, are unprepared for this epidemic. We are, instead, still generally in pursuit of material wealth or financial survival and are financially unconcerned about AIDS. When AIDS starts killing us or a member of our families, only then will we fully understand that AIDS also means "Instant Bankruptcy." *The Wall Street Journal* reported the following heart-wrenching story on August 5, 1987:

"Until AIDS cut his brief career short last January, the 29-year old New Yorker earned $62,000 a year and was rising fast. These days, insurance pays all his medical expenses. But it doesn't pay his rent. Too weak to work, he is spending the last of his $15,000 savings. 'When it is gone, I will probably go on welfare,' he says." The story then cited numerous other examples of young men and women being wiped out financially overnight after they had contracted AIDS.

Our present insurance and medical care systems cannot cope today with the coming colossal financial impact of AIDS. What will happen tomorrow as the numbers soar? No one has the answer to that question. Worse, no one even seems to be thinking about this modern financial and personal scourge in those terms.

As AIDS spreads, there will be fewer people working, fewer goods being produced, less wealth being created, and less credit being spent except for medical care for AIDS victims (and this wealth creation is a drag on the economy, not the beneficial effect of producing new wealth in the form of goods and services).

In 1987, insurance companies estimated their AIDS medical bills in 1991 would be $39 billion. In 1986, they paid out $19 billion in medical claims. It is easy to see that AIDS will wreck all of our insurance companies. The federal Medicaid-Medicare systems are totally inadequate. A year or two more of rising bills and they will be insolvent, too, like the FSLIC is currently.

Cities and states cannot carry higher medical burdens. Many of them are at the financial brink now, even before the present developing depression.

The terribly long sick period of two years plus constant care for an AIDS victim brings in its wake incalculable future costs. Obviously we cannot, as a society, continue the present system of AIDS care. What will we do then? Maybe put active AIDS patients into remote sanitoriums as we did with tuberculosis victims at the turn of the century? We would then let AIDS-infected doctors, dentists, and nurses care for them. My point: as the epidemic grows, a critical stage will emerge. Then the disease starts to be transmitted by other means: coughing, sneezing, close contact with others, etc.

Some think this may already be happening. In any event, this would mean more AIDS-infected people with even higher costs than stated.

How will AIDS affect real estate? Adversely would be putting it mildly. According to the July 7, 1987 *San Francisco Chronicle,* "The AIDS epidemic could take $1 billion toll on the nation's real estate in 1987 because of lost rents, lower property values and depression economic activities. The accounting firm of Deloitte, Haskins and Sells said fear of acquiring AIDS could make it harder to sell some homes or lease business properties, not only in San Francisco, but elsewhere. There is a lot of fear."

There are currently $2 trillion in real estate mortgages outstanding as a potential AIDS related target. Would you buy a home occupied by a person with AIDS? Would you rent it? Most people would respond, "No!"

The vast national real estate market is slowly sinking and it will continue to worsen. Within four to six years, millions of Americans will be active AIDS-sick. Coincident with that, or just beyond, are harsh economic realities: millions of empty homes, parked automobiles, empty offices and hotels, halt of economic activity coming and, with it, a halt of "The American Way of Life."

AIDS will not only adversely affect America's economy, but those of all nations, thus forcing great changes in people's lifestyles and governments.

AIDS will continue to infect and kill into the 21st Century, insuring the above unpleasant events – unless our leaders proclaim war on AIDS now. A cure for AIDS is out there somewhere – we must believe we will find it.

CRITICAL MASS LEVEL

Sooner or later, all plagues in history have reached a "Critical Mass Level." AIDS will be no different. This is the level or plateau where enough people become infected that the responsible organism becomes more virulent and then spreads/infects by multiple routes of transmission. If this happens in AIDS (and it probably already has in some areas of the world), such routes of HIV infection as kissing an AIDS-infected person, drinking from an AIDS-virus contaminated cup, bites from insects carrying the AIDS virus, and eating AIDS-virus contaminated food may not be so crazy after all.

In summary, we all should be as informed about the HIV and the AIDS disease as much as possible and do all we can to contain it. We must both respect and fear this disease, but never stop fighting it. There are more and more AIDS cases being reported daily, and more and more "officials" and "AIDS experts" admitting they really don't know very much about AIDS. The World Health Organization is now admitting that it's time to "dig in," because there are not likely to be any particular breakthroughs against AIDS.

Many experts fear that a cure for AIDS is far in the future, if then, and a vaccine against AIDS is impossible. Whatever the truth is, we must now concentrate on preventing the spread of the disease; because if we don't, we can look forward to AIDS infection of the entire nation in just a few short years.

Make no mistake about it, AIDS is a PLAGUE – a plague that will make all previous plagues look like child's play. I sincerely believe a cure (and possibly a vaccine) for AIDA is eventually probable, but only if we recognize the dangers now and strive to contain the disease to achieve this goal. *The very survival of mankind depends on man's ability to find this cure.*

CHAPTER III
WHAT IS AIDS?

*The wise man's eyes are in his head;
but the fool walketh in darkness:
and I myself perceived also that one event
happeneth to them all – death.*
                               Ecclesiastes 2:14

What is AIDS? Most everyone has heard about it and knows it is a terrible disease, but they really don't know much about the disease itself. The term AIDS ("Acquired Immune Deficiency Syndrome") is "a secondary immune deficiency syndrome caused by a virus and is characterized by severe immune deficiency resulting in opportunistic infections, malignancies, and neurologic lesions in individuals without prior history of immunologic abnormality." (5)

What is a virus? A virus is the smallest of parasites, in some instances, crystallized like, with a central core of nucleic acid and an outer cover of protein. It is wholly dependent on cells (bacterial, plant, or animal) for reproduction. The nucleic acid core (RNA or DNA) represents the basic infectious material that in many cases can penetrate susceptible cells and initiate infection.

In simple language, a virus is a very small living organism that invades, infects, and kills a larger living organism. Viruses infect both man and animal. There are several hundred different viruses that may infect man, AIDS being one of the more recent ones identified. The viruses occurring primarily in man are spread mainly via respiratory and bodily excretions. Their spread is limited by inborn resistance, prior immunizing infections or vaccines, sanitary and other public health control measures, and, occasionally, by chemoprophylactic agents.

There are now three human retroviruses called T-lymphotrophic viruses (HTLV). HTLV types I and II appear to cause some human

T-cell leukemias and lymphomas, and HTLV type III is the cause of AIDS. The "L" in HTLV stands for *Lenti* which comes from the Latin word *Lentus*, meaning slow. After this virus infects its victim, it usually takes five to fifteen years before the symptoms/signs of the disease become evident. The credit for discovering the AIDS virus goes to both Dr. Luc Montagnier of France and Dr. Robert Gallo of the United States; *however, many people argue Dr. Montagnier is the first, true HIV discoverer.*

The AIDS virus has multiple interesting characteristics, all of which contribute to its ability to infect and kill its victims so effectively. This virus can:

- Live for weeks in a dry state (one to two weeks).
- Live in a liquid state for two weeks and beyond.
- Reproduce rapidly (20 times faster than the influenza virus).
- Mutate very rapidly (100-1,000 times faster than the influenza virus), up to 9,000 different types it change to.
- Invade and infect a human body within 24 hours.
- Invade a human body and be dormant (in the skin, bone, brain, or macrophage blood cells) for many years.

This last trait is terrifying. It reminds me of the alien creature in the science fiction movie, "Alien." In this movie, the creature incubated in a human body until it was ready to leave. When ready, it burst out of the human's chest, killing the unfortunate host.

Here, the AIDS virus hibernates in a human being until it is ready to activate itself and begin reproducing more AIDS viruses and killing its own host. In short, such a dormant AIDS virus is like an atomic bomb, ready to explode and kill its unfortunate and unsuspecting victim – *anytime.*

The AIDS virus attacks man in two ways: it attacks the white cells (specifically the T4 lymphocytes) in the blood and the brain. The virus invades the T4 lymphocyte, where it rapidly reproduces itself and destroys the function of the cell. In so doing, the immune system is slowly and eventually destroyed, thus leaving the victim defenseless against the AIDS virus as well as other invading organisms.

Recently, it has been shown that other white cells called monocytes and macrophages are attacked as well. With time, the victim becomes more and more defenseless and susceptible to infection by a variety of other "opportunistic" diseases. These diseases then invade, infect, and eventually kill the unfortunate AIDS-infected victim. The virus itself, however, destroys its victim when it attacks the central nervous system. Here, the virus invades and destroys the brain cells of the victim to the point where the victim eventually becomes helpless and dies. AIDS, therefore, kills in two ways: *directly* and *indirectly*.

There are three stages of the AIDS disease: the first Asymptomatic stage, the second AIDS Related Complex (ARC) stage, and the third full-blown AIDS stage (see Figure 3). Victims of AIDS in the first stage become "blood test positive" from weeks to months after being infected by the AIDS virus. Dr. William A. Haseltime, a leading AIDS researcher at Harvard Medical School in Boston, has stated that "once infected, a person remains infected for the rest of his life. Once infected, a person is infectious. It is not safe to assume otherwise."

Victims in the first stage show no visible signs or symptoms of the disease; however, they begin "shedding the AIDS virus" through various bodily fluids, such as blood, saliva, urine, sweat, and cerebral spinal fluid. Because of this fact, these AIDS victims can spread the disease to uninfected people if proper precautions are not taken. This first stage can last from weeks to years.

The second stage of AIDS is the AIDS Related Complex (ARC), and occurs when an AIDS-infected individual begins to manifest symptoms and signs of the disease, which ones depending on whether the immune system or the central nervous system is attacked. Weight loss, drenching night sweats, persistent diarrhea, swelling of lymph nodes (especially in armpits and groins), chronic fatigue, intermittent fever, malaise, lethargy, rectal warts, oral thrush (yeast infection), or low blood counts (low red cells, white cells, or platelets) are all signs or symptoms when the immune system is under attack.

Chronic memory loss, seizures, loss of muscle control, inability to speak coherently (or at all), psychiatric disturbances, hallucina-

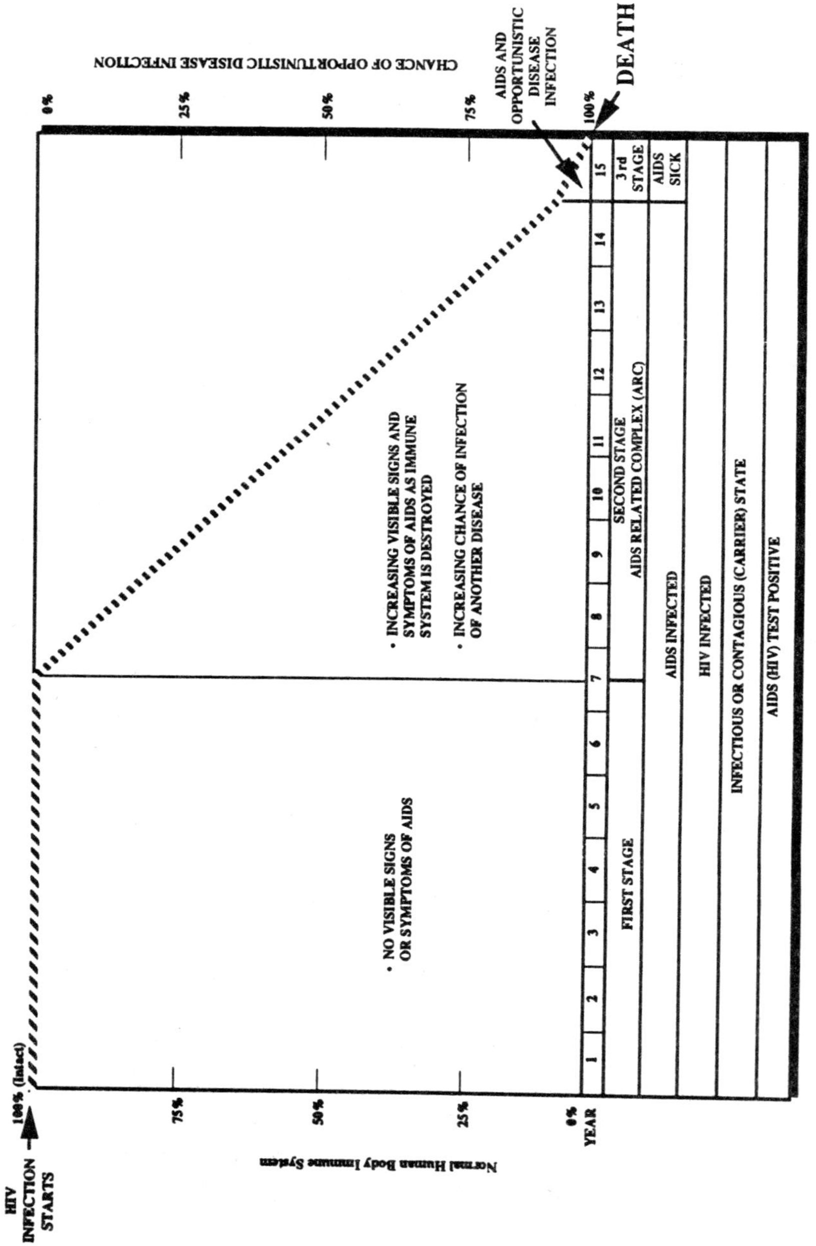

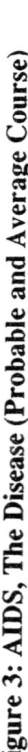

Figure 3: AIDS, The Disease (Probable and Average Course)

tions, and progressive deviations are signs that the central nervous system is being attacked.

Dr. James Staff, Medical Investigator at the National Institute of Health, states that there are over 50 clinical manifestations of ARC. "The number of persons with pre-AIDS or AIDS Related Complex (ARC), however, is estimated by some researchers to be ten times the number of full-blown AIDS cases." (6)

The third stage of AIDS is the full-blown syndrome. These victims are visibly AIDS sick. They have progressed to being infected by certain opportunistic symptomatic diseases (e.g. Pneumocystis Carinii Pneumonia, Chronic Cryptosporidosis, Toxoplasmosis, Tuberculosis, Kaposis Sarcoma, Cystomegalovirus, Herpes Symplex, Herpes Zoster, Cryptococcosis, and Chronic Interstitial Pneumonitis) or by the development of the more advanced central nervous system involvement (e.g. evidence of severe symptoms/signs of meningitis and encephalopathy) or by certain secondary cancers known to be associated with AIDS infection (e.g. Kaponi's Sarcoma, non-Hodgkins lymphoma, or primary lymphoma of the brain).

What is the present curative treatment of AIDS? Simply put – *NONE!* At this writing, the only treatment the medical community can offer is "supportive care." The only advice: "Don't get the disease." All people should practice preventative care, because once infected with the HIV, there is no cure and it is almost 100% lethal.

"More than half of those initially diagnosed with full-blown AIDS (AIDS-sick or third stage AIDS) will be dead in eighteen months. More than 70% will be dead in two years and virtually no one will be alive in five years." (7) Because of the AIDS virus' ability to rapidly mutate from one infectious form to another, it is impossible to develop an effective cure or vaccine. AIDS experts, therefore, have little hope for a cure or vaccine for the disease in the near future. Recently, Dr. Jay A. Levy, a physician and AIDS virus researcher at the University of California at San Francisco says, "I'm an optimist for a vaccine, but we've got a long time to wait. I don't make any predictions, but I'm saying we won't have a vaccine until well past the year 2000."

How does AIDS spread? This one question is causing more discussion, fear, and concern than all the other questions put together. It has been well documented that the AIDS virus is found in the bodily fluids. It has also been shown that the virus can stay alive outside the human body in a liquid (water) or dry state for seven to fourteen days, and still be infectious under certain conditions.

With this in mind, most people agree that a non-infected person can become infected by receiving a blood transfusion with AIDS contaminated blood, by being stuck with an AIDS contaminated needle, or having "unprotected sex" with an AIDS infected partner. What seems to concern most people, however, is the question of whether AIDS can be transmitted by kissing, insect bites, screened "AIDS-free" blood transfusions, casual contact, or even the close nonsexual contact that occurs in the normal day at school, work, restaurants, and home.

Intimate kissing or oral sex (fellatio, cunnilingus) could break the mucosa in and around the mouth, allowing for possible AIDS-infected blood to blood, AIDS-infected saliva to blood, or AIDS-infected vaginal secretions/semen to blood transmission. Any lesion or inflammation in a person's mouth can greatly increase his/her risk of AIDS infection if the AIDS virus is present.

It has been shown that gonorrhea and syphilis can and have been transmitted through kissing; therefore, some experts feel AIDS can be transmitted via this route as well. Representative Dan Burton (Republican-Indiana) stated this fact on the House floor on June 9, 1988. Since it has never been proven that kissing an AIDS-infected or possible AIDS-infected individual is 100% safe, I don't recommend such an adventure.

The blood used by hospitals for transfusions is carefully screened by the Red Cross for the AIDS virus; however, it is impossible to screen all blood. In a new book, Masters and Johnson stated "that 1,600 contaminated blood samples may be escaping each year with almost as many transfusion recipients getting infected as before strict blood-screening tests went into effect." They also stated that the risk of AIDS infection from a transfusion of a single blood component is about one in 5,400.

Obviously, there is little to worry about when receiving a blood transfusion, say many AIDS experts – unless you're the one receiving the tainted unit of blood! I feel a patient who needs blood for medical reasons should be transfused, but needless blood transfusions should be avoided. When possible, one's own blood should be used for transfusions.

When a person accidently gets stuck with an AIDS-contaminated needle, AIDS infection can result. Such infections have occurred, but the probability of infection is considered very low. This being a truism, can AIDS be transmitted by the bite of an AIDS virus carrying insect (mosquitoes, bedbugs, ticks)?

The AIDS virus is *very* small. *Approximately 230 million AIDS viruses will fit on the period at the end of this sentence,* enough viruses to infect every American alive today. Also, the AIDS virus has an extraordinary reproductive capacity and, according to Dr. John Seale, "a single virion (virus) introduced directly into the blood will regularly transmit infections."

Dr. Carolyn MacLeod and Dr. Mark Whiteside, heads of the Center for Tropical Disease in Miami, Florida, say "the amount of blood that is transmitted from a syringe an IV Drug user uses is infinitely smaller than the amount of blood one can receive from a housefly or a mosquito, and yet it is transmitted through these syringes." I believe it possible for AIDS to be transmitted by insect bites, particularly in warm humid areas (e.g. countries near the equator), where people are repeatedly bitten daily by such disease carrying insects.

What about casual or close nonsexual contact? Can AIDS be transmitted this way? Again, I think it is possible even though it has yet to be proven. Logically it makes sense. If one AIDS virus can stay alive seven to fourteen days in a dry or liquid environment, and if it can be activated when coming in contact with human blood (or other such bodily fluids), then the probability is that it can infect an uninfected person under the right conditions.

This being the case, I find it difficult not to warn people that such contact with an AIDS victim might be dangerous to their own health and therefore they should be very careful. This disease is too dangerous, too fatal for any assumptions concerning its transmission.

Remember, no one knows everything about the AIDS virus and disease, especially about all of its modes of transmission.

The diagnosis of AIDS is made on the basis of clinical manifestations described above, the isolation of the AIDS virus from serum, cells or lymph nodes, and the demonstration of antibodies to the AIDS virus in the victim's serum. Once diagnosed, the AIDS patient must be informed and carefully treated.

At this point, I feel it appropriate to excerpt some pertinent and interesting information from a speech to the English House of Commons by Dr. John Seale, Royal Society of Medicine (Third Report From the Social Services Committee, Session 1986-87, "Problems Associated With AIDS," Volume III, Minutes of Evidence [8 April-13 May 1987] and Memoranda). Dr. Seale is considered one of the leading "AIDS experts" in the world.

Introduction

- No politician can make rational decisions to deal with AIDS without a clear understanding of the nature and severity of the epidemic, the means of transmission of the virus, and the prospects for cure or preventive vaccine. The key scientific facts underlying the epidemic are quite simple, though AIDS is perceived to be unusually complex and full of scientific uncertainties. These perceptions have been produced by a few scientists and others who have recklessly minimized the seriousness of the epidemic and have fostered confusion and dangerous misconceptions.
- The most important and urgent task for politicians, both in Government and Parliament, is to force scientists to speak clearly, precisely and honestly about the AIDS epidemic. Half-truths, wishful thinking, flawed scientific hypotheses and deceptions have been perpetrated by scientists, and allowed to flourish as conventional wisdom, aided and abetted by editors of scientific and medical journals. The deceptions must be exposed with maximum publicity.
- The public must be fully informed of the true nature of the threat from the virus which faces us all. Once this is done the

mass of the population will accept measures essential to halt the spread of the virus, even though they will inevitably require severe curtailment of the liberty and civil rights of everybody, just as happens in war-time. The longer the truth is obscured from the public, and the greater the multitude of innocent people who die most horribly as a result, the more ferocious will be the explosion of hatred and revenge against those guilty of perpetrating the deceptions.

- The virus has the properties of a skilled, devious, hidden and implacable invader with the capacity and willingness to kill every man, woman, and child in our country. It may now be spreading amongst us precisely because it has this capacity. It is unwise to assume that such a force can be vanquished without taking actions which the people of Britain accepted as entirely appropriate to fight two world wars; particularly as dissemination of the virus is being actively encouraged by some who wish to destroy our society.

A. The Nature Of The Disease

1. AIDS is a contagious, infectious, communicable disease caused by a lentivirus (slow virus), a member of the family of retroviruses.
2. No lentivirus has been known to affect humans before the advent of AIDS.
3. AIDS is a typical slow virus disease with a prolonged, silent incubation period of great variability, but usually lasting several years, followed by slowly progressive disease always ending in death.
4. An epidemic of a new slow virus disease spreading unchecked is the ultimate virological nightmare, yet in none of the major scientific or medical journals has this been spelled out clearly and the implications discussed.
5. Death is caused by the AIDS virus infecting, and slowly destroying, cells in the brain, lungs, intestine and the immune system.

B. Mortality Following Infection

1. Within five years of infection with the virus, 25 percent of people have developed full-blown AIDS and all of them die. This is the official conclusion of the U.S. Public Health Service recently endorsed by leading scientists from the National Academy of Sciences in Washington.
2. The ultimate mortality within twenty years of infection is unknown as the virus has been spreading for only ten years. The optimistic view held by a decreasing number of virologists is that only 50 percent of those infected will die. Many virologists now accept the pessimistic view, that all people infected with the virus will eventually be killed by it.
3. All virologists are agreed that once infected with AIDS virus, people are potentially infectious to others for life.

C. Failure Of Antibodies Or Vaccines To Protect

1. In all people with antibodies to the AIDS virus, some virus persists in brain and other cells from which it cannot be removed. In contrast to most virus infections, antibodies to a lentivirus do not provide protective immunity; they fail to neutralize or eliminate it. Although many people infected with the AIDS virus look and feel well for several years, destruction of cells of the brain and immune system is progressing slowly.
2. The outlook for a successful vaccine is bleak. None is available for the lentivirus diseases of animals. Search for a vaccine against infectious anaemia for horses for eighty years, and against maedi-visna in sheep for forty years, has proved futile. Indeed, when antibodies to a lentivirus are produced artificially by vaccination, the vaccinated animals die after subsequent infection more rapidly than those which are not. In spite of many successful vaccines, it should be realized that for the majority of viral and bacterial diseases vaccines do not work.

What Is AIDS?   37

D. Bleak Outlook For A Cure

   1. No simple, effective, curative drug, like penicillin, will be available for AIDS in the foreseeable future because once a person is infected, the viral genetic code is permanently inserted into the human genetic code of cells in the brain and other tissues. Any drug which blocks replication of the virus, thereby halting the progress of the disease, will have to be taken continuously for life. All drugs used so far are highly toxic and expensive. If a cheap, apparently effective, drug becomes available it will take several decades to be certain that it is both effective and safe. Nevertheless, many companies will announce "promising" new drugs and "breakthroughs" in the treatment of AIDS for simple commercial motives.
   2. The handling of the recent AZT clinical trials by the U.S. Government was particularly important. The U.S. Public Health Service insisted the trials cease long before any long-term benefit of the drug had been shown, and before the manufacturing company suggested it, thereby misleading the public into believing a "cure" for AIDS was already in the pipeline. Such disinformation weakens the political will to implement the tough control measures required to halt the spread of the virus.

E. Transmission of AIDS – Sexual Intercourse

   1. Scientists and doctors have repeatedly stated as fact that the AIDS virus is fundamentally transmitted during sexual intercourse but is, unfortunately, sometimes transmitted in the blood. This is highly misleading, though published laboratory and epidemiological evidence, and editorials in scientific and medical journals, have been heavily slanted to support this "fact."
   2. In reality AIDS is characteristically a blood transmitted infection, which is only transmitted with difficulty during sexual intercourse compared with the genuine sexually

transmitted diseases gonorrhea and trichomoniasis. All the experimental and epidemiological evidence is consistent with this view.
3. Obviously AIDS is transmissible during sexual intercourse, but so is influenza, granular fever and scabies. Sexual intercourse is only one of many ways by which the virus can be transmitted, and is by no means the most efficient.
4. The illusion that AIDS is essentially a sexually transmitted disease arose from the first observations that AIDS appeared to affect only sodomites with numerous partners. However, sodomy is not sexual intercourse in the biological sense of the words. As we are dealing with a very important biological event, the transmission of a lethal parasite from one human host to another, it is essential that scientists use words describing the transmission with the utmost precision.
5. In biological terms sexual intercourse means the union between male and female which may result in reproduction of the species. In mammals this invariably requires contact between male and female genitalia. Consequently sexual intercourse between two men in the biological sense is impossible.
6. Scientists who state, or imply, sodomy is sexual intercourse without some qualification are being imprecise and misleading, whether intentionally or not.
7. Homosexual men engaged in homosexual activities frequently insert their fingers, fist, penis or tongue into the lower intestinal tract of their partners. These maneuvers transmit any virus which persists in the blood for months or years with devastating efficiency, even though no virus is present in either semen or saliva. This has been shown very clearly with hepatitis B virus which, in prosperous communities, infects the majority of homosexual men within three years of becoming sexually active; whereas hepatitis B infection remains rare amongst heterosexual men and women, even though they frequently change partners.

F. Dysinformation From Scientists

1. The AIDS virus persists in an infectious state (i.e. as cell-free virions) in blood and semen at levels up to 25,000 virions per mililitre, according to the only published paper giving this critically important information. Cell-free virions were detected easily in saliva more than two years ago, but quantitative studies have still not been published.
2. No infectious virion has been detected in semen according to the only two detailed published studies on the subject, which between them included a grand total of merely three men examined. In 10 per cent of 50 infected men, according to another report sent to me personally but which gave few details, cell-associated virus has been detected in a few white blood cells in semen, but never in spermatozoa.
3. Virions have been detected in the vaginal secretions in only trivial quantities – about one per milliliter – indicating that their infectivity is minimal.
4. The scale of the deceptions and misinformation perpetrated by virologists, clinicians, and editors of scientific and medical journals about the infectivity of genital secretions, compared with that of blood, serum, and saliva, has been astonishing. In the presence of a new, lethal virus spreading amongst people, for which no vaccine or cure is in sight, every sane person would assume that scientists have been working flat out to verify precisely how it is transmitted.
5. On the contrary, having assumed for a variety of motives that AIDS is a sexually transmitted disease, like syphilis or gonorrhea, a negligible research effort has gone into the critical matter of transmission. A few preliminary papers were published and their findings have been repeatedly quoted as showing the opposite to what they actually showed. When this was pointed out in letters to the editors of major medical and scientific journals, publication has been refused. No attempt has been made to check, double-

check, and recheck the findings in other laboratories, and in other countries, or to rectify published errors.
6. As far as it goes, the tiny research effort into infectivity of bodily fluids indicates that saliva is more infectious than genital secretions, but that blood and serum is vastly more infectious than either. Consequently the idea that condoms can have any significant effect on the spread of AIDS in a nation is utterly preposterous.
7. Governments all over the world are spending millions of pounds advising their citizens to prevent AIDS by using condoms on the basis of manifestly fraudulent misrepresentation of scientific evidence presented by scientists themselves.
8. The AIDS virus is unusually stable outside the human body. It retains almost all its infectivity after seven days in water at room temperature and some after being kept dry for a week. A virus with this degree of stability, which persists in the blood and is shed in saliva, cannot possibly fail to be transmitted in many ways apart from sexual intercourse.

G. Variable Efficiency In Means Of Transmission

1. A virus which persists in moderate quantities in the blood for years and is shed in small quantities in saliva will be transmitted with far greater ease by some means than by others.
2. Injection of the virus through the skin in hypodermic needles is the most certain method of transmission. This happens when blood-contaminated hypodermics are re-used without sterilization, as is common amongst drug addicts in the West and in health care facilities in less prosperous countries. It also occurs when virus-contaminated blood transfusions and clotting factor are administered.
3. Male homosexual contact of the finger, penis, or tongue with the rectal wall of another man transmits the virus

very easily. Seventy percent of the male homosexual population of San Francisco were infected within six years of the arrival of the virus in the city, and nearly 30 per cent of London homosexuals are already infected. The percentages are raising remorselessly in large cities throughout the western world, unaffected by the highly acclaimed "safe sex" propaganda.

4. Well over 50 per cent of new-born babies of infected mothers are infected.
5. Moderately efficient means of transmission include mouth-to-mouth and genital contact before and during normal sexual intercourse, oral salivary contact between small children, needle-stick injuries to nursing staff, and chance contact of sores or abrasions with blood, serum, saliva or sputum.
6. Inefficient means of transmission include social kissing, inhalation or respiratory aerosols caused by coughing or sneezing and blood sucking insects.
7. Transmission by inhalation is only inefficient because of the relatively small number of virions shed in saliva and bronchial secretions. However, if an AIDS virion is inhaled into the lung it is engulfed by an amoeba-like macrophage on the lining of the alveoli (air sacs). It has been shown repeatedly in the laboratory that the AIDS virus readily infects macrophages, and the virus replicates within them, thereby enabling infection of people to be initiated by this route.
8. Understandably, and wisely, the DHSS has officially advised all British dental surgeons always to wear masks to avoid AIDS virus infection when using high speed drills. These drills make aerosols of saliva similar to those produced by sneezing.
9. Chronic lymphoid interstitial pneumonitis is a well recognized variety of pneumonia caused directly by infection of the lungs with the AIDS virus. It is similar to the pneumonia of maedi-visna in sheep and is particularly common in children with AIDS. When associated with

pulmonary tuberculosis, a very common complication of AIDS, it is inevitable that coughing will produce some aerosols containing tubercle bacilli and the AIDS virus. After the fluid in the aerosols evaporates, the minute dry flakes containing tubercle bacilli and AIDS virus float in the air indefinitely and both remain infectious for days.

10. The normal route of transmission of the maedi-visna lentivirus between adult sheep is by respiratory aerosols when there are crowded closely together in winter shelters. Maedi-visna is not a sexually transmitted disease of sheep.
11. The efficiency of transmission of AIDS virus by biting insects will depend upon the quantity of virons in the blood of the bitten person, the anatomical structure of the biting parts of the insects, their feeding habits and other factors.
12. Infectious anaemia of horses, a lentivirus disease, is characteristically transmitted by large biting insects, particularly stable flies and horse flies. It is not a sexually transmitted disease of horses.
13. The AIDS virus has been shown to remain infectious in the stomach of bed bugs for at least two hours. It has been shown that it can infect the cells of insects, including mosquitoes and cockroaches, both in laboratory cell culture and in intact insects. Replication of the virus in insect cells has not yet been demonstrated.

H. Saturation Of The British Population With The Virus

1. There is a key to estimating how long it will take for the people of Britain to be saturated with the AIDS virus, if its spread is allowed to continue unchecked as at present. This is the application of probability theory to the known facts about the virus, its pathogenesis, the frequently of "contact," and the efficiency with which different "contacts" transmit the virus.

What Is AIDS?

2. The basic facts are that the entire population is susceptible to infection, and once people are infected they remain potentially infectious to others for life.
3. As the number of people infected rises the probability of transmission during any particular "contact" between individuals also rises.
4. Initially the virus was introduced into Britain from the United States by homosexual men who soon infected others by having frequent, efficient "contacts" – sodomy with strangers. As the number of infected homosexuals rises the probability of infection being transmitted during one "contact" rises at first exponentially, but then at a slower doubling rate as saturation with the virus of the homosexual population is approached.
5. Once some intravenous drug addicts were infected, a further, frequent, efficient "contact," self-injection with shared needles, rapidly spread the virus amongst addicts.
6. As a number of infected homosexuals and addicts increased, efficient "contacts" rarely performed – such as receiving a blood transfusion, or clotting factor, or having a baby – infected more and more people.
7. Once a critical mass of infected people has been created by highly efficient "contacts," then "contacts" which are only moderately efficient but occur very frequently – such as normal sexual intercourse or small children playing together – will spread the virus in ever widening circles throughout the population.
8. Finally, highly inefficient "contacts" which occur very frequently indeed, such as coughing and sneezing in public, and being bitten by insects, will infect many people as millions of infected persons interact with the non-infected, and saturation of the entire British population becomes unstoppable.

J. Varieties of Misinformation

1. People with AIDS are categorized as belonging to a small

number of "risk groups" giving the false impression that the vast majority of people cannot get AIDS.
2. AIDS is portrayed as only a behavioral disease caused by sexual and narcotic misdemeanors. This implies that if anyone gets AIDS it is their own fault.
3. Emphasis on transmission of the virus during sexual intercourse, and education as a solution to the epidemic, implies that the disease will disappear with modified behavior. This misses the point that as the epidemic explodes, infection by chance, non-sexual contact, becomes ever more common.
4. By equating sodomy with sexual intercourse the impression is given that homosexuals have just been unlucky to get infected before heterosexuals. In reality homosexual activity has spread the virus through the population at a vastly greater speed than normal sexual intercourse could achieve.
5. The value of blood tests for diagnoses of AIDS virus infection is repeatedly denigrated by those who do not want them introduced compulsorily. In fact the blood test is an unusually reliable diagnostic tool.
6. The suffering of those with AIDS is highlighted while ignoring the suffering of those who will get AIDS in the future if appropriate steps are not taken to stop its spread.
7. The rights of those infected with the virus are stressed, while the rights of the uninfected to be protected from infection with a lethal virus are ignored and glossed over. Protection of the life of its citizens is one of the major obligations of the State.

K. Methods of Control

1. Once the truth is known and publicized the steps required to halt the epidemic become more obvious and less controversial.
2. Speed is of the essence because every day that is lost will increase the human misery which, in any event, will be vast.

3. We are facing a national catastrophe equal to any in the history of the nation. The life of every citizen is at stake. Death from AIDS is a protracted horror unequalled by other diseases.
4. The only way to halt the spread of the virus is to identify all those who are infected by compulsory testing. Government must then take whatever steps are required to ensure that those infected do not pass the virus on to anyone else.
5. The longer this action is delayed, the greater will be the task when it is finally undertaken, and the greater the danger that the spread of the virus will then be unstoppable.
6. The actions required by government are comparable to those taken in waging a war of survival.
7. The war against AIDS is a war of survival. If we lose, Britain and all of her people will perish.

I consider this to be one of the most important articles I have read about AIDS. It is short, concise, and to the point. Even though this report is over two years old, its message is pertinent, loud and clear – the AIDS plague is the worst of all known plagues and is only beginning. Every nation, every person had better recognize these facts and begin protecting themselves from the AIDS virus as soon as possible, or perish from the face of the earth.

STATISTICS IN THE UNITED STATES

What are the statistics of AIDS, particularly in America? At a speech in Santa Barbara, California (May 1988), Dr. John Platt (a futurist and biophysicist) said the following:

(1) World-wide, there is a vast under reporting of the AIDS data.
(2) There are large groups of AIDS-infected people that are not reported, such as AIDS-related deaths (AIDS infected people who die from other causes, including suicides, drug over-

doses, accidents, and various diseases) and the AIDS infected people in the untested population.
(3) The majority of Americans have not been HIV tested, because they do not want to be tested. This greatly complicates the gathering of meaningful data.
(4) Presently the CDC estimates that by the end of 1991, 250,000 cases of AIDS-sick people will be around and 150,000 people will have died from AIDS. Dr. Platt estimates these figures to be very conservative and that this data can be safely multiplied by two to three times, which gives us more than 500,000 AIDS-sick cases by the end of 1991. Dr. Platt estimates two to three million Americans are presently (mid 1988) AIDS infected. In June 1988, Representative Dan Burton (Republican – Indiana) said that most scientists now estimate there are presently four to five million AIDS infected people in America.
(5) This data should be multiplied by a factor of 50 to 80, which would then give the total number of AIDS cases (AIDS-infected only, AIDS-related complex, and AIDS sick). By so doing, Dr. Platt estimates that fifteen to twenty million Americans will be AIDS infected by the end of 1991; however, Representative Burton estimates 20 to 25 million Americans will be AIDS infected by that time.
(6) After 1991, Dr. Platt estimates that the numbers will double every year – 30 to 40 million cases in 1992, 60 to 80 million cases in 1993, 120 to 160 million cases in 1994, 240 to 320 million cases in 1995 – most, if not all, of the people in the United States. If Representative Burton's figures are used, then Dr. Platt's figures are dwarfed – 40 to 50 million in 1992, 80 to 100 million in 1993, 160 to 200 million in 1994, etc.
(7) Presently, under very accurate testing in Massachusetts, .2 % of all mothers having babies have newborns that are AIDS infected. A CDC survey shows this percentage to be .3% in the Midwest and .4+% in "Hot Spots" (areas where AIDS is prevalent, such as New York City, San Francisco, Houston, and Miami).

(8) Dr. Platt estimates that by 1994, in the United States, the total population will decline for the first time in its history, because the total deaths will begin exceeding the total births; thereafter, reliable AIDS documentations will accelerate.

At the Fourth International Conference on AIDS in Stockholm in June 1988, Dr. Lars Olaf Kallings, Chairman, reported: "The whole picture is now even more frightening then we expected." As frightening and depressing as the present situation is, I fear that the future will be worse. In America in particular, I see:

(1) A declining population with a far lower standard of living.
(2) A much simpler lifestyle.
(3) A return to nature.
(4) A closer knit family.
(5) A return to religion.
(6) A "commune-like" relationship and dependence amongst neighboring families.

"Survival" will be the main concern of all peoples. Some present countries will cease to exist, and the remaining (or new ones) will have far different political structures and goals. The primary purpose of governments will be to help people survive – not vice versa as it now is. Politicians, attorneys, policemen, social workers, etc., who are supposed to serve and protect their people, will do so, and those who don't will quickly be replaced. *Survival* will be everybody's primary concern.

What can we expect here in the United States when AIDS reaches plague stage?

(1) A definite change in our government's goals and priorities. Smaller, not bigger government; more concern about its own people than foreigners; more "regional" (than "national") laws; more police-like (than democratic) government; more concerned about protecting human life (than protecting human rights); more concerned with protecting innocent and healthy people (than criminal or sick people).

In short, a government of people, by people, and for people. Everyone will be trying to survive a disease they fear, qand know little about, and has no cure.

(2) The typical American will become more family oriented, as well as more religious. Families will be larger, closer, and stronger. They will grow more of their own food, make more of their own clothes, have more babies, educate themselves, and cooperate with other families with similar goals.

(3) Life in America:
  (a) More rural than urban.
  (b) Cities and towns will become smaller and many abandoned.
  (c) Crime will definitely increase, especially in larger cities.
  (d) People will travel less often and only when necessary.
  (e) Hotels, motels, restaurants, service stations, theaters and other such public and private gathering places will all be adversely affected. Many will cease to exist and the rest will be smaller, cleaner, and safer.
  (f) Because of limited funds and a shortage of health care workers/facilities, health care will be rationed – the AIDS-free sick being treated before the AIDS-sick patients. AIDS-sick patients will be treated in AIDS-only facilities and only by AIDS-infected and volunteer health care workers. Some form of accepted euthanasia will be adopted and practiced.
  (g) Entertainment will change. Areas where large groups of people congregate, such as crowded amusement facilities (theaters, sports arenas, amusement parks, and gambling casinos) will be avoided by most people; thus, the future for such facilities is bleak. The *home* is where most of the future entertainment will be. Television, radio, music, games, cards, small neighborly parties, and barbecues will be the primary form of entertainment in the future.
  (h) Shopping for food, clothes and other necessities will be done on a much smaller scale, primarily by telephone, television, and mail. The large shopping malls and centers of today will be largely deserted, thus becoming the

"concrete pyramids of the 20th century."
- (i) The medium of exchange of the future, at least at the local level, will be bartering, and silver and gold coins. Credit cards, checks, and charge accounts will be but a memory of things past.
- (j) The sexual behavior of Americans will definitely be affected; it is already changing. People will marry more and younger, practice less premarital or extra-marital sex, have less homosexual relationships, practice less perverted sex and divorce less. Practicing or indulging in prostiution will greatly decrease. Loose sex will literally disappear. Gone will be the pick-up bars, "bath" houses, cat houses, massage parlors, and other such places where a more promiscuous and dangerous form of sex is practiced.
- (k) The drug problem of today will disappear, because AIDS will destroy those with the problem.
- (l) Because of AIDS, the practice of homosexuality will literally disappear, at least openly.
- (m) Prostitution, the oldest profession, will become the smallest profession.

Globally, each country will have to fight AIDS the best it can. Countries will help each other, but only after they help themselves first. Business, trade, and travel amongst nations will greatly diminish. Wars will be another memory of the past – all nations will be too plague-ridden and poor to fight anybody.

What does all this mean? Is Mother Nature punishing the human race? Has she forsaken the human race? No, I think not. I think she may be trying to save our planet. Because of man, earth's forests are being depleted, many forms of life have become extinct or are becoming extinct, oceans and rivers are being polluted, the atmosphere is being polluted, the soil is being poisoned and covered with concrete – in short, man is destroying his environment and life-sustaining planet.

The AIDS plague will probably reduce the number of humans to the level it was for thousands of years – 500 (plus or minus) million people. By so doing, our rich life-giving and sustaining earth can then replenish itself. Hopefully, man will have learned from his past mistakes and begin living *with* his environment, rather than against it.

ETIOLOGY OF AIDS

Finally, where did the AIDS virus come from? What is its origin and how long has it been infecting Man? These are $64,000 questions. The truth is, no one really knows! There are many theories and assumptions concerning the origin of AIDS, but none of them have ever really been proven or accepted.

A little study in virology might help answer these questions. AIDS is caused by a virus. "Many viruses grow in animals and many in humans, but most viruses that affect animals don't affect humans. There are exceptions, of course, such as yellow fever and small pox. There are some viruses in animals that cause very lethal cancers in those animals, but do not affect Man or other animals. The bovine leukemia virus (BLV), for example, is lethal to cows, but not to humans. There is another virus that occurs in sheep called sheep visna virus which is also non-reactive in man. These deadly viruses are "retroviruses" meaning that they can change the genetic composition of cells they enter. The AIDS virus is such a virus – a retrovirus. It doesn't occur naturally in any animal." (8)

The following are interesting opinions, facts, and theories on the origin of AIDS:

(1) It appears that AIDS started almost simultaneously in the United States, Brazil, Haiti, Central Africa, and Southern Japan. The first case of AIDS was reported in 1981. Some researchers claim the disease was first recognized in 1972, but the documentation here is vague and suspect. In any event, the question continues to arise, why and how did the AIDS virus appear so suddenly and why in so many places at relatively the same time? The answer is still unknown.

(2) Dr. Robert Gallo, one of the two discoverers of the AIDS virus, told the Rhode Island Society on September 30, 1987,

"This is not a new mutation. My guess is that man was infected with this virus for a long, long time." (9) Dr. Gallo believes that the virus was isolated in small groups of peoples living in deep Africa; but over the last 25 or more years, these rural people went to the cities where they introduced the virus to the urban, susceptible populace. Dr. Gallo's theory is certainly not shared by many people and is just that – a theory.

(3) The theory that the African green monkey is responsible for the AIDS disease is the most often cited cause of origin. As the story goes, an AIDS-infected African green monkey bit a native in Central Africa and the AIDS-infected native then went to town and gave it to a prostitute – not, presumably, by biting her but through sexual intercourse. From this "contact," the disease literally "took off."

Others think the AIDS-infected green monkey spread the disease to man by either biting him or being eaten by him. In any event, one way or another, this poor green monkey is often blamed for the onslaught of AIDS. Kirk Kidwell wrote, "Yet as popular as the green monkey theory became in the news media, most scientists were hesitant to support it. One of the factors arguing most strongly against this hypothesis was the simple fact that AIDS was virtually nonexistent among those Africans having the most exposure to green monkeys, especially certain pygmy tribes in Central Africa who hunt and eat green monkeys." (10)

When one considers the fact that the AIDS virus is not found naturally in man or any animal, or the fact that it is not genetically possible to transfer the AIDS virus from monkeys (when purposely infected by man) to man by natural means, or the fact that it was impossible for the poor little green monkey to travel so fast and at the same time to so many places in the world, just to infect man in 1981 – I think we can exonerate the green monkey theory.

(4) Many experts believe that AIDS is a man-made virus – a hybrid virus that is deadly to humans. "Dr. Theodore Strecker's research of the literature indicates that the National Cancer Institute in collaboration with the World Health Organization made the AIDS virus in their laboratories at Fort Detrick (now NCI). They combined the deadly retroviruses, bovine leukemia virus and sheep visna virus, and injected them into human tissue cultures. The result was the AIDS virus, the first human retrovirus known to man and now believed 100% fatal to those infected." (11)

Some people claim this man-made, man-killing virus was then inoculated into millions of unsuspecting humans around the world when vaccinated with small pox and Hepatitis B vaccines. The AIDS virus was purposely mixed with these vaccines. If all this is true, the question is, why? Why would any health agency be involved in such a diabolical plot? Is all this an offshoot of an experiment in germ warfare that went astray? Is this some type of conspiracy? I don't know if there is any truth to any of these questions, but I certainly hope not.

(5) Could the AIDS virus have come to earth from space? Why not? Meteors and other space debris are constantly bombarding the earth, so the AIDS virus could have literally dropped in on us from space. If so, I'm certainly glad we don't get many other such new-life forms from space!

(6) Could the AIDS virus have been dormant for many years in the frozen polar ice caps, being recently released from melting ice glaciers? This theory is just as logical as the rest.

(7) Could God have created the AIDS virus to protect life on earth from man? This thought appeals to me more than the rest. On this earth, Mother Nature (God) has checks and balances to create, protect and control all forms of life; this

She/He has proven time and time again. Throughout earth's history, many forms of life have either adjusted to the environment or perished. AIDS just may be Mother Nature's vehicle to help or force man to literally limit his numbers and live with his environment, instead of destroying it. *If man cannot do this, he will surely perish.*

All the above theories are possible explanations as to the origin of AIDS. I'm sure there are other such theories, but I'm afraid we will probably never know the real answer. However, as one African AIDS researcher commented at the Third International Conference on AIDS in 1987, *"When there is a lion in your home, you don't worry about how it got in, you worry how to get it out."*

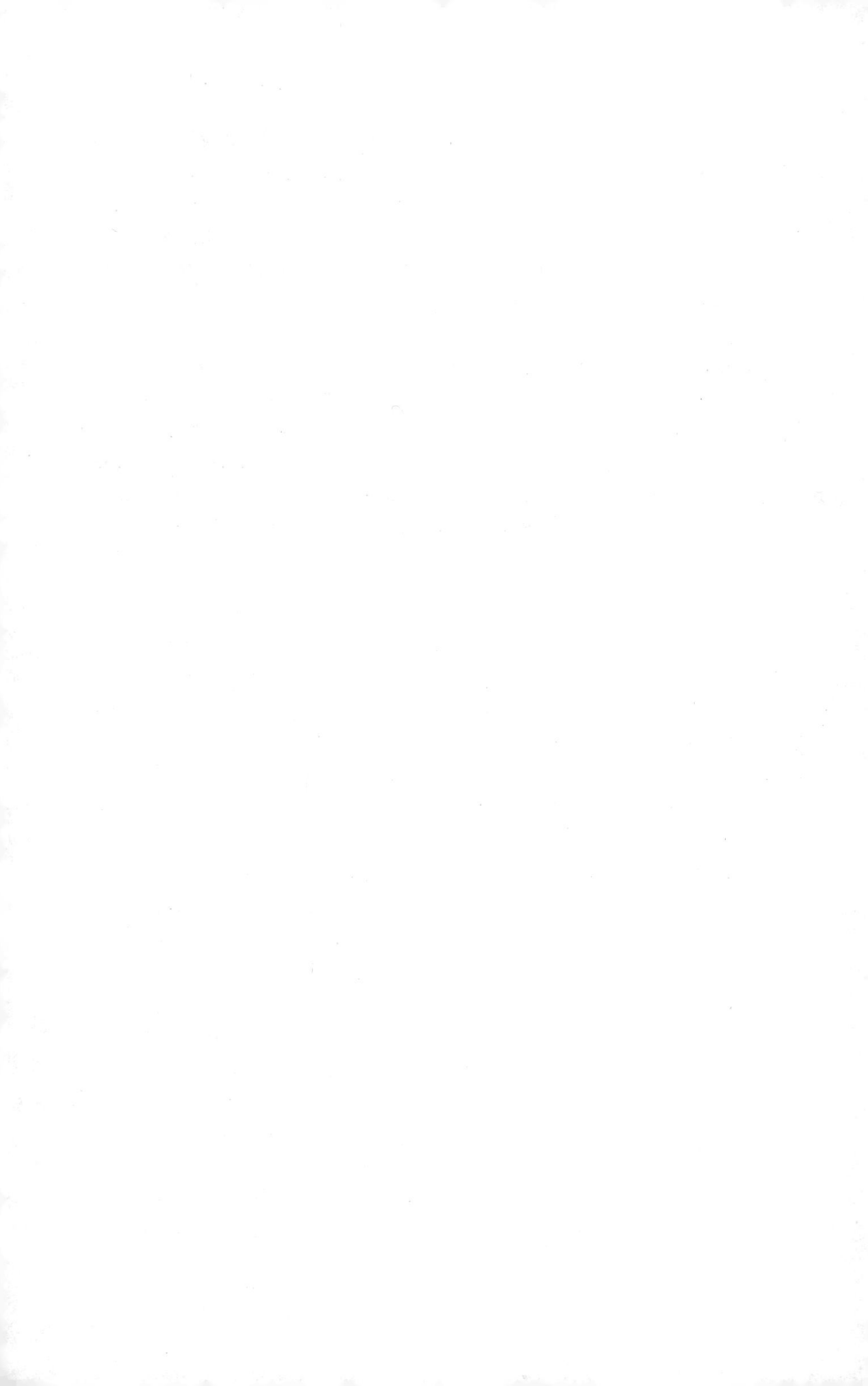

CHAPTER IV

MAN'S FUTURE – AIDS CURE OR EXTINCTION?

> *For wisdom is a defense, and money is a defense: but excellency of knowledge is, that wisdom giveth life to them that have it.*
>
> Ecclesiastes 7:11

Is there a cure for the AIDS disease? Is there a vaccine? If not, will a cure or vaccine ever be developed? Is either or both possible?

Here lies the basic problem in the war against the AIDS virus. Unfortunately, most people "assume" that science will find a cure and a vaccine for this disease. People are constantly bombarded with misinformation and dysinformation by the government, media, medical bureaucracy, special interest groups, and drug companies concerning a possible cure or vaccine for the AIDS disease. The media often makes irrational AIDS news to sell newspapers; the government often distorts, minimizes, or omits the AIDS truth to keep people's hopes up and to prevent a "panic;" the drug companies make millions of dollars by selling useless or exaggerated helpful "drugs" for AIDS; and the medical bureaucracy fears retaliation from the politicians and special interest groups, so it follows the "silence is the best policy" route.

Another dangerous "assumption" is that the search for the HIV-infection cure and/or vaccine is a race, some kind of competitive contest between scientists and nations. A good example of this is the ongoing feud between American and French scientists about which group first isolated the AIDS virus. Scientists around the world are trying to find the answers to these questions. Many of them realize that if they discover any answers first, they'll be showered with publicity and wealth beyond their wildest dreams.

Scientists, governments, and drug companies around the world should be working together, not separately, in a concerted effort to find the AIDS cure and/or vaccine.

I believe an AIDS cure is possible and probable, but not in the foreseeable future. Finding a vaccine, however, is another question. I believe a vaccine is possible, but improbable. There are 9,000 base pairs on the genome of the AIDS virus; thus, there are 9,000 to the fourth power possible different AIDS viruses.

This means there are literally trillions of possible combinations of the AIDS virus, all of which could be as infectious to humans as the other. (12) This virus mutates almost at will; a vaccine against one combination would be useless for another. Already we have recognized many AIDS viruses – HTLV-1, HTLV-2, HTLV-3, etc. How can we develop a vaccine to cover all of these combinations?

This problem is the same we have with the flu viruses – as soon as we have a vaccine for one, another flu strain develops, making the previous effective vaccine useless (e.g., Asian Flu, Hong Kong Flu, etc.).

Other problems of developing an effective AIDS prevention vaccine are the long incubation periods of the disease (up to 15 years), the scarcity of "human guinea pigs," the high cost of the research, the interference by self-serving or special interest groups (such as ambitious politicians, "scoop-minded" news reporters, medicrats) and the bureaucracy of government in general.

In summary, we will probably have a cure, but I'm afraid it will come years from now and after many, many people have died. As far as an effective vaccine is concerned, I seriously doubt one will ever be found for the reasons stated above.

WILL AIDS BE THE FINAL PLAGUE?

Pestilences and plagues are as old as man. Columbus, besides discovering America, is also the scoundrel who brought syphilis to Europe. Some now compare AIDS to syphilis.

Noted historian Barbara Tuchman wrote in her book, *A Distant Mirror,* about the onslaught of The Black Death in Europe around 1350 (though it is rumored to have started in China about 25 years earlier). There is no data on how many died, but it was in the millions. Some estimate that half the people alive, when it started, died by the time it was over. The disease spread by flea bites, a form of blood transmission.

Although the death toll rose like a rocket and then tailed off, people were still dying from it 250 years later. But the Black Death was very different from our modern AIDS plague. You could catch the former at noontime and be dead by the time the sun went down. AIDS, on the other hand, can incubate from five to 15 years before breaking out; but in the meantime, you are infectious and contagious to other people. In other words, you can go about your life in a normal fashion, and then one day it *explodes* in you! Meanwhile, since you are an AIDS carrier, *you have probably HIV infected many other people.*

PLAGUE

What is a plague? Plague is an affliction, any great evil, a calamity, a deadly epidemic disease. Such a disease spreads rapidly among people in a community, often causing a high mortality rate. Plagues have been with man throughout his existence, limiting his numbers and affecting his life.

Because of various plagues in history, wars have been won and lost or not fought at all; nations have been decimated, conquered or even eliminated; and different peoples of the world have been greatly reduced, some to the point of extinction.

Present day Americans, as well as most people of the world, have forgotten the frightful plagues of the past. They can't even imagine the misery, horror and deaths those plagues caused. America has not had a full-blown plague for many years; therefore, today's people have no knowledge of plagues and thus no experience on how to fight one. Most people think that because they live in a world of modern medicine and scientific wonders, there will never be another plague. *Silly people!*

The following is a review of some past plagues that have afflicted mankind:

(1) As a child, I was fascinated by adventurist figures such as Hernando Cortez who conquered the Aztec nation, Francisco Pizarro who conquered the Inca empire, and Captain James Cook who conquered island after island around the world. It never occurred to me, however, to ask myself a few simple questions. How could a few people on a few ships conquer hundreds of thousands, even millions, of people? Why did the conquered peoples usually accept Christianity and give up their own various religions so easily? What happened to the almost extinct pure Hawaiian race (less than 10% remain) or the now extinct Aztec peoples? Now, I ask myself, "How could I have believed such nonsense then?" The answer is easy! *I was uninformed and gullible.*

The true events that led to Cortez' "victory" over the millions of Aztec natives are little known and fascinating. Cortez landed on the Aztec land (Mexico) with five to six hundred men. Thinking these white men were gods, and terrified of their guns, cannons, and horses (which they had never seen), the Aztecs showered the Spaniards with jewels, gold and many other gifts. Because of the Aztecs' reluctance to fight and their apparent great wealth, the fearless Cortez declared war on this nation of millions.

Cortez and company marched in and killed all the way to the edge of the capital city (now Mexico City). Seeing these Spaniards as mortals and not gods, their horses easily killed, and the power of their guns limited, Montezuma and his many warriors attacked. Cortez and his small army were quickly routed and forced into full retreat. When reaching his ships, Cortez noticed the Aztecs were not continuing their pursuit; therefore, he set up camp on the beach, regrouped his men, and enlisted local Aztec-hating native people for his army. Then Cortez again marched on the capital city.

Instead of encountering an expected formidable foe, Cortez found his path littered with dead or dying Aztec Indians. When he reached and entered the capital, he found a raging smallpox epidemic – the Aztec nation was literally dead or dying. The smallpox virus was brought over and introduced to the Western Hemisphere by Cortez' men, the majority of whom were immune to the disease. This virus then infected the entire susceptible Aztec nation and destroyed it, because none of the natives had any immunity to the virus.

It was not Cortez and his small army, but the smallpox epidemic or plague which was the true "conqueror" of the mighty Aztec empire.

Never-before-seen diseases, such as smallpox, measles, chicken pox, and malaria were introduced to the New World by the Old World people (who were immune to these diseases) in the fifteenth and sixteenth centuries. These diseases infected and literally decimated the people of the Western World, because they had no immunity against them. It was these devastating new diseases amongst the susceptible Indians that caused the New World peoples to be so easily eliminated and their literally empty lands thereafter so easily reclaimed by the Old World peoples.

(2) Yellow fever, a very contagious disease caused by a virus, was brought to the New World from West Africa by seafarers. They also brought the vector, a certain never-before-seen mosquito (*Aedes aegypti*), which carries this infectious disease from man to man.

With the yellow fever virus and vector both present, the first epidemic of yellow fever broke out in Yucatan and Havana (Central America) in 1648. This disease not only decimated the local population, but all other peoples coming to this area not having immunity. The French first attempted to connect the Atlantic and Pacific Oceans in Central America by building the Panama Canal (1879-1889), but failed because of the high cost of building the canal and the high mortality rate of their work force by the yellow fever disease. After the French abandoned the project, the United States completed the Panama Canal (1904-1914), but only with very strict precautionary methods for yellow fever, such as successfully controlling the vector (mosquito) numbers and a sizable loss of life.

(3) Malaria, another contagious disease which needs a mosquito to transmit it from man to man, was also introduced to the New World by the seafarers. From China westward, through centuries, this disease caused plague after plague, killing millions of people. Again, when introduced to the New World, it too contributed to the devastation of the various native peoples.

(4) Bubonic plague. Epidemic diseases date back to 200 B.C., according to Biblical and Egyptian text. The first described bubonic plague was the Justian plague of A.D. 542, reappearing periodically thereafter. It probably was one of the ancient plagues as well, but this has never been proven.
Man is infected with this disease by a flea bite, from fleas living on rodents. Occasionally the disease can spread by inhaling the droplets (aerosol) of a cough from an infected person, the disease then being called pneumonic (rather than bubonic) plague.
Bubonic plague started in China, then proceeded to Europe, and finally to the New World. Whenever the disease struck, it struck rapidly and viciously. It is recorded that 10,000 people per day died when it first struck Constantinople and lasted four months. It often killed more than 40% of the population wherever it struck, which then took many years to replace. The plagues of the 6th, 7th and 14th centuries were particularly devastating to Europe. "The Black Death" term was given to this disease because of the misery and death it caused man throughout history. Today, even though a cure does exist, the bubonic disease terrifies everybody when it strikes.

The following excerpts from an epic book, A Distant *Mirror* by Barbara Tuchman (1978), give us some idea of the horrors of the Black Death:

Man's Future – AIDS Cure or Extinction?

- In October 1347, trading ships put into the harbor of Messina in Sicily with dead and dying men at the oars. The diseased sailors suffered pain and died within five days of the first symptoms.
- "So lethal was the disease that cases were known of persons going to bed well and dying before they woke, of doctors catching the illness at bedside and dying before the patient."
- In a given area the plague accomplished its kill within four to six months and then faded, except in the larger cities where, rooting into the close-quartered population, it abated during the winter, only to reappear and rage for another six months."
- "Although the mortality rate was erratic, ranging from 20 percent in some places to 90 percent and total elimination in others, the overall estimate of modern demographers has settled on "a third of the world died then." That would have meant about 20 million deaths. No one knows the truth how many died ... When graveyards filled up, mass burial pits were dug with corpses piled on corpses until they overflowed ... In enclosed places, such as monasteries and prisons, the infection of one person meant the infection of all."
- "In the countryside, peasants dropped dead on the roads, in the fields and in their houses. Survivors, in growing helplessness, fell into apathy, leaving ripe wheat uncut and livestock unattended ... the dearth of labor held a fearful prospect because the 14th century lived close to the annual harvest both for food and next year's seed ... the sense of a vanishing future created a kind of demential of despair.
- "To the people at large, there could be but one explanation – the wrath of God. A scourge so sweeping and unsparing without any visible cause could be seen as divine wrath took many forms. Of all the terrors, mystery of the contagion was the most terrible since, most of the time, no one knew the cause. The apparent absence of earthly cause gave the plague a supernatural and sinister quality."
- "The general acceptance of this view created an expanded sense of guilt, for if the plague were punishment, there had to be a terrible sin to have occasioned it. What sins were on the

14th century conscience? Primarily greed, the sin of avarice, followed by usury, worldliness, adultery, blasphemy, falsehood, luxury, irreligious retribution for oppressing the poor, etc."
- "Efforts to cope with the epidemic availed little, either in treatment or prevention. Helpless to alleviate the plague, the doctor's primary effort was to keep it at bay. Doctors gave attention to diet, bodily health and mental attitude."
- "During the plague, as street cleaners and carters died, cities grew befouled, increasing the infection. Residents of a street might rent a cart in common to remove the water, but energy and will were depressed."
- "Quarantines became popular and Poland established this at its frontiers, giving it relative immunity. In general, Draconian means were adopted everywhere to stop the spread."
- The theory, emotions and justifications of anti-Semitism were laid at that time in the canon law codified by the councils."
- "Since the Jews were damned anyway, they were permitted to lend at interest rates of 20 percent and more, of which the royal treasury took the major share. The Jews loaned, others took the profits. As commerce swelled in the 12th and 13th centuries, increasing the flow of money, the Jews' position deteriorated in proportion as they were less needed. Jews became isolated and expelled from society."
- "What was the human condition after the plague? Exhausted by deaths and sorrows and the morbid excesses of fear and hate, it ought to have shown some profound effects, but no radical change was immediately visible. The persistence of the normal is strong. Behavior grew more reckless and callous, as it often does after a period of violence and suffering. Because of intestate death, property without heirs, etc., a fury of litigation arose. Education was spurred by the concern for the survival of learning."
- "The obvious and immediate result of the Black Death was, of course, a shrunken population which, owing to wars and reoccurrence of the plague, declined even further by the end of the 14th century. The plague laid a curse on the century in the

form of its own backlash...but it eventually receded."
- "It left apprehension, tension, and gloom among the populace."

This is a very good historical account of what the Black Death was like. Few people today know the misery, terror, and tremendous loss of human life those bubonic plagues caused. Fewer yet realize that AIDS, too, is a plague – a plague which will prove far worse than the Black Death. Since most Americans have no understanding of the true horrors of plague, the misery and death toll caused by AIDS will be unimaginable.

These reflections of a few past plagues show what an uncontrolled, incurable, highly infectious, contagious, lethal disease can do to susceptible peoples and societies. AIDS is just this kind of disease, but worse. Past plagues infected, killed and left rapidly, but *AIDS does not*. AIDS infects and manifests itself slowly, usually years later. It is 100% fatal and thus far, incurable. How it spreads from person to person and why it mutates (changes its form) so often and rapidly is not fully understood. It is feared as, the HIV mutates more and more, its virulencewill tend to increase, thus infecting and killing many more people. AIDS is a new disease and appears to be in its initial stages of infecting man. In the near future, I believe AIDS will prove to be the worst plague ever to affect mankind.

CHAPTER V
AIDS RISK/ PRECAUTIONS

All things have I seen in the days of my vanity:
there is a just man that perishes in his righteousness,
and there is a wicked man that prolongs his life in his wickedness
Ecclesiastes 7:15

Which people are most likely to be exposed and infected by the AIDS virus? These people are grouped together into what are called "high risk groups." Homosexual and bisexual males, drug addicts (primarily intravenous [IV] users), prostitutes, hemophiliacs, and people practicing bisexual and heterosexual promiscuity are all considered high risk groups. These groups are usually found in the inner-city communities (usually Hispanics, Blacks, and prostitutes) who have high rates of IV drug use and sexually transmitted diseases.

The Merck Manual (Fifteenth Edition) states the following: "In the U.S.A. and Europe, statistical data on persons with AIDS are remarkably similar. Using data up to the beginning of 1986 from U.S.A., 90% of patients were 20 to 40 years old, 93% were men, and 94% could be placed in groups that suggest a possible means of the disease acquisition: homosexuals or bisexual men, 74% (8% were also IV drug users); heterosexual IV users, 17%; persons with hemophilia, 1%; heterosexual sex partners of persons with AIDS or at risk of AIDS (e.g., spouses of persons with AIDS, prostitutes), 1%; and recipients of transfused blood or blood components, 2%. Of the 6% unaligned to a high risk group, many could not be fully investigated."

If you are not a member of one of the above high risk groups, it does not necessarily mean you are safe from possibly contracting an HIV infection. The following excerpts from *The AIDS Cover-Up* (1986), by Gene Antonio are interesting:

- "In the U.S.A., male homosexuals comprise over 3/4 of all AIDS cases."
- "Less than 1% of all AIDS are linked directly to heterosexual relations, but this may soon change. It is increasingly being recognized coitus is not impervious to AIDS transmission."
- "6% of AIDS involve persons with no known risk factor."
- "Among female prostitutes, the high frequency of sexual encounters, combined with the exposure to large numbers of anonymous partners (thirty to forty per week is not uncommon) results in bodily trauma and a high incidence of venereal disease. The resulting genital lesions and sores provide ports of entry and exit for the AIDS virus. These diseases may also provide co-factors which are believed by some researchers to help trigger reproduction of the virus and development of the syndrome."
- "Data obtained from Africa and here in the United States indicates that bisexual and heterosexual promiscuity are viable means of spreading AIDS on a vast scale. In Africa, infected female prostitutes and their patrons have been cited as major sources of AIDS transmission."
- "Upwards of 85 percent of the United States urban drug-addicted population is infected with the AIDS virus as well. Within this group of an estimated 250,000 persons, are thousands of infected women, many of whom support their drug habit through prostitution."
- "Upwards of one and a half million homosexual/bisexual men are presently infected with the AIDS virus."
- "The apparent, present lack of evidence concerning non-sexual, non-blood transmission related means of transmission is not a firm guarantee of actual or potential lack of risk."

Another important group of people who are at great risk for AIDS infection are health care workers. Physicians, nurses, hospital employees, medical/dental office employees, and dentists are often exposed to people who are HIV infected.

Of this group, workers in hospitals are at greatest risk. The hospital emergency, surgical, and obstetrical departments are the most likely departments to come into contact with the AIDS virus. Because of this fact, I believe more and more health care workers will leave the profession, and less new workers will enter the medical field. Shortages of these workers is already appearing and is one of the reasons the quality of medical care delivered is deteriorating.

The present "fear of AIDS" in this profession is very real and is causing great concern. Because politicians and medicrats aren't directly exposed to the AIDS virus, they are minimizing the AIDS risks *for everybody else*. However, most of the "hands on" health workers know that this disease is contagious, has no cure, has no vaccine, is 100% lethal and is very little understood. They fear the AIDS virus and take the disease most seriously. The question many now ask is, what's more important, their line of work or their lives?

What about pregnancy? Can a pregnancy be affected by the AIDS virus? Yes. While only 7% of AIDS-sick patients reported are women, this figure is rapidly increasing. 17% of all female AIDS cases occurred in the first quarter of 1988. (13) As stated earlier, Dr. John Platt notes "that under very accurate testing in Massachusetts, 2% of babies delivered had AIDS. In the Midwest, a CDC (Center for Disease Control) survey showed the number was 3%. In hot spots for AIDS like Miami, New York City, San Francisco, Houston, the percentage was 4% plus."

Yes, the AIDS virus does affect both the pregnant mother and her baby. It appears the fertility rates, as well as the pregnant patient's health are essentially unaffected when the female is early AIDS infected; however, in the later stages of the disease, the deteriorating health of the victim does adversely affect the pregnancy.

"The clinical course of early AIDS infection in pregnant women is not much different from that of non-pregnant seropositive women." (14) Of course, the pregnant female is just as contagious as when not pregnant, but pregnancy itself does not appear to worsen or help the course of the AIDS disease. The baby's fate, however, is quite different. When an AIDS-infected female (early or late in the disease) conceives, carries, delivers, and rears a baby, the outcome is usually disastrous.

"Among children there is a substantial risk for transmission from parent to offspring, particularly in the prenatal and perinatal period." (15) From the AIDS battlefield in Newark, N.J., James M. Oleske, a pediatric immunologist from the University of Medicine and Dentistry of New Jersey reports that "the vast majority of pediatric AIDS cases nationwide are now acquired prenatally – that is, from early pregnancy through the time of birth – through infection of the mothers with human immune deficiency virus (HIV). What we're seeing more and more of in Newark, and the same will be seen elsewhere," Oleske says, "are women who are infected although they are not drug users, but they were exposed to high risk males."

"Because approximately half the children born to HIV carriers are expected to develop fatal AIDS, this represents an area of great concern," he says. Previously, blood transfusions accounted for the majority of pediatric AIDS cases nationwide. By 1991, Oleske predicts, the cumulative number of infected children will range from 10,000 to 20,000, most with symptoms, and one of every ten to fifteen U.S. hospital beds will be occupied by a child with HIV infection. (16)

Because the AIDS virus can cross the placenta, the baby is AIDS infected in more than 50 percent of the time. Since the AIDS virus has been demonstrated to be present the mother's breast milk, this mode of transmission has also been implicated.

Because of the poor chance for a good baby outcome, I believe all pregnant patients should be tested for AIDS disease. If the test is positive, the patient should be immediately informed and given a choice of whether to carry and deliver the baby or to have an abortion.

AIDS-infected females should be well informed what pregnancy means to them and their babies. AIDS-infected women should practice effective birth control and even be encouraged to be sterilized, when possible. An AIDS-infected pregnant patient is not only a danger to her herself, but to her baby, to her relatives and friends, to her obstetrician and his office staff and to her hospital's obstetrical/surgical departments.

The whole issue of AIDS in pregnancy is frightening and depressing, but it's just another system (man's reproductive system) which AIDS is attacking. We are just beginning to see the adverse effects AIDS will have on pregnancies, newborns, attending physicians, and others in the obstetrical field and health facilities.

I believe this problem, AIDS in pregnancy, is much worse than reported and is worsening by the day. I believe 65 to 100% of the babies born from these unfortunate mothers will be AIDS infected and eventually die. The health care costs and problems that will soon manifest for the care of AIDS-infected pregnancies will be unimaginable. Make no mistakes about it, we are just beginning to see the developing disaster AIDS will cause in man's reproductive life cycle.

PRECAUTIONS AGAINST AIDS

What precautions can one take to prevent becoming infected with HIV? Truthfully, no one really knows how to prevent the spread of AIDS! If the answer were known, AIDS would not be the problem and threat to mankind that it now is.

The best prevention is to assume that there are many ways to become infected with the AIDS virus, only some of which are known today. Since all the ways the AIDS virus infects are not known, we must be "on guard" at all times. The following are must precautions:

(1) Read this book, understand, and remember it. AIDS is contagious and 100% lethal. It is the plague of the 20th century – the Plague of Plagues. Therefore, don't underestimate it or assume anything about it.

(2) Educate yourself and your loved ones about AIDS. This is extremely important. This is not as simple as it sounds because AIDS is an extremely complicated disease. Every day, more news about the disease is known and circulated

by the media. The more one knows about AIDS, the better his chances are to avoid infection. Evaluate all AIDS information carefully, discarding the nonsensical or false.

(3) Know who the "high risk groups" are. If you are in any of these groups, be very careful. If not, be careful when in contact with a person in these groups.

(4) Practice "safe sex." Do not have sex with an infected person or a person you don't know unless you use a condom and/or diaphragm and you realize your chances of becoming infected is greatly increased. Don't practice anal sex. Know your partners and talk to them about AIDS.

(5) Do not inject drugs (heroin, speed, cocaine, etc.) with needles and syringes used by others.

(6) Use disinfectants. While the AIDS virus is able to stay alive outside the body in ideal conditions, it is easily killed with any good disinfectant, including soap and water, hydrogen peroxide, rubbing alcohol, and household bleach (one part bleach to nine parts water).

(7) Accept blood transfusions only when necessary and only if properly screened for AIDS and prepared by appropriately housed blood banks.

(8) Don't assume AIDS is primarily a sexually transmitted disease. Always keep in mind that other modes of becoming infected are possible and even probable. Don't become a statistic of some other future-proven route of infection, such as mosquito bites, "casual contact," or kissing.

(9) Remember that AIDS is still primarily confined to gay and bisexual men in the United States at this time, but heterosexuals are not immune to the disease. The virus does not prefer one human to another. It will infect both men and women

AIDS Risk/Precautions

given the opportunity. *Don't give it that opportunity!*

(10) AIDS-infected people are just as infectious as AIDS-sick people. Treat both the same – very carefully.

(11) When in public, cleanliness is the best precaution. Patronize only clean restaurants, theaters, and other such public or private establishments. Use only clean public toilets and drinking fountains, and try to avoid such facilities as often as possible. Try to stay out of congested areas when possible, as coughing, sneezing, and spitting may increase your chances of infection. Common sense here can prevail.

(12) Don't go to the hospital unless absolutely necessary and only consent to surgical procedures or blood transfusions when necessary.

(13) Visit your doctor if you suspect you may have been infected with the AIDS virus. After testing you, he will tell you if you have AIDS or not. If you don't, consider yourself lucky and take the above precautions to heart. If you do, begin immediate treatment and get counseling for yourself and advice on how to help prevent infection to others.

All of the above precautionary measures can help one's chances of escaping AIDS infection; but, remember, infection is still possible. The more we learn about the disease, the more precautions we will be able to ascertain.

CHAPTER VI
POTPOURRI OF AIDS: PART I

Vanity of Vanities, saith the Preacher; all is vanity
Ecclesiastes 12:8

From *All Fall Down,* William Campbell Douglas, M.D., 1987:

- The innocence and playfulness of children, even in the face of grotesque situations and death, is noted in the games they often devise and play. "Ring around the rosey, pocket full of posies, ashes to ashes, we all fall down" was a children's verse describing the worst plague in recorded human history, the Black Death of the Middle Ages. The typical little red boils of the plague were surrounded by a red ring ("ring around the rosey"). Infected people smelled terrible so the victims carried flowers in their pockets to disguise the smell ("a pocket full of posies"). Ashes were mixed with water to serve as an ointment ("ashes to ashes"). The dying would, as humans are prone to do, just keep going until the end and then drop dead on the street ("we all fall down"). Modern children dealing with today's Black Death – Kaposis Sarcoma which blackens the skin, and other deadly varieties of AIDS, may not be as poetic, but, they too, make a game of impending death. In New York they have a game called "AIDS." When a child is tagged, he has "AIDS" until he tags another child. History does repeat. (1)

My Comment: I've been singing this lyric since I was a little child and never knew its meaning until recently. More interestingly, none of my friends knew its meaning either. Isn't human behavior predictable – we often do and say things we know nothing about.

From the *San Jose Mercury News,* Santa Clara County, California, August 20, 1988:

- A study by the Hudson Institute (a non-profit research and public policy center based in Indianapolis), doubles the estimates of Americans with AIDS. The article stated: "Twice as many Americans might be infected with the AIDS virus than the government estimates, and the virus might be much more prevalent among heterosexuals than widely thought, researchers reported Friday."
- A "best guess" at the number of AIDS-infected Americans at the end of last year was 1.9 million and 3 million, with the most probable range between 2.2 million and 2.6 million people.
- The Hudson Officials said the institute's study suggested AIDS might be spreading much faster than had been suspected and could have much more sweeping policy implications.
- George Keyworth, Hudson research director, said "If there is a larger pool of infected people, then these are important new implications for national health policy – not only in terms of the strain on medical treatment resources, but also in terms of potential spread of the disease in coming years; and these are equally important implications for individual behavior in the face of increased hazard."
- The Hudson Officials said perhaps the most alarming conclusion of their study was that the virus appeared to be much more widespread among heterosexuals than commonly thought – particularly among those who do not use intravenous drugs. Many heterosexuals, they said, mistakenly think they are not susceptible to AIDS and have become "complacent" in taking precautions against contagion.
- A breakout of the disease into the non-monogamous heterosexual population is more than a theoretical possibility," said Kevin Hopkins, a Hudson AIDS researcher. "According to our study, such a breakout into the mainstream heterosexual

population is unavoidable unless dramatic behavior changes or medical progress takes place soon."

My Comment: Where are those "AIDS Experts" now, who told us that the heterosexual rate of infection was low and we had nothing to worry about? This article proves two things – AIDS is on the march and, almost everyday, some "AIDS Experts" are proven wrong. Why do they persist in misinforming the public about the dangers of AIDS? One would think that after being proven wrong so many times, they would stop making incorrect assumptions or ridiculous statements about the AIDS virus and its behavior.

From *The New American magazine,* "Heterosexuals And The AIDS Epidemic," Vol. 4, No. 10, May 9 1988:

- Dr. Mathilde Krim, founding chairman of the American Foundation for AIDS Research, criticized the work (CRISIS: Heterosexual Behavior in the Age of AIDS by sex researchers William H. Masters, Virginia F. Johnson, and Dr. Robert C. Kolidy) as "needlessly alarming" and "a very serious setback to AIDS education." She reproached the three authors for promoting "senseless hysteria" and suggested that they were "commercializing on AIDS and the fear of AIDS."

My Comment: These kinds of irresponsible statements from supposedly responsible leaders lull the nation's people into a state of "AIDS complacency."

From the *San Francisco Examiner,* "AIDS Workers Struggle With Burnout," August 28, 1988:

- The latest casualties of the AIDS epidemic are not those struck down by the fatal syndrome, but the doctors, nurses, attorneys, social workers, and volunteers who stand by their sides.
- Battling burnout, they work long hours at a frantic pace against an incurable disease . The feeling, psychiatrists say, is like combat fatigue. But there's no coming home from this war.

- We've felt an ocean of grief" said Alison Moet, head nurse of San Francisco General Hospital's inpatient AIDS ward, a five year veteran of the unit. "We've seen so many people be so young, watched their fine minds and talents struck down. How can it not affect us – individually and as a community?"
- Young and idealistic, they once believed they could quickly conquer AIDS if only they worked hard enough. But five years after establishing a network of innovative organizations – the Shanti Project, The AIDS Foundation, San Francisco General Inpatient AIDS Unit, and the AIDS Mental Health Project – the AIDS epidemic is killing more people than ever: three to five San Franciscans every day.
- The workers say they feel dangerously depleted, physically and emotionally.
- The signs are unmistakable, say mental health workers. Once energetic workers become lethargic, distracted, and disorganized, others are overly stressed and agitated. Their conversations develop a sharp and anxious edge, Moet said.
- As the death toll mounts, the City worries it will be unable to attract and retain the talented workers and volunteers it has relied on in the past.
- In emotional self-defense, Hally Smith of the Shanti Project stopped attending funerals and memorials, except those of loved ones. "You're asked to get close to a person who has only a short time to live. Then, when that passage takes place, it is devastating," Smith said. "There is grief overload."
- Trained to heal, workers are frustrated by an illness that allows no healing. "We need to adjust our image of the benevolent and powerful medical profession, well prepared for all crisis," McKisick has written in a book, *What To Do About AIDS* (U. C. Press).
- AIDS support groups must plan to protect their staffs, Nickens said. "Otherwise, there is burnout and high turn over - you just run through your staff."

My Comment: This article points out that the AIDS patients are but some of the victims. The misery this disease can cause never seems to end, *it only goes up, up and up!*

From the *Los Angeles Times,* "AIDS Toll in S.F.:City Under Siege," August 22, 1988:

- About 4% of the City's residents – including a staggering 50% of the estimated 42,500 to 69,100 gay men – are infected with the AIDS-causing human immune deficiency virus. Barring a cure of effective treatment, all can expect to die, most within 10 years.
- "Nearly one person in 20," John H. Jacobs (executive director of the San Francisco Chamber of Commerce) said shaking his head in horror, "I was in World War II. You could do better than that in a city under attack."
- A city under attack. A war. A natural disaster. A holocaust. These are the images leaders in business, politics, medicine, labor and the arts conjure when reflecting on the present and future of AIDS upon this city of 750,000. Already, with more than 5,000 diagnosed cases, 3,000 deaths and an estimated 30,000 people infected with the virus but not yet ill, no facet of life – from the tourist trade to apartment vacancies – is untouched.
- The past is bleak enough, with more San Franciscans dead of AIDS than from all the wars in this country, combined and doubled. AIDS has already claimed more lives than the great earthquake and fire of 1906, which killed 2,010 of the city's 450,000 inhabitants. But seven years after the first recorded AIDS death here, a painful realization is seeping in. This is only the beginning.
- Businesses are braced for skyrocketing medical expenses and potential labor shortages. Health coverage has become a major element in labor negotiations. Political analysts suspect gay political influence will wane as more and more gay men succumb.
- "All the mechanisms we have used to keep the awful truth at bay are breaking down." said Dr. James W. Dilly, executive director of the AIDS Health Project. He echoed the fear of

many who believe the city is ill prepared for "the overload of grief" it will face as the AIDS death rate doubles to six people a day by 1993. "I don't think there will be a pall cast over the city," Major Agnos insisted, convinced of the resilience of his constituents. "But it will certainly be something that all of us feel and carry with us because it is going to be the biggest human tragedy in the modern history of this city."

- By 1993, 12,349 to 17,022 San Franciscans will either have AIDS or dead from it, the Public Health Department said in a report issued in March. The range reflects uncertainties over treatment advances.
- No other city approaches San Francisco per-capita rate of infection. San Francisco has about three times more AIDS cases per-capita than New York and 10 times as many as Los Angeles.
- Because the short-term outlook for any treatment breakthroughs is bleak, city officials are gearing for the worst. The $90 million spent in the fiscal year just ended in government and private money to care for people with the disease could rise to $376 million a year by 1993. Where AIDS patients require roughly 140 hospital beds now on any given day, as many as 440 beds a day will be needed in five years, the Department of Public Health predicts.
- "The clock is ticking," said Dr. David Werdegar, San Francisco Health Department chief. "I have the feeling that the public forgets that there is a time dimension – that a great many people got infected in the early 80s and (the time when they will become sick) is getting closer."
- Indeed, many people find it difficult to look unflinchingly into the future. "It is very hard to speak rationally about how it will feel," said Supervisor Harry Britt, who is gay.

My Comment: This is a powerful and frightening account of the adverse effects AIDS is having on the city of San Francisco. The AIDS threat is *adversely* affecting business, housing, medical expenses, labor, health insurance, politics, hospital beds and, of course, AIDS victims themselves. San Francisco truly is a city in distress and in the early stages of an epidemic with all its attributes present – fear, grief, pain, concern, anxiety, and danger.

I live and practice near San Francisco and, because of the AIDS disease, I know of more and more people in the surrounding communities who are avoiding the city. When I now visit the city, I see more and more restaurants almost empty, theaters half full, and shops empty. In short, a once prime tourist-filled city is now a shadow of its former self. This city is beginning to resemble the cities of the "Black Plague or Death" times, as described in the history books.

From the *Monthly AIDS Update* newsletter, "A Biblical and Medical Analysis," by Ed Payne, M.D., Editor:

- "AIDS is our number 1 health problem," says Otis R. Bowen, Secretary of Health and Human Service.
- "AIDS is the third most pressing problem facing the country today, after the federal deficit and drug abuse." Survey of company executives by *Fortune Magazine* and Allstate Insurance Company.
- All Americans will be severely impacted by AIDS whether threatened by infection with its conservative virus or not. For example, one percent of all death payments from life insurance are AIDS related. That figure doesn't sound like much except that an increase to 4-5 percent could threaten the benefits of all policyholders.

My Comment: I would think the opinions of the above responsible people would awaken or alarm most of us as to the importance and dangers of the AIDS disease, but I'm afraid not.

From the *Wall Street Journal*, "AIDS Virus in Infected People Mutates at a Dizzying Rate, Two Studies Show," August 4, 1988, page 20:

- The AIDS virus, which long has confounded Scientists with its ability to vary geographically now has also been shown to

- mutate swiftly and extensively within individual patients.
- Two studies of infected but healthy carriers, done by teams of researchers at the University of Alabama and national Causes Institute, clues to the dizzying variability of the virus that causes acquired immune deficiency syndrome.
- The reports, published in today's edition of the British Journal Nature, also raise renewed questions and concerns about the prospects of developing a vaccine against the virus, given its power to change and thus dodge the body's immune defenses.
- In their tests, scientists found one patient harbored 17 different mutants, all apparently descended from a common virus. Certain genes were 3% to 8% different from one mutant to another.
- "What that's saying is that during the rational course of infection with the AIDS virus, people are actually infected with a complex mixture of genetically related but distinct viruses. This mixture evolves over time," explained George M. Shaw, co-author with Michael S. Saag of the University of Alabama report.
- In its second study, Amanda G. Fisher and Flossie Wang-Stool in the laboratory of Robert Gallo of the National Causes Institute suggested that the genetic variability of the AIDS virus (and its mutants) may affect its infectiousness and its "preference" for attacking one type of cell over another.
- Dr. Shaw said the real impact of such mutation on the course of the disease, on the body's response, remains to be discovered in future studies. "The important question is: What's the biological significance of this variation?" he said.
- "There's so much yet to know about the complex interaction between the virus and its host – man," Dr. Shaw said. "So much that we don't even begin to know."

My Comment: This article puts it nicely: the AIDS virus spreads and mutates very rapidly and we really know very little about it. People who work with the AIDS virus and AIDS-infected people are informed, but since so little is actually known about the AIDS problem, no one should be considered an "AIDS expert." The only

AIDS experts are the qualified, responsible people working with AIDS, who are the first to admit they don't know most of the answers about AIDS and the first to recommend caution and respect for this terror.

From the *San Jose Mercury News,* Santa Clara County, California, "AIDS found in Relatively Few Prostitutes,"August 20, 1988:

- AIDS testing of female prostitutes and their customers - groups under close scrutiny or potential carriers of the deadly disease among heterosexuals – indicates that infection among prostitutes is not as widespread as some experts had expected.
- An equally important finding is the scant evidence of female prostitutes passing AIDS virus to their customers. Two studies that tested 627 New York City men who visited prostitutes found only three cases in which the virus was thought likely to have been caught from a prostitute. "I don't know of any proven cases of female prostitutes infecting clients," said Dr. William Darrow, an AIDS epidemiology official at the Federal Centers for Disease Control in Atlanta.
- Although health officials still are concerned about AIDS among prostitutes, some had feared that the problem was greater than the latest studies show, in light of the frequent sexual contacts by prostitutes. Indeed, the AIDS infection rates for prostitutes are lower than for groups regarded as being high risk.
- A crucial factor may be in the sexual practice of prostitutes. Most told researchers that they require customers to use condoms, and that the customer's most frequent request is to perform oral sex, which has not been proven to be a frequent mode of AIDS transmission.

My Comment: There are many who say the "oldest profession in the world" is the cause of everything bad and sinful, but apparently the AIDS disease may not be one of them.

From *The Futurist,* "The Social Consequences of AIDS," by Edward Cornish, November-December 1987:

- The impacts of AIDS will be increasingly pervasive. Governments – national, state, and local – will have to cut funding for other programs in order to provide for AIDS victims. Life insurance companies may have to raise their rates, especially for younger people. Individuals will modify their lifestyles to avoid contracting the disease.
- The impact of the new plague (AIDS) will enter peoples lives in countless other ways such as:
- Ethnic and religious groups that are promiscuous will be affected disproportionately, and their numbers may decline. Already there is concern about the Eskimos due to their relaxed sexual mores. By contrast, groups practicing strict fidelity and producing many children (e.g. Hutterites and Orthodox Jews) may gain in numbers.
- People will become more cautious about physical contacts of many kinds. Kissing, hugging, even handshaking may become less casual; some people may even adopt the Oriental custom of bowing as a substitute.
- Mothers will be less willing to let their children play outside, fearing all kinds of risks such as children finding and playing with discarded medical or personal items with blood on them.
- Clothing may become more modest as people downplay their sexuality. Public sunbathing may become less popular.
- Special AIDS institutions (hospices, etc.) will develop, despite protests against "AIDS colonies."
- Many medical professionals will move to other occupations or seek other duties out of fear for their personal safety. (Some health workers have already contracted the AIDS virus from patients.) The nurse shortage could intensify.
- Separating boys from girls in schools may come to be viewed as a sensible measure to reduce the likelihood of sexual contact.
- Restrictions on travel may increase, as nations try to protect their populations.
- Euthanasia may become tolerated or even encouraged for AIDS victims due to the heavy cost of caring for them, their suffering, and the dismal outcome of the disease.

- Drug use may decline. Since intravenous drug abuse often leads to exposure to AIDS, public opinion may support strong measures to curb drug trafficking. Malaysia and Thailand now punish drug dealers by hanging.
- Illegitimate births may decline. Fear of AIDS will probably reduce pregnancies among unmarried women.
- People's health may improve – if they don't get AIDS. Measures to prevent AIDS may reduce the incidence of other sexually transmissible diseases. Curbs on drugs may reduce hepatitis and many other health problems.
- Medical research will boom. The spillover of new findings will benefit almost all areas of medicine.
- Research into human sexuality will intensify. Psychologists, sociologists and others will be funded to discover the causes of sexual behavior, such as homosexuality and promiscuity.
- Marriages may become more stable since spouses will feel less free to "play around."
- Even a short list such as this shows that AIDS is a major social force that knows no boundaries and that will greatly alter the human future. As futurists, we are challenged to anticipate the impacts of the disease and to suggest strategies for coping with it.

My Comment: This is an excellent article on the probable effects of AIDS on our society. Anybody who thinks the future will be much like the past, both socially and economically, is in for a rude and frightening awakening.

From the *Los Angeles Times,* "Children Born With AIDS Face a Brief, Bleak Future," By Larry McShane, April 10, 1988, Associated Press:

- Recent State Health Department figures indicate that the potential numbers of AIDS-infected newborns is growing at a startling rate. One in 61 babies born in New York City last November carried antibodies to the AIDS virus, which means that they had been exposed to the virus.

- About 40% of those children will develop AIDS in some form; 25% to 30% of those children will be dead before their second birthday. Most of them were born to mothers who used drugs intravenously.
- Dr. Stephen Joseph, the City Health Commissioner, put the number of children born in the city with AIDS antibodies last year at about 600; for 1988 the projection is 1,000. Between 1980 and 1986, the total was only about 250 children.
- But even in Massachusetts, a state not known for large outbreaks of AIDS, one in 476 child-bearing women tested positive for AIDS antibodies, according to a study reported recently in the *New England Journal of Medicine*.
- Nationwide, there were 865 cases of pediatric AIDS reported as of February 29, with 111 diagnosed in just the first two months of the year.

My Comment: What a frightening development! As time goes on, more and more women become infected with the AIDS virus. Since most of these women are in their reproductive years, it stands to reason many will become pregnant and usually produce AIDS-infected babies. Most of these poor babies are "born dying." What a tragedy!

As an obstetrician, I have been trained to look for problems before they occur in childbirth and believe me, *AIDS is the "problem of problems!"* I think AIDS in pregnancy will become a nightmare. Right now, I feel all pregnant women should be AIDS tested in early pregnancy and if infected, be given a choice of having the baby or having an abortion, and being sterilized thereafter. Unfortunately, I am presently in the minority on this point. In the near future, AIDS in pregnancy will prove to be a national disaster.

From the *Dallas Times Herald,* "State report doubles AIDS projections," by Nora Zamichow, August 19, 1988:

- In just seven years, the number of Texans diagnosed with AIDS will jump nearly sevenfold to 30,000, almost double the number of cases experts had predicted, according to a state

task force report scheduled to be released today.
- And by the end of 1992, another 15,000 Texans will fall prey to the fatal disease – bringing the total projected total to 45,000 AIDS sufferers – a tenfold increase over the current number of cases.
- "An epidemic compels a well-planned, efficient, and coordinated response. Unfortunately, Texas' response to the HIV epidemic has evolved in a haphazard manner, without a strategic plan guiding the state's activities," said the report.
- Texas is fifth in the number of AIDS cases reported in the nation and, according to the report, Texas' share of the national total of AIDS cases will increase from 7% to 10%.
- "These new numbers drive home the fact that the epidemic isn't going to peak and be over in 1991 – which is what a lot of people thought," said Buck Buckingham, director of Dollar AIDS/ARM Network. "The epidemic is going to continue to grow through most of the decade, and we are woefully underprepared to deal with the projected increases."
- The report also said:
    1) Discrimination against people with AIDS is common and "costly" for taxpayers since it often results in loss of jobs and housing.
    2) Texas is "poorly prepared" to meet the needs of infants born with HIV infection.
    3) Drug treatment programs are "woefully inadequate" in trying to stem HIV transmission by intravenous drug users and hundreds of drug addicts are unable to receive treatment at all.
    4) A lack of statewide coordination has hindered Texas' response to the AIDS epidemic.

My Comment: This article reinforces my belief that the AIDS disease is spreading much faster than projected and due to the lack of an effective "Federal Universal AIDS Policy." States are free to determine their own AIDS policy, resulting in a hodge-podge of rules and regulations across the nation for the management of the HIV and AIDS disease. No wonder AIDS is spreading faster than projected.

From *Awake,* "AIDS, A Global Killer," October 8, 1988:

- Surgeon General of the United States, C. E. Koop said: "No previous disease has been at once so mysterious, so fatal, and so resistant to therapy and vaccine development." He stated: "We do not yet have a cure, nor do we have a vaccine – and we probably won't have one generally available before the end of the century. Make no mistake about it, AIDS is fatal and spreading." Dr. Koop also said: "I have been a surgeon for almost 50 years, and I have never seen such a threat as AIDS." The publication, *AIDS and the Third World,* said "Many medical experts, and a majority of virologists, now believe that the death toll among HIV-carriers will approach very close to 100%. The belief that all will eventually die is based partly on the fact that as every year goes by, more people who contracted the virus three or four or five years ago, do indeed, develop the disease. And it is based partly on the studies of the HIV virus itself." Of course, such views are estimates. Only time will tell if they will be realized in actual fact.
- In fact, *The Futurist* states: "AIDS may kill more people by the end of this century than have been killed by all our wars (of all the nations)." In Africa, few, if any, wars have ever done what AIDS is now doing. Britain's *New Scientists* observes: "AIDS is running rampant through Africa." An article in *Politician of Denmark* said: "Uganda's chief AIDS official states, "Unless something changes, every second adult in this country will be HIV-positive in the year 2000! Almost half of all AIDS cases in Africa are women in their child-bearing years. Children account for one of every five AIDS cases in Rwanda. In Zambia, 6,000 babies will be born with AIDS this year. Among 800 prostitutes tested in Nairobi; nine out of 10 were infected with HIV. And these women sleep with an average of 1,000 customers per year."
- "If we do nothing, the continent will die," says Pieter Piot, a

Belgian expert. Jonathan Mosin, who heads WHO campaign, states: "The alternative is to give up on Africa, as if the world were not a single planet. But the epidemic cannot be stopped in any one country before it is stopped in all of them."

- Thus, many medical authorities feel that a global AIDS catastrophe has already begun. U.N. Secretary-General Javier Perez de Cuellar calls it a "global conflict" that "threatens us with all the consequences of war."
- In some ways, it is worse than war. Why? Because no end is in sight, the casualties continue to mount, and the "wounded" are not recovering.
- In Africa, AIDS is widespread among heterosexuals. As many women as men have it.
- While the spread of AIDS among heterosexuals in Europe, the United States, and elsewhere, is not yet as rampant as in Africa, it is increasing in that group, too. So more and more women and men who are not homosexual or bisexual are getting AIDS and passing it on to others. A report stated, "AIDS has become the Number 1 killer of women aged 25-34 in New York City." And sadly, a large number – some say about 50% – of women carrying the AIDS virus are giving birth to babies who have the disease.
- The *Medical Post of Canada* reports: "Dr. Thomas Peterman, a medical epidemiologist with the AIDS branch of the Center for Disease Control estimated that 12,000 Americans became infected with HIV (AIDS virus) from contaminated blood transfusions from 1978-1984." Many of these blood recipients have died or are dying. Various hospitals have advised those who received blood transfusions before new testing methods were introduced in 1985 to get checked for AIDS.
- In one study of married men who got AIDS from blood transfusions, it was found that 14 percent of their wives also had the virus.
- A medical report by specialists at Mainz University in the Federal Republic of Germany states: "Transfusion medicine has to accept the fact that absolutely HIV-free blood no longer exists."

My Comment: Anybody who isn't a little concerned about AIDS after reading this article, is probably unconcerned about almost everything else in their lives. The main points here are that the AIDS disease is very contagious, lethal, and global. A cure or vaccine for AIDS are not in sight and the mounting toll in human lives will be unimaginable. Also, this disease will most definitely adversely affect the social, economic, and political fabric of every country in the world.

From *The New American,* "Heterosexuals and the AIDS Epidemic," by Kirk Kidwell, May 9, 1988, Volume 4, No. 10:

- The AIDS epidemic has broken out of the homosexual world in which it was cast and is now running rampant among heterosexuals, according to a recent book written by sex researchers William H. Masters, Virginia E. Johnson, and Robert C. Kolody.
- "Contrary to claims by various government agencies and public health experts that infection with AIDS virus is still largely confined to the original 'high risk' groups (gay and bisexual men and intravenous drug users)," the researchers write in their new book *Crisis: Heterosexual Behavior in the Age of AIDS,* "the epidemic has clearly broken out into the broader population and is continuing, even now, to make silent inroads of infection while many maintain an attitude of complacency, not realizing that they too, are at risk."
- Masters and Johnson also say that the number of infected Americans is closer to three million, "most of whom are otherwise healthy and unaware of their infected, contagious state." Further, they believe 200,000 (6.7 percent of those three million AIDS carriers) are non-drug abusing heterosexuals.
- "AIDS is breaking out. The AIDS virus is now running rampant in the heterosexual community. Unless something is done to contain this global epidemic," the Masters and Johnson team warns, "we face a mounting death toll in the years ahead that will be the most formidable the world has ever seen"
- Surgeon General C. Everett Koop has called the Masters and

Johnson book "irresponsible" and accused them of using "scare tactics."
- "AIDS is not exploding into the heterosexual community," Dr. Robert Wionslow, assistant secretary for health at the U.S. Department of Health and Human Services, assured the American public.
- A study published in the January 1, 1988 issue of *The Journal of the American Association (JAMA)* found that eight percent of wives of spouses infected by contaminated transfusions became infected with the AIDS virus over a period of two to three years. In another study, published in the February 6, 1987 issue of *JAMA,* 12 of 17 husbands (76 percent) and 14 of 28 wives (50 percent) were infected through sexual contact with their infected spouses.
- Surveys of blood banks, which test all donated blood for AIDS, found only 0.02 percent of donors (one in 5,000) are infected.
- A New York City survey reported in the *Annals of Internal Medicine* (October, 1987) suggested high existing levels of HIV infection in women in their middle and late twenties.
- Masters and Johnson write: "The somewhat chilling conclusion we have reached in this: AIDS virus has certainly established a breakhead in the ranks of heterosexuals, and because heterosexuals who have larger numbers of sex partners are most likely to be infected, the odds are that the rate of spread among heterosexuals will now begin to escalate at a frightening pace."
- Dr. William A. Haseltime of Harvard School of Public Health told the Washington Post (March 15, 1988): "Many experts fear that, if AIDS virus has gained a 'beachhead' in the heterosexual population of the United States, the experience of Africa could be repeated here. We don't understand the conditions for the heterosexual spread in Africa enough to predict that it could not happen in our major urban centers as well.... The potential is there, and the burden of proof would be placed on those who claim it will not spread. It is foolhardy to think that what happened in Africa could not happen here."
- One of the lessons of the African experience with AIDS is

that those who are sexually promiscuous are at the highest risk of acquiring HIV infection.
* The association between promiscuity and AIDS suggests that AIDS will become an increasing problem among promiscuous heterosexuals.
* A U.S. Army study by Robert Redfield found that 55 percent of the spouses of patients in the later stages of HIV infection became infected, whereas, only 16 percent of the spouses of patients in the earliest stages become infected. Consequently, according to transmission in Africa, "more heterosexual transmission will occur as more heterosexuals enter the more infectious stage of HIV infection." (AIDS, December, 1987)
* Dr. James Goodert of the National Cancer Institute concluded that "it may be possible to prevent HIV transmission and subsequent AIDS by taking appropriate steps to warn seronegative partners of seropositive individuals that the risk of transmission may increase over time."
* Thus, it is crucial for America to treat AIDS as the public health crisis it is and to implement those public health control measures that have traditionally been applied to sexually transmitted diseases: testing, infection reporting, contact tracing, and criminalizaton of knowing transmission of the AIDS virus. Whether the AIDS epidemic becomes as serious a problem for the entire United States population as some experts fear, will depend to a great degree on how quickly and aggressively American society responds.

My Comment: It's no wonder people are confused after reading articles like this. Why do some AIDS experts tell us that AIDS is a plague and a danger to man's very existence, and others tell us just the opposite? Who's right? Actually, it doesn't really matter. What is certain is that AIDS is "on the march" and is a mystery even to the experts; therefore, we have no choice but to treat the AIDS virus and disease as a potential deadly plague, the worst possible scenario. If we listen to the responsible AIDS experts (who are trying to warn, protect, and educate us from/about this disease), we have nothing to lose and our lives to gain. We have no choice; treat

AIDS as if it is the "Black Death," or worse!

From *Hippocrates* magazine, "The Doctor," by Stephen S. Hall, May/June 1988:

- Now 32 years old, his promising career suddenly in ruins, his aspirations no greater than to turn 33, Hacib Aoun, M.D. (a surgeon who became infected with AIDS after a contaminated needle stick during surgery) has had ample opportunity to contemplate the role of the doctors in the face of AIDS. Sometimes, watching television, he hears experts debate the ethics of refusing treatment. Often, with controlled fury, he enters that debate, lecturing at Yale, Harvard, Dartmouth. He finds it difficult to believe that there can be even two sides to the issue of a doctor refusing to treat a patient who needs it.
- Dr. Aoun says, "I think physicians have to make an important decision early on, very early on, in their careers, if they're going to go on with medicine for what it is. It's taking care of ill people. It's taking care of people who have nobody to care for them, provide for them. I guess that decision means taking some risks, but if you're going to be a physician, be it completely."
- As long as there has been pestilence, there have been fearful doctors who have found ways to discharge their obligations somewhat less than completely.
- During the Black Death of 1148, which claimed 100,000 lives in Venice, artisans and young people were forced to care for the dying because "many doctors fled," as one historian writer stated, "while others shut themselves in their houses." In the London plague year of 1665, the vast majority of physicians reportedly deserted the city. Each generation of physicians has encountered diseases that made it weigh mortal fear against moral obligation – bubonic plague, leprosy, yellow fever, tuberculosis, polio, and now AIDS. Countless numbers, too, have perished fighting the good (and short-lived) fight. The entire faculty of the school of medicine in Montpellier, France, valiantly treated plague victims in 1348; the entire faculty died.

- AIDS may finally take a smaller toll than the plague, but doctors are nevertheless, wary. Arthur Caplan, a biochemist at the University of Minnesota, says, "I don't think it's a majority of doctors, but it's a real problem. Every day there are medical students who don't want to see patients who have AIDS. Every day there's a dentist who won't take them. Every day there's a nursing home that won't take them. It's serious."
- The number of actual incidents of refused treatment is probably low, but the degree of reluctance is not. Peel away the protective gowns and masks (if you can find a pair, so scarce have they become during the current nationwide shortage), and underneath you will find considerable fear of exposure. Interns and residents suffer AIDS anxiety by day, AIDS nightmares by night.
- Risk of exposure is everywhere. A study at John Hopkins Hospital showed approximately 3 percent of patients coming to the emergency room tested positive for the AIDS virus. Interns and residents once wore patient blood as a badge of honor, a show of commitment. Now it's a fool's badge of courage.
- Surgery and obstetrics pose, perhaps, the greatest exposure to blood and bodily fluids. In the usual course of labor and delivery, an obstetrician will handle, at least, a liter of blood and amniotic fluid, often more, to say nothing of membranes, placentas, umbilical cord, and, of course, the baby. "In the case of emergency," says Bethesda, Maryland, obstetrician and gynecologist, Lewis Townsend, "You're up to your elbows in blood and you're trying to save their lives. There's blood just everywhere." In the operating room, a persistent risk is the patient who may have been infected via previous transfusion. According to the Center for Disease Control, an estimated 12,000 people in the United States have been infected through blood transfusions.
- A report issued by the Center for Disease Control on May 22, 1988, described how three health care workers apparently became infected with the virus when their skin or mucous membranes came into contact with the blood of infected patients.

The three were the first health workers reported to have contracted the virus through only limited contact with small amounts of blood.
- The May 22, 1988, message passed down to its scary essentials, is this: If AIDS-infected blood happens to insinuate itself into any break in your skin, be it a paper cut or acne, or a rash, or a needle stick, or if it splashes into your mouth, there's a chance you could get AIDS.
- The number of health care workers who have been infected by AIDS patients is believed to be low, and the rate of infection for highly exposed workers is very low, but not zero!
- No one knows the number of health care workers who have become infected on the job.
- Society has long assumed that refusal to treat, covert or blatant, violates the oath that doctors take when they graduate from medical school. Society is wrong.
- There is no language in the Hippocrates oath that obligates doctors to treat every patient who comes along. Even if there were, AIDS would prompt some physicians to rewrite that section. "When I took the oath, I agreed to treat patients. I didn't agree to commit suicide," is the hyperbolic view of one surgeon. Sentiment like that will probably prompt the American Medical Association to draw a somewhat deeper ethical line in the dust last December, when it declared that doctors "may not ethically refuse to treat a patient whose condition is within the physician's current realm of competence solely because the patient [tests positive for the AIDS virus]. According to physician Alan R. Nelson, Chairman of the Board of Trustees of the Medical Association states, "The AMA has a long-standing policy that says that physician and patients have the right to choose each other. But we don't emphasize that in the instance of a physician's refusal to care for a person with AIDS."
- Surgeon General C. Evert Koop (last September) ripped "the unprofessional conduct of a fearful and irrational minority" who refuse to treat patients with AIDS, while testifying before the presidential commission on the AIDS epidemic.

- Arnold S. Relman, physician and editor of the *New England Journal of Medicine,* weighed in with this comment to the *Journal Surgical Practice News:* "[Doctors who] are not willing to accept the risk, and who are going to pick and choose the patients they are willing to serve on the basis of minimizing personal risks to themselves, I think, ought not to be in the practice of medicine." The Health and Hospitals Corporation of New York City, which runs the city's hospitals, such as Bellvue, decided last August that any physician who refused to treat an AIDS case would be fired.
- "Yes, there are risks," Aoun (a surgeon who got infected with AIDS by sticking his finger with an AIDS contaminated needle during a surgical procedure) says, shaking his head, "Jesus Christ, can you imagine what will happen to these patients with AIDS if physicians, in general, start taking similar attitudes?"
- Dudley Johnson, M.D. (a cardiac surgeon) admitted to a local newspaper (March 1987) that since 1985, he screened all his patients for AIDS antibodies and that he refused to operate on some of these patients. This was the first time a physician publicly admitted he refused to treat an AIDS infected patient, which has caused Dr. Johnson much criticism amongst the media, many colleagues, and the public. Editorials denounced him, people sent hate mail. Surgeons silently applauded him. As one doctor puts it, "He was brave enough to say it publicly, and put up with the public scrutiny." Another said , "At least now, the issue is out in the open."
- In an admittedly unscientific sampling, more than 90 percent of Johnson's fellow surgeons who responded to a *Surgical Practice News* questionnaire said, they didn't feel Johnson's position was irrational.
- "There's one hundred percent mortality [with this disease]," Lorraine Day, M.D. head of orthopedics at San Francisco General Hospital) told the San Francisco Chronicle newspaper. "We're talking hardball here."
- Many doctors are emotionally burned out by the experience of treating young patients who will never be cured, and there are

reports that medical school students are choosing less dangerous specialties, that prospective interns are avoiding certain teaching hospitals with high AIDS caseloads. That message, in turn is not lost on public health officials. Surgeon General Koop recently acknowledged that refusal to treat AIDS patients "threatens the very fabric of health care in this country."
- Four out of five dentists refuse to treat AIDS patients, according to a recent American Dental Association survey.
- Dentist, hygienists, and their clients risk infection when tainted blood and saliva splattered into the eye or mingle with cuts – or even, long nails – on ungloved hands.
- By May 1986, only 29 U.S. dental workers – all but one from high-risk groups – had been diagnosed with AIDS.
- The Dental Association delegates in 1987 passed a resolution that "vigorously opposes any government mandate directing who a private practicing dentist may or may not treat."

My Comment: This article relates some of the more important problems AIDS is causing in the health care field – primarily the reluctance of physicians/dentists to treat AIDS-infected patients and the growing fear and risk of AIDS-infection by physicians, dentists and other health care workers. Dr. Aoun (the AIDS-infected physician by a contaminated needle) had the right *before his infection* to treat or not treat any patient he wanted to, no one was interfering with that right. Unfortunately, he got AIDS-infected by one of his patients. However, no one forced or coerced him to treat that patient, who was later found to be AIDS-infected. He alone made the choice to treat that patient. After Dr. Aoun became infected, only then, did he start advocating that other physicians/dentists should not have that same right.

Of course, there are plenty of people who support his philosophy, especially people who do treat AIDS-infected people. I sympathize with Dr. Aoun, but I don't agree with him. No health care worker should have to care for anybody they don't want to care for, and no patient should have to have a health care worker they don't want. If it is any other way, the practice of medicine would be hazardous to all concerned and the quality of health care delivered will definitely deteriorate. There is no question about it, today more and more health care workers, including physicians and dentists, don't want anything to do with AIDS-infected patients because they fear for their lives and the lives of their loved ones. *This is not a matter of morality or ethics, it is a matter of life or death and facing reality.*

From *Contemporary OB/GYN* magazine, "Managing AIDS in pregnant patients," by Howard L. Minkoff, M.D., September 1988:

- A large number of studies have demonstrated a 20% to 50% risk of perinatal transmission (a newborn baby born with AIDS, from an AIDS-infected mother). The prognosis for the child diagnosed with HIV disease is extremely poor. Most children born with HIV die within the first few years of birth.
- "Infection control in the era of AIDS" by Philip B. Mead, M.D. Universal precautions for physicians are listed:
  (1) Use gloves when touching blood or body fluids, mucous membranes, or non intact skin, and when handling items or surfaces soiled with blood or body fluids.
  (2) Use a mask and eye protection during procedures that may generate splashing or droplets in the air, such as when spraying aerosols.
  (3) Use a gown or plastic apron when splashing of blood is likely.
  (4) Wash hands carefully as they become contaminated with blood or body fluids.
  (5) Take extraordinary care in handling needles and other sharp objects.
  (6) Dispose of sharps in puncture-resistant containers.
  (7) Make sure emergency resuscitation devices are available to minimize the need for emergency mouth to mouth resuscitation.
  (8) Exclude from patient care all personnel with exudative lesions of weeping dermatitis until those conditions have resolved.

My Comment: AIDS infection in pregnancy is definitely increasing. Because of political interference, legal obstacles, and the threat of costly lawsuits, AIDS testing of all pregnant women or newborns is not being done today. All pregnant women and their babies need to be tested for AIDS and, if positive, appropriate medical measures be instituted. In the near future, the numbers of AIDS cases in pregnancy will explode, which will result in yet another AIDS nightmare for the nation to deal with.

From *The McAlvany Intelligence Advisor* monthly newsletter, by Donald S. McAlvany (editor), September 1988:

- America and the entire world are faced with the greatest medical crisis since the Black Death plague which wiped out over one-third of Europe's population several hundred years ago. The AIDS plague, the severity of which has consistently been covered up by the American and other governments to avoid a panic, is already at epidemic levels and will within a few more years be pandemic. The economic, political, and sociological implications of this plague are horrendous and will change the course of the U.S. and world history for centuries.
- What is AIDS? AIDS is actually a family of viruses related to HIV (HTLV-3), Hepatitis B, Herpes Type 2HSV, and Epstein-Barr virus (which causes mononucleosis – the so-called "kissing disease"). There is not one AIDS virus but thousands (i.e., 9,000-2) or perhaps millions is accurate. AIDS is the most rapidly mutating virus in history and therefore (according to Surgeon General Koop) it will be difficult, if not impossible to ever find a vaccine cure.
- It is more likely that it came from mass vaccinations with contaminated vaccines by the World Health Organization in Africa in the 1960s. The vaccines are made by taking a virus of a disease and injecting it into an animal or a tissue culture of an animal part. Once the disease is fully developed in the animal or the tissue culture, they take the serum from the animal and generate the vaccine. But, if the animals or their parts which were injected with smallpox or Hepatitis B vaccine

were already infected with other viruses, those viruses could have crossed with the injected viruses to create a third virus (i.e., AIDS).
- On May 11, 1987, *The London Times* (one of the most highly respected newspapers in the world) carried a well researched and documented story which accused the World Health Organization of having triggered the AIDS pandemic with its mass smallpox inoculations in Africa and the Third World in the 1960s. (There was a total blackout of this story in the major media in America.) The greatest spread of the AIDS infection coincides almost perfectly with the areas which had intense immunization programs, with the number of people inoculated as follows: Zaire: 36,878,000; Zambia: 19,060,000; Tanzania: 14,972,000; Uganda: 11,616,000; Malawi: 8,118,000; Rwanda: 3,382,000, and Burundi: 3,374,000.
- Brazil, the only South American country covered in the smallpox eradication campaign has the highest incidence of AIDS in that region. About 14,000 Haitians stationed in Central Africa at the time of the program received the WHO vaccinations and shortly thereafter AIDS broke out in Haiti. Part of the voodoo rituals in Haiti are anal intercourse (which is also practiced widely throughout Africa). The virus infestates in the intestine, and hence, spread quickly in Africa (where promiscuity is the norm – i.e., several different sexual partners per day) and in Haiti. American homosexuals (especially from San Francisco) have used Haiti as a playground for decades, picked up the virus there, and quickly spread it throughout the homosexual community of America.
- Many of the world's leading AIDS researchers now quietly admit that the WHO inoculations of 97 million Africans and millions of Brazilians for smallpox, and millions more for Hepatitis B, were probably done with contaminated vaccines and, therefore triggered the world AIDS pandemic. (Editor's Note: See an excellent article, "WHO Murdered Africa" by William Campbell Douglas – Health Freedom News – September 1987.)
- How Widespread is the AIDS Pandemic? The Atlanta based

Center for Disease Control (CDC) (which has consistently played down and understated the number of AIDS virus infections and AIDS disease cases, while minimizing the ways in which the virus can be contracted) has recently quietly admitted that 3 million Americans are now infected with the virus. CDC is desperately afraid of causing a panic and so is participating with the U.S. government cover-up of the extent and severity of the plague. Interested readers should get Gene Antonio's excellent book, *The AIDS Coverup*. Private AIDS researchers and scientists who have no such constraints believe that the number of Americans now infected with the virus is closer to 8 million. So, between one out of thirty and one out of eighty Americans are already infected with the virus. All will eventually contract the disease and die.

- Regardless of which estimate (3 million, 8 million, or something in between) is correct, the ominous fact is that the number of cases of infection is doubling each year. If the CDC estimate is correct (and if that doubling rate continues), within 6 years and 3 months (1995) every American could be infected with the virus. If private estimates are correct, within less than 5 years (i.e., by the end of 1993) all Americans could have contracted the virus. (Editor's Note: I believe that rate will slow down because, as the epidemic worsens, more people will come to understand it and will take strong measures to protect themselves.)
- Recent reports estimate that 380,000 people in Los Angeles are infected by the virus with larger numbers in New York and larger numbers percentage-wise in San Francisco. At least 5,000 gay men have died in New York City, and areas of Greenwich Village and the Upper West Side are beginning to look like "the day after" as businesses, restaurants, clubs, clothing stores, etc. are shutting down.
- In June 1987, 50 AIDS experts met near Geneva and concluded that 75 million (or one-third of the population in southern Africa) already have the virus and will have the disease within 4-5 years. Similar groups in Western Europe have estimated that 300-350 million black Africans in sub-Sahara Africa

will be dead from the disease within a decade. In Africa whole villages have been wiped out. The disease is also spreading into the South African population via migrant workers from countries to the north.

- What are the methods of transmission? The official government line is that AIDS can only be spread by sexual intercourse (homosexual or heterosexual) with an infected person, by a contaminated blood transfusion, or by using a contaminated IV needle. The government (led by the Surgeon General and the CDC) dogmatically maintain that the AIDS virus cannot be transmitted casually and hence they claim that the virus can be contained if "safe sex" (i.e., the use of condoms) is employed, if clean needles are used by drug users, and if the blood blanks are cleaned up (and they claim that they have been). These explanations are over simplistic, defy logic, and defy the facts.
- AIDS is a virus like the common cold virus or the myriad of flu viruses we have seen in recent years. Those viruses are spread by sneezing, coughing (i.e., from pulmonary sources), from kissing and other forms of close contact. Why then not the AIDS virus? The outbreak of Legionnaires' disease at an American Legion convention in Philadelphia in the early eighties is an excellent example of an airborne virus. That virus, which proved fatal to over 30 people, was introduced through the heating/air conditioning of the hotel and was inhaled into the lungs. (A few researchers believe that could have been a test case germ warfare attack.)
- The AIDS virus has been found by researchers in every form of body fluid: semen, blood, tears, perspiration, urine, saliva, etc. If the virus is in those fluids, why wouldn't it be transmitted in those fluids as it is widely understood to be in blood and semen? Elderly couples and parents and children whose only form of sexual contact has been kissing, are known to have infected one another with the virus.
- The CDC and Surgeon General dogmatically maintain that AIDS cannot be transmitted by insects. But most, if not all viruses can be transmitted by insects (i.e., mosquitoes, flies,

cockroaches, ticks, fleas) to both humans and animals (i.e., the bubonic plague via fleas, malaria via mosquitoes, the polio virus via flies, Rocky Mountain spotted fever via ticks, etc.) What is the difference between a mosquito (a live flying needle) and a metal needle? Only the size of the needle, and a virus is sub-atomic in size and thus quite capable of passing through a mosquito's beak.
- In the 1950s in Australia there was an explosion in the rabbit population. An eradication program was initiated by infecting thousands of rabbits with a highly infectious virus. For many months the results were disappointing – only a few thousand rabbits died. Then suddenly millions of rabbits began to die, and in a brief period almost a billion rabbits perished. Research was done to find out why so many rabbits died so quickly, and the conclusion was that the virus was spread by mosquitoes which normally preyed on the rabbits. Mosquitoes would bite infected rabbits and then bite and infect uninfected rabbits. Millions of infected flying needles wiped out most of the Australian rabbit population literally overnight.
- Numerous AIDS researchers have concluded that the virus can exist on a dry surface for two weeks (this has been widely reported) and in liquid indefinitely. No known chemical substance (i.e., chlorine, antibiotics, chemotherapy, radiation) will kill the virus – only a temperature above 169 degrees will destroy it. Another fallacy is that AIDS is sexually transmitted by homosexuals, and that it is now spreading faster among heterosexuals (which are, of course, a much larger group). Additional evidence that AIDS can be transmitted casually is the fact that over 6% of the reported cases were not homosexual, IV drug users, recipients of blood transfusions, promiscuous or associated with any "high risk" group or behavior. The origin of their infection is a total mystery. That group is growing!
- If, indeed, the AIDS virus can be transmitted casually, as a growing body of evidence seems to suggest, there are a number of areas where a person has a growing risk of exposure which should be avoided:

A. Extra- or pre-marital sex (hetero- or homosexual).
   B. Kissing strangers (where they and their background are not well known).
   C. Uncovered toilet seats.
   D. Salad bars.
   E. Public swimming pools.
   F. Steam baths and jacuzzis.
   G. Discos and public bars.
- Why will the AIDS Virus Spread so Fast? The government inspired cover-up of the severity of the crisis (to avert or postpone a panic in the hope that a cure will be found before the extent of the crisis is known), and legislation to protect the victims from discrimination is going to accelerate the spread of the disease. Several reasons for the rapid spread of the disease are:
   A. America is a Promiscuous Society. Many gay men have sex with anywhere from 12 to 200 lovers per year. Many heterosexual men have sex with 5-12 partners per year, and the great majority of single Americans from 15 to 60 years of age are very sexually active. (The new book by Masters and Johnson confirms these trends and warns of the rapid spread of AIDS among heterosexuals.)
   B. Millions of People are Carriers of the Virus (and thus can infect others) but don't know it. In addition, early stage infections don't show up on blood tests, so even tested people can be carriers, give infected blood, etc.
   C. Intentional Infecting. Many people in high risk groups feel the government is not doing enough to find a cure, so if they can spread the disease faster, then the government will do more. The "Doc Holiday Syndrome" is also present, whereby some dying and embittered AIDS victims decide to try and take as many people with them as possible.
   D. Government Misinformation. The government (via the CDC and Surgeon General) is telling people that they are safe if they practice safe sex, use condoms, avoid using dirty needles, etc. They are misrepresenting the

ease with which the disease can be transmitted via heterosexual sex and casual transmission as described in Section A-4 above. The government has declared the blood banks safe, but private medical researchers believe there is a 20% chance of AIDS infection via blood transfusions.
E. Americans are a Transient People. We travel a great deal, eat out a lot, spend a great deal of time in airports, rail and bus stations, frequent public restrooms, exercise at public health clubs, fly in small enclosed capsules (called airplanes) where the air is recirculated and breathed over and over, etc. In short, our chances for exposure are high, and at this writing, there is absolutely nothing to prevent or slow down the spread of the virus.

• Whether from germ warfare, the World Health Organization, or just spontaneous outbreaks (the "signs of the times"), there is a viral onslaught against Americans which could take a heavy toll over the next few years. (Remember, one in thirty Americans may already be infected with the AIDS virus.) There are few precautions and measures which concerned Americans might take to protect themselves and their families.
1. Isolation from people is a form of protection from AIDS, but is impractical. Nevertheless, as the virus takes on pandemic proportions, people in small towns, rural areas, or farms will be much safer than people in large cities.
2. As Much as Possible, Avoid High Risk Transmission Areas, including public swimming pools, steam baths, jacuzzis, salad bars, discos and other night clubs, uncovered toilet seats, highly crowded areas such as subways, etc.
3. When in Large Crowds or Public Places, Wash Your Hands Frequently with hot water and soap – especially before eating. If you have shaken hands with a number of people, always wash your hands before touching food.
4. Airlines Tend to Have High Numbers of a Certain High Risk Groups Serving Food. Either refrain from eating

(the food is usually bad) or order a vegetarian meal in advance – which usually comes wrapped in saran wrap. Forego ice in drinks. It is often touched by hands.
5. Avoid Unmarried Sex – and if you're single, know a lot about who you're dating or kissing. Always get an AIDS blood test before marriage. (Many states require these now.)
6. Don't Stick Fingers, Pencils or Other Objects in Mouth (i.e., This writer's teenage daughter chews the end off of every pen she gets hold of. If the habit is unbreakable, boil the object first.)
7. If You Exercise at Health Clubs, Take Certain Precautions: wear gloves when you lift weights or use nautilus or other exercise equipment. A long sleeve sweatshirt is also advisable. There is often perspiration on such equipment. Wear rubber thongs in showers.
8. In Hotels/Motels Avoid Taking Baths – Take Showers Instead. Bath tubs are often not well cleaned from last occupant.
9. All Meat Should be Cooked to 169 Degrees to Kill Any Virus. If a cow is bitten by any AIDS infected mosquito the virus can be in the meat. Likewise if a milk cow is bitten, the virus can be transmitted through milk. Boiling milk or heating meat to 169 degrees kills the virus. (Pasteurized milk is only heated to 142 degrees.)
10. Many Restaurants Employ Large Numbers of a Certain High Risk Group as Food Servers or Preparers – avoid such restaurants. Ethnic restaurants (i.e., Jewish, Arab, Chinese, etc. should be much safer in this respect. And remember, Federal laws prohibit restaurants from "discriminating" by not hiring, or firing someone with AIDS.
11. A Nutritional Diet, Vitamins and Food Supplements, Adequate Rest and Exercise, Reduction of Stress and Good Hygiene will help to keep the body detoxified and the immune system up.

My Comment: Besides being an interesting, provocative aron AIDS, it emphasizes the seriousness of AIDS and how widespread it is. The author bravely contradicts the "AIDS experts" time and time again, supporting his position with facts and common sense. Such articles are purposely withheld from the general public. No one has the right to purposely endanger the health of the general public. By misinforming or not informing (whichever it is) the general public about the horrors of AIDS, untold numbers of innocent people will unnecessarily become infected and die. The quicker our political and medical leaders openly admit we have a lethal plague on our hands, the quicker we can take appropriate precautionary measures and, hopefully, find a cure and/or vaccine.

From the *San Francisco Examiner,* "MDs and AIDS" (Letter to the Editor), by Jean K. Haddad, M.D., October 2, 1988:

- It is true that a few physicians have voiced support for Proposition 102, a proposition that states AIDS will be treated like other contagious diseases, such as syphilis and gonorrhea, and which will be voted upon by California voters on November 8, 1988, but it is important to note that no AIDS experts are among them.
- Physicians with experience in AIDS research, treatment, and policy appear to be uniformly opposed to Proposition 102.
- Therefore, the San Francisco Medical Society joins the California Medical Association, California Nurses Association, and virtually all knowledgeable health officials in urging a "no" vote on 102. (Jean G. K. Haddad, M.D., President, San Francisco Medical Society)

My Comment: This letter is inaccurate for a number of reasons:

   a) Far more than a "few" physicians actively oppose this proposition, especially physicians exposed to AIDS-infected patients.

   b) The author refers to "AIDS experts" and implies that, since they do not support the proposition, we should vote against it. In reality, "AIDS experts" know very little about the AIDS virus and disease – AIDS is still a mystery to *all* of us.

c) Many members of the organizations the author cites as not in favor of the proposition do not share that position. In fact, these organizations never polled their members to see who was for or against this proposition. Therefore, the organizations cited misrepresented many of their own members to the public, hoping to persuade the public to vote the way they want them to.

From the *San Francisco Examiner,* "AIDS WEEK," by Bruce Hilton, October 2, 1988:

- Hours before the deadline the House and Senate voted to continue to provide thousand of low-income AIDS patients with the life extending drug AZT.
- About 6,000 people – not poor enough for Medicaid but unable to pay the necessary $7,200 a year – faced a possible cut off of AZT if the legislation hadn't passed.

My Comment: This is only the beginning of the unbearable costs that will be incurred by the government for treating AIDS patients. The costs will be far too high for most people; therefore, the government (the taxpayer) will have to step in and pay the medical bills. When these costs becomes too high, we can expect many changes in the manner AIDS-infected people are medically cared for. Some of these changes will not be popular or pleasant.

From *Health Freedom News,* "AIDS Vaccine...A Cure as Deadly as the Disease," by Maureen Kennedy Salaman, January 1988:

- When catastrophe strikes, all of the pretty words, all of the good intentions, all of the philanthropic goals sported by bureaucrats, bankers, and politicians suddenly disappear. What

you're left with is the greed that has been lurking beneath the surface. It could be the greed for money; it could be the greed for fame; it could be greed for power; it could be all three. But when the going gets tough, when the worst that can happen does happen, you get to see everyone's true colors.
- Well, after five years of withholding the truth from the American public, and a ludicrous campaign by Surgeon General Koop to "condomize" America, it seems that the bureaucrats are starting to wake up. AIDS is the greatest health problem this country has ever faced.
- Instead of concern and compassion, we are seeing politicians grabbing for the limelight. Each one tries to outdo the other with congressman, after congressman, attempting to show that he or she is on the cutting edge of AIDS research and legislation.
- Have any steps been taken to protect the public? No, in fact, we hear more about the rights of AIDS victims than we do about the right of the American public to protect itself from this deadly virus. Our leaders have granted AIDS the full protection of the Constitution, while denying that same protection to the citizenry.
- Has medical science reacted any better? NO! We've seen their true colors. Instead of working together with scientists from around the world to, (1) tell the people the truth about AIDS, and (2) search for a way to keep the epidemic from spreading, our medical scientists have struggled against each other. Their goal is to grab the headlines, to try and become the next Jonas Salk.
- How have the major drug companies reacted to the AIDS epidemic? In one word: greed! Each is racing to develop the first effective AIDS vaccine. If the drug companies have their way, we'll all be vaccinated with some sort of untested potion. After a minimum test period, the drug (AZT) was tried on humans, because the drug companies said, it wasn't fair to withhold the drug from dying AIDS patients. Fairness had nothing to do with it. Greed was and is the motivating factor. A year's supply of AZT for one patient is $7,000 to $10,000.

This, in spite of the fact that AZT has never been proven to work, and has serious side effects – including anemia and kidney damage.
- Let me be the first to tell you: there can be and will be no AIDS vaccine. A perfectly good example of the futility of finding a vaccine for a mutating virus is the so-called flu vaccine.
- So there you have it – the facade of compassion, caring, and scientific humanism has been shattered by the greed, the pain, and the anguish created by AIDS. Each day lost searching for the billion dollar vaccine means the epidemic grows stronger. Each day without a sane government policy to protect those of us not infected means another day of risk for unsuspecting schoolchildren and those unfortunate enough to require blood transfusions.

My Comment: By stressing the danger of the AIDS virus and exposing some of man's selfish, adverse behavior in the fight with AIDS, Ms. Salaman is one of few who is courageous enough to speak out about the failure of our leaders to wage an effective war against AIDS. So far, self-serving politicians, medical leaders, and various organizations across the country have been successful in suppressing such articles as this one. Again, the public needs to be informed about what AIDS is and how to protect itself from it.

From the *Gilroy Dispatch,* "War on AIDS Mishandled from Beginning for Political Reasons," by Dan Walters, October 1988:

- The discomforting conclusion that Randy Shelts (author of *And the Band Played On*) reaches, bolstered by exhaustive research, is that what should have been treated as a very serious public health matter was, instead, mishandled for political reasons.
- There's been no shortage of legislation purporting to deal with AIDS. Literally hundreds of AIDS bills have been introduced. The liberals insist on treating AIDS differently from other public-health problems; the conservatives, almost gleefully,

demand draconian measures that amount to punishment. The money for AIDS research and treatment, in the meantime, has been caught up in the bitter infighting over the state budget.
- There's absolutely no reason why AIDS should not be treated like any other infectious, deadly and/or venereal disease.
- There also should be a hard-nosed resolve that AIDS, first and foremost, is a threat to the entire population and thus should be confronted without regard to political agendas, whether of the left or right.

My Comment: This article appeared in the small town newspaper of Gilroy, California – not one in a large city. Why? Why aren't such provocative articles found in all cities, thus available to everyone? Why doesn't the public demand it? Why doesn't government listen, let alone follow, such advice?

From *Straight Talk,* newsletter, "Telling It Like It Is," by Tom Anderson, September 29, 1988:

- AIDS attacks the brain and controls the nervous system (as well as other organs); dementia is common, but this is not advertised by medical officials. If the public were aware of this, there would be justified outrage over laws prohibiting the firing of anyone having AIDS such as pilots, bus drivers, teachers, etc. (*First AIDS Report,* 5-6/88) Comment: We strongly favor the factual publication on AIDS. There are some better. *Daily News Digest.*

My Comment: One of the most dangerous and least known characteristics of the AIDS virus is that it attacks not only a victim's immune system, but his central nervous system, as well. When the central nervous system (CNS) is attacked, the victim's brain slowly deteriorates until the victim becomes helpless and dies. Worse, a victim does not know he is AIDS-infected because there are no physical signs or symptoms. Only after the victim shows serious mental problems and abnormal behavior do people suspect the victim is ill and dangerous to himself and others.

This is but another reason why all people must be tested for the AIDS disease. It frightens me that people in sensitive or important occupations such as airline pilots, politicians, and surgeons may be CNS AIDS infected and inadvertently cause great harm to other people. What if an AIDS-brain-infected airline pilot crashed his airplane, killing many or all of his passengers? Or imagine a CNA AIDS-infected President of the United States or Russia starts behaving, saying, and doing strange things because of the AIDS virus!

AIDS central nervous infection should definitely be suspected if a person is acting strange or irrational. To me, this characteristic of the AIDS virus, to attack the victim's brain, is reason enough to test all people routinely for the AIDS virus.

From *Special Symposium Review,* World Health Communications, Inc., "HIV Disease Management and Issues," Vol. 1, No. 1, April 1988:

- What are the clinical perimeters that predict rapid progression to AIDS in an HIV-infected patient? The answer is that HIV-infected patients with the following constitutional symptoms or one of the minor opportunistic infections have a high probability of progressing to AIDS within six to twelve months:
  - Unexplained weight loss
  - Persistent fever
  - Persistent diarrhea
  - Oral candidiasis
  - Oral hairy leukoplakia
- Does neurologic disorders in an HIV-seropositive patient predict rapid progression to AIDS? The answer is that it is difficult to differentiate those alterations in mental function – memory changes, confusion, fatigue – that are due to depression or sleep disturbances from those that are directly caused by HIV. With objective evidence of HIV-related encephalopathy, however, early neurologic dysfunction can predict rapid deterioration of a patient's status.

My Comment: These signs and symptoms are extremely common in everyday life, as well. I see many patients every day who complain or have one or more of these signs or symptoms. Because they are so common, there is no effective way by which to determine who should and should not be AIDS tested based on signs and/or symptoms; therefore, *everybody* should be tested for AIDS – frequently – if AIDS is ever going to be diagnosed and contained.

From the *San Francisco Chronicle,* "AIDS in the Workplace: From Fear to Compassion," by Lloyd Watson, September 21, 1988:

- When the bank's (Bank of America) first employee AIDS case was reported in 1983, the employee was asked to stay home until B of A determined whether the disease was contagious under normal working conditions. "We consulted with UCSF and the Center for Disease Control (CDC) in Atlanta," said Beck (bank spokesman). "When we learned that the person was no hazard to her fellow workers, we made an ad hoc decision that has set the pattern for us."
- The infected employee came back to his job, and B of A began an employee education program that continues to this day.
- "We know we've had over 50 AIDS cases," said bank spokesman Beck, "but we don't know the exact number. Not all employees have reported their illness."
- All, however, have been encouraged to continue to work. "It's good for them," said bank spokesman Beck. "It's good for their families. And it's good for the bank."
- "We've seen an amazing transformation from fear to compassion."

My Comment: I believe that employers need to at this point understand and respect the AIDS virus and take all precautions to protect their AIDS-free employees and customers. If the country's hospitals and medical profession would take the initiative to adequately protect their health care workers and patients, it would set a safe and appropriate example for the rest of the business world.

From *California Physician,* California Medical Association's monthly magazine, "Educating Physicians about AIDS – Let's do it Ourselves," by Laurence P. White, M.D., August 1988:

- California physicians are better informed about AIDS than physicians in any other state. That is encouraging and only what we would want and expect. The bad news is that California physicians are not well informed about AIDS and its transmission, despite the fact that 40 percent of all AIDS cases occur in this state. Just half of California's primary care doctors have seen or recognized a patient with AIDS or have read any scientific papers on the subject.
- We need urgently to convince physicians that AIDS concerns us all, and that we need to put aside our fear and learn a great deal more about AIDS and people with AIDS.
- Knowledge also teaches us to be less fearful of our own safety.
- The health care workers most closely associated with AIDS patients seem to have the least fear of such accidental infection.
- Such education has its own rewards – it is difficult to imagine anything more fascinating than the chance to study an entire new disease as it appears and unfolds. Our lifetime will not offer such a challenge again.
- CMA must convince its members to inform themselves thoroughly about AIDS and to learn about the disease, the immune system, treatment, and controlling the spread of infection.
- The choice is simple. Do it ourselves or be required by others to do what we should have done ourselves. We must remember that ignorance is the enemy – not homosexuals, drug abusers, or the state. We have the ability to make things better ourselves.

My Comment: I read such articles all the time and always, they turn me off and anger me to no end. If our medical leaders truly believed this, they would have taken the above suggestions and insured that the public and the medical profession was well educated of all aspects of the AIDS virus and disease, instead of letting the politicians and medicrats dictate to and control them. As a result, misinformation, complacency, and ignorance abounds and the AIDS virus continues to spread.

From *Human Sexuality* magazine, "Nursing Homes Preparing to Accept AIDS Patients," by Robert C. Marlow, MBA, April 1988:

- There appears to be a legal mandate for nursing homes to accept these patients and some states, most notably Minnesota, have begun to enforce the laws prohibiting discrimination against HIV-infected patients. I anticipate that more states will follow Minnesota's lead.
- The American Health Care Association and its state affiliates are actively involved in dealing with the need for nursing homes to prepare for the eventuality of being asked to accept patients who are HIV-seropositive.
- Frequent educational sessions regarding infection control, in general, and AIDS, in specific, are necessary to keep nursing home staff members fully informed regarding the actions that they need to take to protect themselves from AIDS and to dispel the myths that surround this disease syndrome.
- The adoption of universal blood and body fluid precautions should serve to lessen the anxiety of employees caring for AIDS patients for the first time.
- It is not necessary for nursing home personnel to acquire major additional expertise in order to provide long-term care to AIDS patients.

My Comment: If the AIDS disease is primarily a disease of young and "high risk" people, why do nursing homes have to prepare to take care of AIDS patients, especially such large numbers of them? Of course, it's because the AIDS virus does not distinguish its victims by age that it can and will begin to spread to others outside of the high risk groups. We are not only going to need more nursing home beds, but hospital beds, as well.

This article states that adoption of the "universal blood and body fluid precautions" should lessen the anxiety of the employer and that no further training or expertise by the nursing home personnel (to care for AIDS patients) is necessary. This advice is not only false, but dangerous to the health of those employees. The AIDS virus must be feared and respected at all times; whoever works in an environment where the AIDS virus is known to be present must know how to protect him/herself.

From *National Geographic,* "Fleas: The Lethal Leapers," by Nicole Duplaix, May 1988:

- The deadly tentacles of plague reached across the Mediterranean from Africa during the first pandemic, beginning in A.D. 541. This disease of rodents, carried to man by fleas, reached Constantinople within a year; 10,000 died there daily as the infection peaked.
- Cities were abandoned, agriculture declined, populations plunged, trade faltered. After 200 years, plague mysteriously vanished from Europe. Six plague-free centuries passed. In 1346 it returned, traveling in the wake of caravans and ships that plied trade routes between Asia and Europe. The unwanted import landed at ports like Marseille and Genoa and pushed inland. Cities suffered most; the contagion spread quickly in crowded, filthy conditions. By 1352, 25 million people had died in Europe alone.
- Death's scythe cut across all levels. Peasants dropped dead in fields. In England three archbishops of Canterbury died within one year. Fear suspended other emotions. "This disease is making us more cruel to one another than we are to dogs," English diarist Samuel Pepys wrote in 1665. Corpses were dumped in pits, in rivers, at sea. "Father abandoned child, wife husband, one brother another .... And I, Agnolo di Tura ... buried my five children with my own hands," recorded a chronicler in Siena, Italy. With few to work fields, peasants could demand higher wages; cracks in the manorial system widened. Added di Tura: "So many died that all believed that it was the end of the world."
- When plague entered the human population, the consequences were catastrophic. The first outbreak may have been a scourge that struck the Philistines in the 12th Century B.C.; the Old Testament account mentions "mice that mar the land."
- Later three plague epidemics – so vast they were called

pandemics – ravaged the world. The first struck in A.D. 541, swirling around the Mediterranean in a deadly maelstrom for more than two centuries, killing as many as 40 million people and weakening the Byzantine Empire. "The bodies of the sick were covered with black postules ... the symptoms of immediate death," wrote Procopius, historian of Byzantine Emperor Justinian. At its peak in Constantinople, he reported, the plague killed 10,000 people a day.
- The second pandemic came in the 14th Century, when lucrative trade routes opened across Asia. Caravans and ships brought more than silk and jewels. In October 1347 vessels sailed into Messina, Sicily, with crews dying from a mysterious disease. No one noticed that shipboard rats were also ill.
- The next five years were so devastating that they became known as the time of the Black Death. By 1352, plague had killed 25 million people in Europe alone.
- Feverish victims suffered excruciating swellings in the groin or armpit – the buboes. Most died within five days. Sometimes the infection spread via the bloodstream to the lungs; then death came in three days or less. This was pneumonic plague, the deadliest form then and today.
- Looking for scapegoats, Europeans massacred Jews, suspecting them of poisoning the water. Neighbors turned on neighbors, parents turned on children. The sick were walled up in their houses and later quarantined on islands. To no avail. So many died so quickly that cities dug plague pits for the corpses. With no escape, no cure, "there was no one who wept for any death, for all awaited death," wrote Agnola di Tura, a chronicler in Siena, Italy.
- "The worst thing was finding no explanation for the greatest natural disaster Europe had ever known," Professor Henri H. Mollaret and Jacqueline Brossollet, plague historians at the Institut Pasteur in Paris, told me.
- The church saw the plague epidemic as a manifestation of God's wrath. A committee of doctors at the University of Paris pronounced that it was the sinister result of the conjunction of Saturn, Jupiter, and Mars. A common belief that plague

was caused by "corrupt vapors."
- As the sweeping scythe of plague turned bustling towns into sepulchers and emptied the countryside, it reshaped European society. With few serfs left to till the land, survivors could negotiate for wages with landlords. The breakdown on manorialism and the evolution of an economy based on many sowed seeds of capitalism.
- The spreading stain of plague tainted the world yet again when the third pandemic erupted in China in 1855. Reaching Chinese ports in 1894, it was carried around the world. That year Dr. Alexandre Yersin, a Frenchman sent to plague-riddled Hong Kong by the Institute Pasteur, identified the plague bacillus. The next breakthrough came in 1898 when Frenchman Dr. Paul-Louis Simond discovered that fleas transmit plague from rats to man. Because of the virulence of the pneumonic plague that overwhelmed Manchuria in 1911, a doctor examining a patient wore a gown and mask. But plague remained untreatable until the advent of sulfa drugs in the 1930s and effective antibiotics in the 1940s.
- Plague struck without pattern, skirting one area only to bludgeon another. Busy ports such as Venice, Marseille, and Barcelona endured dozens of outbreaks. England took 200 years to recover from its 14th Century death toll. In the Great Plague of 1665 at least 68,000 Londoners died. Survivors cowered behind shuttered windows as the body collectors cried, "Bring out your dead!"
- In man, plague enjoyed an unwitting ally. Families crowded in houses where rats were tolerated and hygiene did not exist. People wore the same underclothes day and night. Fleas and lice thrived and went along when the clothes of the dead were sold or passed on.
- As the second pandemic raged and waned through the centuries, chroniclers came tantalizingly close to the mysterious cause of the disease.
- In the late 1800s, the third pandemic spread plague around the world. It lingers today. Carried out of China's Yunnan Province in 1855, plague traveled slowly east; by 1894 it reached

Hong Kong, where it killed some 10,000 people. In this charnel house a young French bacteriologist unmasked the pestilence.
- As Hong Kong's death toll mounted, hundreds of ships docked and departed with their familiar complement of rats. Steamships now carried the disease even faster, before unsuspecting crews became ill. Plague fanned out to where it had been unknown: Japan, Australia, southern Africa, and the Americas.
- India, the site of earlier outbreaks, was especially hard hit: six million died in a decade. Once again the Institute Pasteur sent help, this time Dr. Paul-Louis Simond.
- "Plague mistakenly still carries a terrible stigma, something governments feel they should be ashamed of," said Dr. Norman G. Gratz, the World Health Organization (WHO) official in Geneva in charge of keeping tabs on plague control around the world.
- The United States once did the same. When plague came ashore in San Francisco on June 27, 1899, political leaders, protecting business interests at the expense of disease control, overrode health officials and denied its presence. The governor decreed it a felony to publicize its existence. By 1904 more than 100 people had died of "syphilitic septicemia," the official pseudonym of plague.
- Western Americans still pay for the deceit. Infecting one wild rodent population after another, the disease made a macabre march inland. Today 13 states live under its cloud. A result: Forty Americans contracted plague in 1983: six died. Last year there were 12 cases; two victims succumbed. Most cases occur in Arizona and New Mexico. Here plague-prone ground squirrels and prairie dogs live as close as one's back yard.
- Like control, plague treatments have greatly improved. "The slower bubonic form is easily cured with antibiotics," said Dr. Thomas Kereselidze of WHO. "But pneumonic plague, infecting the lungs, is fatal 95 percent of the time. The patient must be isolated and given antibiotics very quickly if he is to survive. Worse, the patient only has to cough or sneeze to transmit it to others."

- No one believes that plague will ever be eradicated. "There is a vaccine, but it is not totally effective and lasts only six months," explained South Africa's Margaretha Isaacson. Yet in plague-rife Vietnam only few vaccinated U.S. soldiers contracted the disease. Wiping out the rodents that harbor plague is impossible – and undesirable during outbreaks of the disease. "If you killed all plague-carrying rodents," said Dr. Isaacson, "their fleas would seek another host, and it could be you! Rodent control should be practiced when there is no danger of depriving infected fleas of their hosts."
- Three pandemics, killing more than 200 million people.... Only disease-carrying mosquitoes have caused as much misery as this fascinating order of insects aptly called Siphonaptera – "wingless siphons." Yet for generations we have not only tolerated these pests, we have used them for entertainment.

My Comment: This is a fascinating and accurate account of the Black Death. Like the bubonic plague, the AIDS plague is a mystery, infects and spreads rapidly, and kills humans. Both plagues adversely affect man's social, economic, and political behavior. As in the days of the bubonic plague, AIDS greatest ally today is man himself. Today, we are denying that AIDS is a plague for political, business, and self-serving reasons. As a result, the disease is spreading around the world, rapidly and effectively. Use the contents in this article to help you foresee what the course and effects of AIDS will probably be. Hopefully, it will cause you to seek ways to protect yourself and your family from the AIDS virus and the problems it will cause.

From *America's Promise Newsletter,* October 1987:

- What do experts predict? Their predictions vary in degree but, regardless, all are of such magnitude as to be beyond the comprehension of the human mind. It may be for this reason that an enraged and alarmed populace has not demanded action by their leadership. We can deal with the lessor catastrophes such as cancer, floods, or hurricanes, but our minds have diffi-

culty dealing with AIDS as a reality because of its awesomeness.
- The predictions of Dr. Robert Redfield of Walter Reed Army Medical Center is that 10 million Americans may be infected by 1991, four years away.
- However, statistical expert, Donald E. Babcock, Ph.D., predicts 23 million deaths within four years, 1991. The number infected but still alive could be ten times as much, or 230 million ... meaning everybody.
- British expert, Dr. John Seals, gives the human race 50 years before it becomes extinct.

My Comment: These ominous predictions should jolt everybody. Since there is no cure or vaccine against AIDS, and since people are still complacent about the disease and its implications, I think the AIDS virus will continue to infect mankind possibly until extinction. Before this happens, hopefully, people will realize the AIDS threat and begin to seriously fighting it.

From *The Spotlight,* "Gann Beats ACLU; Puts AIDS on Ballot," by Fred Blahart, August 29, 1988:

- Paul Gann, best known as the author (along with Howard Jarvis) of California's precedent-setting Proposition 13, has proposed a proposition for the state ballot that would require doctors who detected antibodies of HIV (AIDS) virus or the AIDS syndrome itself, to report it to the Health Department as a communicable disease.
- "We've got to do something to stop the spread of AIDS and this is a start," Gann told *The Spotlight.* "I call it common sense."
- "If people with AIDS and others testing positive for HIV can be identified, they can be contacted and warned," Gann explained. Also, the Health Department can seek out persons with whom the infected person has had contact.
- "If doctors can't report AIDS and HIV, then there is no way to stop the spread of AIDS," he said.

- In California, doctors must report cases of gonorrhea, a usually curable venereal disease, but can't report the presence of HIV antibodies. "If we're going to have a chance to stop this disease, HIV must be detected and reported," Gann said.
- "Once a person has AIDS, he usually becomes too sick to spread the disease. But carriers of HIV spread the virus, and HIV causes AIDS. We've got to detect and report HIV and AIDS," he said.
- "AIDS is always fatal," Gann said. "This isn't going to help me. But, I have friends and relatives it will help. It will help everyone in California."
- Gann sees this as a survival issue. "Why should this be an avid rights issue?" he asked. "If someone is spreading AIDS, that person has already violated his responsibility to society. Freedom and responsibility go hand in hand."
- "If you give someone AIDS, you've committed murder," he said. "It may take 10 years for the person to die, but AIDS is always fatal."
- Gann said that no one wanted to take the responsibility of trying to stop the disease. Since he is already infected and there is no cure, he cannot be influenced.
- "In this case, death and taxes go together," Gann said. "Every AIDS patient will cost the taxpayers $100,000.

My Comment: Mr. Gann is a true humanitarian. AIDS-sick and dying, he is still concerned about the future health and welfare of his fellow man. He helped draft and correlate a petition which would help control the spread of the AIDS virus and disease. The drafting of the petition was the result of the failure of the California Legislature to pass effective Legislation to protect the people of California from the AIDS virus. It was defeated by California voters in the November 8, 1988 presidential election.

In general, the AIDS-uninformed electorate was aware of the importance of this proposition, but was successfully manipulated into defeating it. Many opposed the proposition, but I feel that the failure of the California Medical Association (CMA) to support it caused its defeat. For the CMA to publicly and officially come out against this proposition, without first polling all of its members, was not in the best interests of the California public. Already, another such petition is being drafted for the next election, because many people know such legislation is desperately needed to control the spread of the AIDS virus.

From *All Fall Down* (AIDS and the End of Civilization), by William Campbell Douglas, M.D., 1987:

- The AIDS epidemic promises to become the greatest natural disaster since the great flood.
- 2.45 percent of pregnant women at King's County Hospital in New York are now positive for AIDS. AIDS has increased fivefold in two years in straight-laced Switzerland! They have an estimated 20,000 carriers (*AMA Medical News*, 2/13/87). A burn victim in England has caught AIDS from a skin graft (*American Medical News*, 3/13/87).
- Never before in history has there been a plague to which no one develops any immunity. AIDS in itself is not a disease. It's a deficiency which enables almost any deadly disease to do you in.
- People give little thought to how delicate the social fabric really is. A major assault on this delicate balance, such as AIDS, affects everyone. If 10,000,000 are sick and dying, it will take 50,000,000 of the worried well to take care of them. Many people are refusing to take care of AIDS patients. When St. Vincent's Hospital in New York went to Britain to recruit operating room nurses, it had no takers for fear of AIDS. Who is going to take care of these dying and suffering people?
- Listen to an expert, Mindell Seidlin, director of the Bellevue AIDS program: "The medicines they receive are big guns with a lot of side-effects and toxicity. They receive many diagnostic procedures. They are weak, debilitated, can't feed themselves, they need help to the bathroom, and have severe diarrhea. And 30 percent develop dementia."
- Eventually, because of shortages, antibiotics will be withheld from AIDS patients. There will be protests (at first) of dis-

crimination and euthanasia. But what do you do if half the people in the lifeboat are obviously dying and the boat is sinking because of overload?
- During the first great plague, physicians fled from the centers of pestilence just like everyone else. The great physician, Galen, put it bluntly: "Flee the plague and live to treat another day." And that's exactly what he did. A surgeon in Wisconsin has refused to perform heart surgery on AIDS-infected persons. This rejection will spread as more health care workers refuse to risk their lives for a person doomed to die.
- The ancient physician, Rhazes, was more poetic that Galen:
  "Three little words the plague dispel:
  quick, far and late, where 'ere you dwell.
  Start quick, go far and right away,
  and your return till late delay."
- There will be so many AIDS-positive people within 2 years that it will be impossible to incarcerate and maintain them. The reduction in the productive work force and the cost of housing and feeding them would quickly bankrupt the nation.
- Over 5 percent of all AIDS-infected people work in hospitals (*Newsweek*, 9/24/87).
- AIDS-infected people tend to carry other highly infectious diseases such as a virulent form of tuberculosis, a deadly hepatitis, and torula histolytica, a uniformly fatal type of meningitis. The CDC, Surgeon General Koop, and the politicians are endangering all of us through their refusal to face the reality of this devastating plague.
- Last year Brazil denied any AIDS. Now they are third in cases per capita and climbing.
- If experts think that you can't get AIDS from casual contact, then why are hospitals trying to get rid of employees who have AIDS? Do they know something we don't? AIDS-related job discrimination is skyrocketing (*American Medical News*, 2/27/87).
- Blue Cross is worried about going broke. One official stated that "we are deeply worried" and that the cost for claims will be into the billions by mid-90's. "By 1995 we could be paying

more for treatment of AIDS than we pay out today for all health care claims."
- Did you know that all full-blown AIDS patients, no matter what their age, are rewarded with Social Security Disability? Soon the debate as to whether Social Security is bankrupt will end. There will be no Social Security.
- Ninety percent of U.S. homosexuals now have AIDS (*Conservative Digest,* February 1987). Ninety percent of those have hepatitis. So what is the chance of you contracting hepatitis and AIDS in a restaurant in San Francisco, Atlanta, New Orleans, or New York where restaurant work is the number one means of employment for homosexuals?
- There is going to be a vicious backlash against homosexuals. Any man who shows signs of femininity is going to be avoided like the plague (which he probably has). The "gays" are definitely going back into the closet. San Francisco Mayor Dianne Feinstein, New York City Mayor Koch, and Surgeon General "Chicken" Koop are committing political hari-kari. If AIDS doesn't get them the voters will.
- What else can be done? A lot, but don't believe all that propaganda about a vaccine. The common cold is a virus and they haven't found a cure for that. In fact, they haven't found a cure for any virus. Like cancer, there will be a lot more money made in "treating" rather than curing. The AMA is going down the same old drug trail it went down with cancer. The result will be the same: the squandering of millions of dollars on useless and toxic "chemotherapeutic" drugs. As with cancer patients it's really chemo-euthanasia.
- Even more preposterous is the situation in Bibb County, Georgia. AIDS-infected children are put into classes heretofore reserved for gifted children, thereby exposing the county's gifted children to an even higher probability of contracting AIDS! Ask your school board if they are planning to place your kids next to a sneezing, coughing, AIDS-infected child. If so, get him out of there. Find a private school that is not run by politicians.
- This plague of the late 20th Century is going to bring cata-

clysmic social change. People will no longer worry about "the bomb" or the communists. They will be too concerned about the silent killer within.
- Casual sex, homosexuality, and pornography will no longer be tolerated. *Playboy* and *Penthouse* magazines will only be a bitter memory. Because the prisons will be the last great reservoir of AIDS, crime will plummet. Even a dumb thief will not want to risk death for stealing an automobile. The churches will prosper. We are going to be yanked back to a Victorian Age – whether you like it or not.
- There is already a vicious variant of AIDS that you probably haven't heard about. AIDS-Induced Brain Disease: AIDS-IBD. It is peculiar (and horrifying) because the psychosis may be the only manifestation of AIDS. The average incubation is 15 years and may be as long as 30. (I don't understand how they know the incubation is 30 years if the disease was only discovered in the late 70's. Have they kept the lid on this for 30 years?) So even if public health officials were considering quarantining AIDS victims, these people would go for years undetected, spreading their insanity to others.
- At the present rate of infection we could soon have tens of thousands of these demented people attempting to poison the water supply, driving amok on the highways, sabotaging aircraft, and killing without provocation.
- You think that's irresponsible? The CDC doesn't even report AIDS-IBD although these people are just as infectious as any other AIDS patient. They don't report stage II, AIDS Related Complex, either.
- But statistical expert Donald E. Babcock, Ph.D., says these figures are grossly inaccurate. Using the official data, he predicts 23 million deaths within four years, 1991. The number infected but still alive could be 10 times as much or 230 million – meaning everybody. As all AIDS-positive individuals will eventually die, probably within 10 years, modern civilization and possibly the human race could disappear within two decades.
- Preposterous? British expert Dr. John Seals has stated that the

AIDS virus might "render the human race extinct within 50 years" (*The New American,* January 10, 1987). He may be optimistic. I always wondered how civilizations, like the Incas, just disappeared. I think I am beginning to understand.
- Richard Viguerie points out that AIDS is the "first politically protected disease in the history of mankind." He added: "We have a sick public health community that has been frankly intimidated by the homosexual lobby."
- Koop is guilty of criminal negligence when he tells the American people that you can't catch AIDS from saliva and other body fluids. Dr. William Haseltine: "Anyone who tells you categorically that AIDS is not contracted by saliva is not telling you the truth. AIDS may, in fact, be transmitted by tears, saliva, bodily fluids, and mosquito bites." But Koop implies: Use a rubber and everything will be okay.
- Dr. Koop's promotion of condom usage among teenagers is not only immoral but totally unrealistic. There are reported cases of AIDS from kissing. Deep kissing or "French" kissing is no different from the insertion of any other body part into an orifice of another person. Are they going to wear condoms on their tongues?
- The enormity of Koop's lies are revealed by what the real doctors in the field are reporting. Dr. Fischl, head of AIDS research at the University of Miami, reports that 17 percent of the spouses of AIDS victims, although they used condoms, have already become infected with AIDS.
- Koop has the doctors confused too. A poll by *MD Magazine* revealed that only 28 percent favored quarantine to stop the spread of AIDS, and they were unsure of what they really believed about the disease. Koop has the doctors so confused that they don't think the insurance companies should be allowed to check for AIDS before issuing a policy and they think "education" is the answer!
- Koop and others even lied to us about the basic biology of the virus. They said the virus was "fragile." It is actually one of the toughest of organisms. The Pasteur Institute and the U.S. Naval Institution of Health have reported that the deadly virus

- can live in dry conditions for as long as 10 to 15 days at room temperature.
- Do you know what a fomite is? A fomite is any non-food thing that may harbor a disease. This would include towels, clothing, plates, cooking utensils – practically anything. No wonder the Pasteur Clinic instructed all nurses to burn their clothes and any linen or kitchenware touched by Rock Hudson.
- There was a lot of press a few months ago about the tragic case of a young boy contracting AIDS from a blood transfusion. The publicity concerned his being denied the right to attend school with his peers. The courts forced the school to take him back.
- In all the publicity there was never a word about the fact that the child with AIDS was being put at great risk. In a crowded school environment he is constantly exposed to all of the childhood diseases from measles to mumps, any one of which could kill him. This is another example of how the medical bureaucrats and the courts are obsessed with rights rather than common sense.
- The business community is living in a dream world. Control Data Corporation is typical. Bob Jones, director of their health services, said, "We wouldn't have a policy on AIDS any more than we'd have a policy on heart attacks." Stockholders please note.
- Ford Motor Company says that it has "no reason to believe" that any of its 382,000 employees has AIDS. Sell short.
- The insurance companies aren't dumb. When the District of Columbia banned insurance companies from testing for AIDS, in effect tying the AIDS can to their tail, they simply abandoned Washington. Eighty percent of the 600 insurance companies doing business there have left. The rest are sure to follow.
- Bank of America rep. Nancy Merritt says proudly, "We have taken a stand." That stand is to favor the AIDS-infected person over employees who refuse to expose themselves to the danger of hepatitis, tuberculosis, and AIDS. Two pregnant women refused to work with an AIDS victim. Bank of America said quit if you're going to be so "irrational," so they did. Can

you imagine two pregnant women being told that they must work with an AIDS-infected person? But that's San Francisco.
- You might say that *Business Week* sets the tone for American companies. *Business Week* is bullish on a cure. They say "an intense research effort is making headway," and "AIDS remains unusually hard to get." They are still telling their readers that "outside the body the virus is fragile" and "it can't be spread through food or water." All of the above are untrue.
- A recent Harris poll confirms that American business, like *Business Week,* has its head planted firmly in the sand. Only 14 percent of executives polled are greatly concerned about AIDS, and only 9 percent have considered testing prospective employees for AIDS.

My Comment: Articles like this are powerful, alarming, and convincing. Dr. Douglas' facts are well documented and his analogies reasonable. I agree with most of its contents and all of its goals – to alert and educate the people of the AIDS plague. Dr. Douglas also writes a newsletter called *The Cutting Edge,* a monthly newsletter which keeps his readers current about the *real* AIDS threat. Until such information is widely circulated, the public will continue to be complacent, AIDS-ignorant and, worst of all, vulnerable. People have a right to this information and the right to judge for themselves whether they eventually take precautions against the AIDS virus or not.

CHAPTER VII
POTPOURRI OF AIDS: PART II

> *Then I said to myself, "What befalls the fool will befall me also; why then have I been so very wise? And I said to myself, that this is also vanity."*
>
> *Ecclesiastes 2:15*

From the *Gilroy Dispatch*, "AIDS Initiative Would Relax Confidentiality Protection for Carriers," by Mary Anne Talbott, October 21, 1988:

- Doctors at Wheeler Hospital have decided to back a controversial AIDS-related ballot initiative, despite strong opposition to the measure from the California Medical Association.
- "There's a feeling among doctors that they have been left out of decisions having to do with public health matters," said Bryon Arndt, medical staff president.
- Their position is at odds with the CMA, which issued a minipoint statement in opposition to Proposition 102. The CMA warns the measure will diminish the blood supply, discourage voluntary AIDS testing, and could cost the state as much as $1.75 billion to implement in the first year.
- "At superficial glance, it looks kind of reasonable," said Roger Kennedy, Chairman of the Santa Clara County Medical Society AIDS Task Force. "I guarantee you there will be more AIDS if Proposition 102 passes."
- Ken Todd, medical relations manager for the CMA, called the position of Wheeler's doctors "misguided," and said there have been no other reports statewide of any medical staff taking a position one way or the other on Proposition 102.

My Comment: I'm proud to say that I work in the hospital and am a member of the medical staff mentioned in this article. This small medical staff took the time to address this AIDS proposition and had the courage to go public with its decision, to support Proposition 102. Because these physicians are better informed about the AIDS virus/disease and because they work directly with patients, they acted responsibly.

It surprised and upset me that we were the only medical staff in California to take such a position, and that we were criticized by officials of the CMA for doing so. *This is the best example I can give of the difference between physicians who work directly with patients and those who do not.*

This typifies the seriousness of the AIDS problem in the United States; not only is the general public complacent and uninformed about AIDS, but so is most of the medical profession. This is a ridiculous and frightening situation.

From *Department of California Health Services,* "Increase Noted In Cases of Congenital Syphilis," Number 90-88 for immediate release, September 14, 1988:

- A significant increase in reported cases of infectious syphilis has public health officials worried about the spread of sexually transmitted diseases, including AIDS, in babies born to unsuspecting mothers.
- Dr. Kenneth W. Kizer, Director of the California Department of Health Services, today reported that congenital syphilis whereby a child is infected prior to birth, has increased threefold since 1983.
- California physicians reported 72 babies born with congenital syphilis in 1987, compared to 19 in 1983. Since the first of January 1988, 56 additional cases have been reported, which will result in a projected 50 percent increase over 1987 if this trend continues through the end of the year.
- Congenital syphilis in newborns, however, usually results in much more serious complications than in adults, since the infection is present during a critical stage of physical development.

- Behavior that places individuals at risk for syphilis may also lead to exposure to HIV infection. Therefore, officials fear that more neonatal AIDS cases also could occur in California.
- Even though an infected child may show no signs of the disease at birth, the syphilis infections can produce crippling complications later in life.
- In order to detect early syphilis, and thus avoid congenital syphilis cases, efforts are being made by state and local health agencies to increase testing for syphilis in public and private medical care settings. Based upon their patient's sexual history and clinical findings, and the sexually transmitted disease rates in the community, physicians are encouraged to test for syphilis. Recommendations also call for routine syphilis testing of pregnant women during the first and third trimester, as well as at the time of delivery.
- If syphilis infections are not treated properly, damage can occur to the brain and spinal cord, heart, and other tissues. Mothers infected with syphilis may give birth to deformed, blind, or stillborn babies.
- The counties of birth for the 72 babies having congenital syphilis in 1987 are shown on the table below. Fifty-four percent (39) of the babies were born in Los Angeles County:

County	Number of Births
Los Angeles	39
Alameda	8
San Diego	5
Long Beach	4
San Mateo	3
13 other counties	18

My Comment: The California Department of Health Services appears to be more concerned about the rise of a few syphilis cases than they are *the much more rising AIDS cases in pregnancy and newborns*. Syphilis does occur in pregnancy and does cause many problems for the fetus and newborn; however, the AIDS virus is much more serious, since the mortality rate is almost 100 percent and there is no cure. Physicians have been routinely testing pregnant patients and newborns for syphilis for many, many years; this, unfortunately, is not true for AIDS. The number of HIV-infection cases in pregnant women and newborns is rising almost daily throughout the country. Why is there such concern for a few cases of a controllable and curable disease like syphilis, and so little concern for an uncontrollable, incurable and lethal disease like AIDS? What happened to our common sense? Why doesn't the American College of Obstetrics and Gynecology come forth and aggressively begin protecting our women in childbirth, *by insisting the mandatory HIV testing of all pregnant women?* This insane attitude of indifference and/or ignoring the AIDS virus' attack on man's reproductive system must stop and be addressed as soon as possible.

From the *San Francisco Chronicle,* "Religious Leaders Oppose Proposition 102 – AIDS Law Punishes the Few," by Dan Lottin, October 20, 1988:

- In an unusual show of political unity, the top six religious leaders in Northern California yesterday condemned Proposition 102, the November ballot initiative that would require doctors to report patients who test positive for the AIDS virus.
- Bishop Melvin Talbert, "It does not protect the whole, but punishes a few."
- Bishop William Swing, of the Episcopal Diocese of California, cited evidence that mandatory testing and reporting discourages possible AIDS patients from being tested.
- "AIDS would be driven underground, thus increasing the spread of the virus, not containing it," Swing said.
- The Rev. James Emerson, Moderator of the Presbyterian Church in San Francisco, said the AIDS reporting requirement of Proposition 102 conflicts with the patient confidentiality requirements of doctors and members of the clergy.
- "If that law passes and I was in that position, I would consider it a morally required act of civil disobedience to violate that part of the law," Emerson said. "There is a right to the seal of

the confessional that applies to us all."
- The press conference was organized by the San Francisco AIDS Foundation and Californians against Proposition 102. In addition to the religious opposition, the measure is opposed by the California Medical Association, the American Foundation for AIDS Research, the California Nurses Association, the League of Women Voters, and California Democratic Party.

My Comment: I'm not sure if these people really think they are trying to contain the AIDS disease and thus help the people or if they are really trying to win an election – defeat Proposition 102. I feel that they don't have the best interests or welfare of the populace in mind but, for their own personal reasons, are trying to persuade the California voters to vote against the proposition. They will use anything – politics, fear, human rights, morality, civil disobedience, violating the law, confidentiality – to sway the voter to vote their way. *What will these religious leaders think and do later, when their churches are half or more empty, because most of their members are either AIDS-sick or AIDS-dead?*

From the *San Francisco Chronicle*, "AIDS Patient Gets Custody of Son," by Bill Gordon, October 20, 1988:

- A gay man with AIDS has won custody of his 9 year old son in the nation's first court test involving a parent who has the fatal disease.
- A San Bernardino County Superior Court judge awarded custody of 9-year-old Shawn Wallace to the boy's father, Artie Wallace, 32, until the end of 1989 when his ability to care for the boy will be re-evaluated.
- Wallace reported no significant problems in caring for his son. A former nursing home attendant, he was diagnosed as having acquired immune deficiency syndrome in July 1986.
- "He knows that I have AIDS," he said of Shawn. "He understands that. He is aware that someday it's going to kill me."
- In thousands of similar cases, visitation, and custody rights face legal threats because a parent has AIDS, is infected with

the AIDS virus or is a homosexual, a high risk group for the disease. Archtenbrish, directing attorney of the Lesbian Rights Project public interest law firm, said she hopes the Wallace case will be viewed as a precedent.

My Comment: Insanity and irresponsibility at the highest level – the California legal system. What about the welfare of the child? Doesn't his wants, needs and health count? Doesn't the fact that he is a minor and can't adequately defend or speak for himself, as to what is or is not good or safe for him, matter? Again I ask, where are the infectious disease physicians? When will they speak up? *Will it be when all of us are HIV infected?*

From *Medical Aspects of Human Sexuality*, "AIDS Confidentiality verses the Duty to Warn": by Harold I. Schwartz, M.D., November 1988:

- When a patient infected with the AIDS virus behaves in a way that recklessly endangers others, the clinician may have a conflict between the professional obligation to protect the patient's confidentiality and the duty to protect those whom the patient may endanger. Precedent for the "duty to protect" stems largely from the *Tarasoff* case. In this 1976 California case, a psychologist was held liable for his failure to warn a homicide victim when he knew (or reasonably should have known) that his patient intended to kill her.
- Although a few courts have rejected the *Tarasoff* doctrine, it is widely accepted now as the standard of care. This doctrine was initially conceived as a "duty to warn," but the court ultimately stated that there was a "duty to protect," acknowledging that mere warnings might not be sufficient and that specific actions such as efforts to hospitalize involuntarily a patient who is threatening violence may be required in order to protect potential victims.
- The relevance of the *Tarasoff* doctrine to the AIDS dilemma is clear. In a case filed in 1985, a man who claimed to have been Rock Hudson's lover sued Hudson's estate and two phy-

sicians for failure to warn him that Hudson had AIDS at a time when it was known that he and Hudson were sexually intimate. Since the estates of AIDS patients are usually quite small at the time of their death, it is likely that similar cases will focus on the physicians who knew of a certain patient's diagnosis but took no action to protect individuals known to be sexually intimate with that patient.

- Opposed to the "duty to protect" those who may be endangered, there is the physician's obligation to protect the AIDS patient's confidentiality. The risks of discrimination that accompany the diagnosis of AIDS are abundantly clear. Improper disclosure of the diagnosis could have dire consequences for the patient and thus lead to a suit for breaching confidentiality. It has been argued that any policy that leads to a breach of confidentiality could deter AIDS patients from being tested and counseled, thereby creating an even greater threat to public health. Therefore, a number of states (e.g., California) have enacted statutes or regulations that expressly forbid disclosure to anyone of an individual's HIV status. Public health laws that require reporting and contact tracing of patients with diseases such as syphilis, do not apply in states (e.g., New York) where AIDS has not been declared a sexually transmissible disease.
- Although confidentiality is a vital concept in medical practice, the weight of legal and ethical arguments clearly points to the physician's duty to protect others in certain circumstances. The American Medical Association has firmly endorsed this position.
- In this situation, a clinician should make every attempt to persuade the patient to inform his wife of his HIV status, and to engage in safe sex practices. If this effort fails, the physician has an obligation to warn the spouse. In states that prohibit the disclosure of an individual's HIV status, a clinician should make a report to public health authorities, although he/she may conclude that the obligation to protect others has not been fulfilled if these authorities refuse to act. Although there is some risk of liability in any breach of confidentiality, the

clinician has a greater ethical and legal obligation to protect identifiable victims of reckless behavior.

My Comment: No wonder health professionals are retiring early and the health training schools (medical, dental, and nursing) are having difficulty filling their quotas! Such insane doubletalk from both our lawmakers and medical leaders is ridiculous. By treating AIDS as a political and medical problem instead of the lethal plague it really is, health professionals are placed at great risk – both medically and legally.

Until the government recognizes AIDS as a medical disease and not a political one, and until the medical profession not only accepts its moral, ethical and legal obligations concerning AIDS, *but its responsibility to protect the public from the HIV as well,* I believe the health-care professionals will continue abandoning their careers, resulting in a terrible shortage of these much needed workers. With the number of AIDS cases rising by the day, this will surely add to the disaster.

From the *San Jose Mercury News,* "Incinerator At Hospital Shut Down," by Jack Foley, December 5, 1988:

- A hospital incinerator used to burn contaminated medical waste in downtown Gilroy was shut down last week after neighbors complained about a towering column of smelly, black smoke drifting over homes.
- The incinerator, which was within 50 yards of homes, has been used for at least 10 years to burn such contaminated medical waste as linens, bandages, dressings, and human tissue, (Administrator) Walser said.
- The burning usually does not create thick black smoke or odors and goes largely unnoticed by residents, according to fire officials.
- A county health official said Friday that burning those kinds of materials does not pose a health threat and, in fact, is one of the best ways to dispose of it.
- Lee Esquibel, chief of the Santa Clara County Health Depart-

ment's Environmental Unit, said recently formed county committee is exploring new policies for the disposal of medical waste following heightened concerns about the problem after medical waste washed up on East Coast beaches earlier that year.
- According to Lee Esquibel, hospitals can burn anything they want in their incinerators as long as the burning does not create a nuisance, or harm or endanger anyone.
- Walser said that although it was believed Wheeler had a valid permit to burn and was meeting current regulations, that too was uncertain after a visit Friday from the air quality inspector.
- The agency may put tighter restrictions on future use of the incinerator or order it shut down permanently, he said.

My Comment: This article reports a very dangerous and overlooked health problem – the inadequate disposal of contaminated, toxic, and infectious garbage from health provider facilities (hospitals, physician and dentist offices, medical clinics, etc.). There are no federal regulations or policies for the safe removal of such dangerous waste from such facilities. This garbage contains unsafe material, including contaminated needles, used culture plates, urine, feces, blood, pus, body organs, skin, amputated limbs, dirty bandages, infectious organisms, etc., all of which endangers the health of the general public. The point here is that much more research is needed to prove, one way or another, if the HIV can be killed by such incineration. If so, no problem; but if not, *we have a big problem.*

Much of this garbage comes from patients who suffer from contagious diseases or infections, including AIDS. This, in addition to the early 1988 situation of contaminated medical garbage that washed up on the beaches of the East Coast (which was AIDS contaminated), cannot be allowed to continue if we are to contain the AIDS virus, let alone other infections. The federal government must quickly pass mandatory regulations for the safe disposal of *all* toxic, contaminated, infectious medical waste from all health care providers and facilities in all states of the union.

From the *San Francisco Chronicle,* Fear of AIDS, Editorial page, December 21, 1988:

- Startling evidence that much of the country – even including professional jurists – is still woefully ignorant about the contagion of AIDS, is revealed by the decisions of three Alabama judges to force defendants with the fatal disease to enter their guilty pleas and receive their sentences by telephone.
- The judges variously explained the unprecedented measures by declaring that they either personally feared infection or their court officers did.
- One of them, Judge Jack Montgomery in Birmingham, later changed his mind after talking to his wife and said that he will allow AIDS-infected defendants to come into his courtroom. "I'm putting my professional thoughts above my personal thoughts," he said.
- Earlier, he had acknowledged that he is aware of medical findings by the U.S. Surgeon General and the federal Centers for Disease Control that AIDS is a relatively difficult disease to contract.
- "Call me paranoid if you want to," said Montgomery, "but they haven't proved it to me yet."
- So far, each of the judges has conducted, by telephone, one case involving AIDS.
- The nation's courts are in need of sensible guidelines in dealing with AIDS-infected defendants, or other courtroom personnel, to assure full protection of everyone's legal rights. And the first directive should specify that although AIDS is an infection disease, it is not spread by casual contact or in the same manner as a common cold or measles.
- The Alabama judges are caught up in an unreasonable fear of something that to them, unaccountably, is still unknown.

My Comment: No matter how hard the "AIDS experts" try to convince people that AIDS has "legal rights" and that it cannot be spread by casual contact, many people still use their common sense to guide them when dealing with the AIDS virus. The AIDS virus is a mystery to everybody, and infection by it is literally a death sentence. It is these facts which concerned the above judges. No one should be forced, manipulated, intimidated, or ridiculed to face this virus or its victims – unless they voluntarily want to do so. When will we learn that no one can legislate fear away? Why? *Because fear is one of man's primary defense mechanisms.*

From the *Journal of American Medical Association,* Letter to the Editor, December 23/30, 1988, Volume 260, No. 24:

- To the Editor – We read with great interest the article in the May 27 issue of *JAMA* by Dr. Levy about the importance of human immunodeficiency virus (HIV)-infected cells in transmission of acquired immunodeficiency syndrome.
- It has been reported that the vertical transmission of HIV infection from an infected mother to her newborn is presumptively possible via breast feeding, owing to the isolation of retrovirus from cell-free human breast milk. Although this evidence in no way excludes HIV transmission through the acellular fraction of milk, it does suggest that the risk, if there is one, is likely to be small. This is because of the presence in human milk of a wide range of factors active against free viruses and because oral infection with HIV can occur only in the event of mucosal ruptures. Transmission, therefore, might occur by two different mechanisms: by penetration of retrovirus through oral and gut lesions of mucous membranes or, more frequently, by direct interaction of the infected mothers' colostric cells with mucosal cells of the host.
- The possibility that breast-fed infants acquired HIV infection from mothers via infected colostric leukocytes cannot really be excluded. This is because there are 1,000 to 2,000 x 10s/L viable macrophages, as well as T and B lymphocytes, normally contained in colostrum and human milk ingested by the neonate. Even though transfer of maternal cells through the infant gastrointestinal tract occurs, it would not be expected that the foreign cells could survive for a long time in the host, though it is likely the foreign cells can persist long enough to transmit HIV.
- Thus, several studies support the possibility of postnatal transmission of acquired immunodeficiency syndrome to infants

by breast-feeding. This mechanism is suggested by the finding of free virus in human milk, but infected colostric cells could transfer HIV by direct interaction with mucosal cells of the infant. (Pietro Cocchi, M.D., Cesare Cocchi, Jr., M.D., University of Florence, Italy).
- In reply: I appreciate the comments by Dr. Robbins and Drs. Cocchi and Cocchi. Because the major source of HIV transmission in seminal fluid is infected cells, my remark about nonoxynol 9 has been documented only on infectious virus, not on infected cells. In fact, there have been no clinical studies showing that this compound helps prevent HIV transmission. Thus, one cannot assume that nonoxynol 9 is an effective means of protection against the sexual transmission of acquired immunodeficiency syndrome.
- The presence of HIV in milk has been reported. It can be found as free virus as well as associated with infected cells. Nevertheless, the level of infectious virus appears to be low. Certainly, newborns with a less developed gastric mucosa may not have sufficient acid to kill virus or virus-infected cells. Therefore, the greatest risk for infection by HIV from milk would be to the neonate shortly after birth. As suggested by Drs. Cocchi and Cocchi, transmission could occur by contact of infected cells with the infant's mucosal lining. This route appears to be a major means of maternal transmission for human T-cell lymphotropic virus type I. (Jay A. Levy, M.D., University of California, San Francisco).

My Comment: This excellent and informative article shows the great risk breast-fed newborns of AIDS-infected mothers are in. Newborns can become infected by the AIDS virus through contaminated breast milk. The AIDS disease in pregnancy is rapidly becoming one of the most important health problems of the nation, and the number of AIDS-infected pregnancies will soon dwarf all the other numbers of contagious diseases in pregnancy – gonorrhea, syphilis, etc. – together. The baby is at great risk from day one of its life, both in the uterus and after delivery. For these reasons, I believe all pregnant women should be tested for AIDS, and if

AIDS-infected, treated appropriately. To provide such care, these pregnant women should be recognized as being high risk, and then treated in facilities that specialize in the management of HIV-infected pregnancies. The most "overlooked" important fact is that the longer the fetus is subjected to the HIV in utero, the more likely it will be born with a congenital anomaly or HIV infected or both! *A very frightening point.*

From *American Medical News,* "People with AIDS get Mixed Sympathies," December 9, 1988:

- While the American public has sympathy for people with AIDS, it has little for those from the two groups at highest risk of contracting the disease – homosexuals and intravenous drug users, a New York Times/CBS poll has shown.
- Only 36% of the 1,606 telephone respondents said they had "a lot" or "some" sympathy for "people who get AIDS from homosexual activity," while 26% had sympathy for "people who get AIDS from sharing needles while using illegal drugs."
- By contrast, 75% said they had sympathy for people who have AIDS, and 19% said they had "not much" or "no" sympathy.
- Support also was swayed by the amount of sympathy respondents expressed for AIDS patients. Of the 19% who had little or no sympathy, 66% opposed free distribution of needles, while of the 75% who had sympathy, 49% supported the proposal.

My Comment: The interesting point here is that most of the American public has sympathy for HIV-infected people, but not if they are homosexual and intravenous drug users. If the complacent, AIDS-uninformed public feels this way today, how will they feel or respond tomorrow, when they are AIDS-informed and the AIDS plague is raging? How will they feel when they find themselves HIV-infected or fearful of contracting AIDS? Who will they blame for the spread of the disease or for the unnecessary deaths caused by the disease?

A review of history of past plagues shows that a public under siege by plague is usually fearful, apprehensive, violent, depressed, and angry at the responsible people who caused or helped spread the disease.

From *The Gilroy Dispatch,* "Cost of AIDS Treatment Criticized," Washington (AP), November 15, 1988:

- AIDS victims are being deprived of the best possible treatment because drugs cost too much, experimental therapies are not widely available.
- The report issued by the House Government Operations Committee says it is "appalling that despite the fact that AIDS must be considered the single most compelling challenge to public health in recent U.S. history, unfortunately, neither the president nor the secretary of (health and human services) has articulated any national leadership policy for the epidemic..."
- The committee says AIDS victims are being exploited through "the unnecessarily high cost" of drug treatments. Long distances from clinical trials deny many patients access to experimental drugs, it says. In addition, women, children, and intravenous drug abusers are often denied participation in such trials, it says.

My Comment: The true cost of AIDS treatment is but in its infancy; when the AIDS plague is raging and AIDS-infected and AIDS-sick people are all around us, the medical costs will be astronomical. The nation must begin preparing now for this soon-to-come unbearable and horrendous burden of AIDS medical costs. If the present system of medical care and funding for HIV-infected people is not changed soon, the present system of medical care for all people will be destroyed and national bankruptcy inevitable.

From the *San Francisco Chronicle,* "Survey Says Teenagers Misinformed on AIDS," Associated Press, December 2, 1988:

- A new federal survey of high school students, reported yester-

day, shows that many teenagers are misinformed about AIDS.
- The national Centers for Disease Control and local school officials surveyed students in the ninth through 12th grades last spring about their knowledge of AIDS and their own personal risks. The surveys were conducted statewide in eight states as well as in seven big city school systems, including San Francisco.
- Surveys were also conducted in Chicago, Los Angeles, New Orleans, New York City, Seattle, Washington, D.C., as well as in the states of California, Kentucky, Michigan, New Jersey, New York, Ohio, Pennsylvania and Washington.
- Findings did not differ greatly from survey to survey, and misinformation was widespread. For example, more than 70 percent of the students responding in Chicago, Los Angeles, New Orleans, and New York believed – wrongly – that someone can be infected with AIDS by giving blood.
- "They clearly know the primary sources of HIV (AIDS virus) transmission, but when it does come to things like blood donations ... mosquitoes, and public toilets, there are a whole lot of misconceptions," Laura Kann, a researcher with the Atlanta-based health centers said.
- In another example, more than half the students responding in Los Angeles and New Orleans believed – wrongly – that AIDS can be contracted by using a public toilet. And more than 70 percent of the teenagers responding in Los Angeles believed – again, wrongly – that AIDS can be transmitted through insect bites.
- On the other hand, at least 84 percent of all the students responding knew that using drug needles can spread AIDS, and at least 88 percent knew that they could get AIDS though sexual intercourse.

My Comment: This study documents my concern of the widespread misinformation about the AIDS virus and AIDS disease. Because of this misinformation, most people of all ages don't know what is true or false, dangerous or safe, real or unreal about the AIDS problem. Even this article, which is reporting about AIDS misinformation, reports in a very irresponsible and slanted manner. There is no conclusive proof that AIDS cannot be contracted through a mosquito bite or by using a public toilet. To categorically state that this belief is "wrong" is irresponsible and dangerous.

From the *San Francisco Chronicle*, "AMA Calls Disposal of Waste 'Irresponsible'," United Press International, Dallas, December 8, 1988:

- The American Medical Association's house of delegates yesterday acknowledged that infectious medical waste is "polluting the environment" and threatening beaches, but it said existing laws should be able to control the problem. The report, adopted as policy by the nation's largest physician-membership organization, stated that federal and state laws "if adhered to and properly enforced" should be adequate to protect the public and environment.
- "Irresponsible, uncontrolled waste disposal is polluting the environment and threatening the use of vast recreational areas of the nation's coastlines," the report said, citing several well-publicized examples.
- The report said U.S. hospitals generate 750 million to 800 million pounds of waste a year, and 15 percent of it is infectious. Each hospital bed in the country, the report added, creates about one and a half pounds of infectious waste per day.

My Comment: While the AMA recognizes the problem of the irresponsible disposal of infectious and toxic medical waste in this country, its statement that "existing laws should be able to control this problem" is nothing more than a cop-out. Again I say, the AMA should lead the country in this war against AIDS, not follow it. It should not tolerate or allow the government and special interest groups to endanger the public; and it should insure that everything possible is being done to take care of the AIDS infected and, especially, protect the AIDS free people.

From *Physicians Financial News*, "California Voters Reject

Initiative on AIDS Reporting, Tracing," by Elizabeth S. Weinstein, December 15, 1988:

- California's Proposition 102, the highly controversial ballot amendment that would have reversed the state's policies on AIDS testing and reporting, suffered a nearly two-to-one defeat in November 8th's election. The proposition was defeated in all 58 counties, including the home county of Republican Congressman William E. Dannemeyer, who sponsored the initiative.
- The proposition, which had been called "a meat-ax approach to public health" by Bruce Decker of the "Stop Dannemeyer – No on 102" committee, would have repealed segments of California law that protect the privacy of people with AIDS. The proposition would have required physicians and testing centers in California to report to the health department the identities of anyone who tested positive for the HIV virus. It also would have established mandatory contact tracing of the sexual partners, or needle-sharing partners, of people with AIDS.
- "This is clearly a reaffirmation of California's rejection of what the health-professional community has – virtually unanimously – called irresponsible," says Mr. Decker.
- California voters did, however, approve Proposition 96, which permits law-enforcement officials and emergency workers to demand AIDS testing of people charged with certain sex crimes and assaults.
- The California Medical Association (CMA) opposed 102 from the start, and raised money to fight it, "although we had put so much money into fighting LaRouche that we didn't have much left over," says Dr. Laurens P. White, the Association's president, referring to two earlier proposals for similar legislation put forth by Lyndon LaRouche, seen by many as a right wing extremist.
- But Proposition 102 had considerably more support than Mr. LaRouche's bills ever did, and many people were surprised when 102 was defeated. Some pre-election opinion polls had

reported 58 percent of Californians in favor of the amendment, as opposed to 31 percent against.
- Rep. Dannemeyer says that voters were swayed by "outrageous, excessive cost estimates" for the proposed changes, when they got to the polls and read through the proposal – some, perhaps, for the first time. He also says that voters were unduly influenced by CMA's opposition to the measure.
- "The public in California has not yet come to appreciate the fact that the CMA and the CNA (California Nurses Association) are dominated by the political left," says Mr. Dannemeyer. He also blames Surgeon General Everett Koop, whom, he says, came out against 102 after publicly supporting increased testing and contact tracing elsewhere. Rep. Dannemeyer calls Dr. Koop's support "an irresponsible act of duplicity."
- Opponents of 102 called its mandatory reporting and tracing both counterproductive and unnecessary. In addition to fining doctors $250 for not reporting actual HIV carriers, the proposition – if it had become law – would have required them to report names of people whom they "reasonably suspected" might have the virus.
- One outspoken supporter of 102 was Paul Gann, a 76 year-old who contracted AIDS after a 1982 blood transfusion. Mr. Gann was already well known for sponsoring a conservative tax-cutting proposal 10 years ago. Many opponents maintained that Mr. Gann's support of Proposition 102 amounted to little more than a crusade against homosexuals.
- The fact that Mr. Gann contracted AIDS was "a great tragedy," says Dr. White, but it would not have been prevented by the legislation of Proposition 102. "Unhappily, the transfusion took place before there was a blood test for this virus," he says, adding that there are about 150 other Californians who became infected the same way.
- In addition to the CMA and the CNA, opponents of 102 included both California senators, all the state's major newspapers and AIDS service organizations around the country. Over 100 Northern California corporations contributed funds to the "No on 102" campaign. Besides attacking the proposition for being

discriminatory and unnecessary, a common rallying point was the threat it presented of driving AIDS underground, says Maureen Anderson, spokesperson for the CNA. If those who suspected they had the virus were denied anonymity, they would stop coming forward for testing, she says. "And basically this would lengthen the AIDS epidemic."
- "There is plenty of evidence that people do not want test results to be known," says Dr. White. "All our research is based on anonymous testing." The proposition would have terminated confidentiality at blood banks, which could have meant "the end of cancer research and heart surgery," he says.
- In addition, says Dr. White, the bill's provision for mandatory contact tracing "way overshot the mark." As a result of legislation that will go into effect in January, physicians are allowed to inform a patient's spouse, sex partner, or needle-sharing partner if the patient tests positive for AIDS. They are also permitted to share information about patients' HIV status with their physician colleagues.
- Rep. Dannemeyer calls California's existing AIDS policies "politics, not public health" – the same charge that is frequently leveled against his own proposals. "There's a network of physicians who are disgusted with the leftward tilt of Organized Medicine" in California, he says.
- But the only apparent such network was a group of doctors who dissented from the CMA's stand on 102, calling themselves "California Physicians for a Logical AIDS Response." While members of this group (who did not respond to repeated requests for an interview) reportedly are intent on changing the state's legal stand on AIDS, they are criticized by many for being uninvolved in both the treatment of the disease and its prevention. "They have no special experience in AIDS treatment or virology," says Dr. White, but were recruited by politicians for their conservative ideology.
- Mr. Decker says he is relieved at the rejection of 102 that voters accomplished at the polls, but his enthusiasm is tempered with wariness. "I'm getting tired of fighting these things," he says. "The message just isn't getting though to these AIDS

charlatans" – those activists who are not involved in either AIDS treatment or education. "I would hope that they would see this and just back off."

My Comment: This article is full of information and misinformation. The defeated Proposition 102 is accurately explained. When first introduced to the California electorate, the polls showed the voters in favor of it by a two-to-one margin; but after the opponents finished frightening, confusing, and misinforming the voters, it was defeated by a two-to-one margin.

Dr. White, the CMA president, made some very irresponsible and incorrect statements, especially when he stated "passage of Proposition 102 could have meant the end of cancer research and heart surgery." Hogwash! The CMA in general, and Dr. White in particular, were used by the opponents to incorrectly state that "the California health professional community has – virtually unanimously – called Proposition 102 irresponsible." Since the CMA never polled its own membership on this issue, I feel it was an irresponsible statement on their part.

Also irresponsible are the statements of Maureen Anderson, spokesperson for the CNA. She attacked the proposition by saying it was discriminatory and unnecessary, and it would drive AIDS underground thus lengthening the AIDS epidemic. More hogwash! Obviously, Dr. White and Ms. Anderson don't appreciate AIDS as a terrible, contagious medical disease, which threatens the entire world.

The remarks of Rep. Dannemeyer, sponsor of Proposition 102, are excellent. He, like I, blame the outrageous and false charges against Proposition 102, and the influence of the CMA's opposition, as the main reasons the voters were misinformed and confused and thus voted down Proposition 102.

Because of Proposition 102, the California Legislature was forced to pass legislation before the election in an attempt to ease some of the ridiculous and restrictive confidentiality laws concerning AIDS. I feel this new legislation, which became effective January 1, 1989, was hurriedly devised and passed; thus it is inadequate and confusing and will cause more problems than it will solve. All this was done purposely, before the election, to help defeat Proposition 102 – by saying it was now not needed. This is a good lesson on how to use politics to help sway voters, one way or another. Finally, I, like my other colleagues who see many patients every day, am definitely not an "AIDS charlatan," an activist who is "not involved" in either AIDS treatment or education. Because of such outspoken, unrealistic, AIDS-ignorant, people, the medical profession's hands are and will remain literally tied for the proper prevention, research, diagnosis, and treatment of the AIDS plague.

From the *AIDS Advisory*, "New AIDS-Related Laws Take Effect January 1," Volume 2, Number 1, January 1989:

- During its 1988 session, the California Legislature enacted a number of laws pertaining to HIV testing and disclosure of such test results. These laws take effect January 1, 1989.
- New legislation requires the physician treating a patient to obtain informed, rather than written, consent from the patient. As a consequence, the consent standard for HIV testing is now consistent with that utilized for most other medical procedures.
- In order to obtain a patient's "informed consent," a physician must disclose all information which is "material" to the patient's decision whether to proceed. Material information is defined as "that which the physician knows or should know would be regarded as significant by a reasonable person in the patient's position when deciding to accept or reject the recommended procedure," supplemented as necessary in cases in which "the physician knows or should know of a patient's unique concern or lack of familiarity with medical procedures." This standard does not require a warning for every possible risk, and the physician is not required to give a "mini-course in medical science." However, the patient must be given enough information to make a knowledgeable decision regarding the recommended medical procedures. Generally speaking, to give informed consent, a patient must be informed of:
    1. The nature of the treatment;

2. The risks of the treatment;
3. The expected benefits of the treatment; and
4. Any alternatives and their risks and benefits.
- In order to satisfy the informed consent requirement, a physician must also determine that a patient's consent is both competent and voluntary. First, the patient must be capable of making the particular medical care decision at issue. That is, it should be clear that the patient understands the nature and consequences of a decision to accept or to forgo a particular diagnostic or therapeutic medical procedure. Second, the consent must be voluntary, rather than coerced. Therefore, while a physician should provide sufficient information to permit the patient to make an informed decision, the physician should not exert improper pressure to obtain the patient's consent.
- The patient's medical record should contain specific evidence that the patient's consent was competent, voluntary, and informed. Physicians would be well-advised to carefully document in the patient's medical record that the physician provided the above information to the patient and that, during the ensuing discussion, the patient appeared to understand the information conveyed. Such documentation should be consistent with established medical record-keeping standards.
- Although the law does not require it, a physician may still wish to obtain the patient's written consent to the HIV test, bearing in mind that such a writing does not relieve the physician of his/her duty to ensure that the patient's consent is truly informed.
- There are three exceptions to the rule requiring "informed consent" that might be relevant in this context:
    1. Emergency situations where the requirement is impracticable.
    2. Cases in which the patient has requested that he or she not be informed.
    3. Situations in which the physician can prove that under the circumstances it would be reasonable to believe that "the disclosure would have so seriously upset the patient that the patient would not have been able to dispassion-

ately weigh the risks of refusing to undergo the recommended treatment."
- Under the current conditions, probably only the second exception will apply; it is unlikely that the first or third exceptions will be appropriate in this situation.
- First, emergency care usually must be provided immediately. Under existing technology, HIV antibody test results are not available for a number of hours after testing. A physician cannot delay necessary treatment until he/she has obtained the results of an HIV antibody test.
- Second, in most cases, the physician will not need the results of an HIV antibody test in order to determine the appropriate course of immediately necessary treatment for an emergency patient. Therefore, it will generally be neither feasible nor necessary to test such a patient for HIV antibodies without prior consent. The health care team should presume that an emergency patient is HIV positive and implement appropriate infection control procedures. Testing may be performed after the physician obtains the patient's informed consent, or the consent of an incompetent patient's legal representative, after the emergency has passed.
- Third, a physician should generally presume that a patient's best interests will be served if the physician seeks the patient's informed consent to, and therefore participation in, decisions regarding particular medical interventions.
- Under the new law, HIV test results may be disclosed to members of the health care team without the patient's written consent. HIV test results may be disclosed through the patient's medical record or otherwise, without the patient's written consent, to the following specific categories of persons:
    1. The patient's health care provider, which includes virtually all licensed health care providers and health care facilities, including physicians; podiatrists; dentists; optometrists; paramedics; chiropractors; marriage, family and child counselors; clinical social workers; licensed health facilities; clinics and home health agencies. (The term "health care provider" does not include a Knox-Keene health

care service plan.)
2. An agent or employee of the patient's health care provider if that person provides direct patient care and treatment.
3. A health care provider who deals directly with donated human body parts.
4. The patient or an incompetent patient's legal representative.

- Although HIV test results may be placed in the patient's medical record, the physician would be well-advised to take special precautions to ensure that such information in the medical record is not inadvertently released to unauthorized persons or entities. Existing law imposes a variety of civil and criminal penalties for negligent or willful disclosure of HIV test results without written consent to unauthorized persons or entities, i.e., those not listed above.
- The 1988 legislation requiring that the results of premarital HIV tests be placed in a special part of a patient's medical record has been eliminated. Now, premarital test results are to be treated in the same manner as other HIV test results: They can be placed in the medical record and disclosed without patient consent to the categories of persons specified above. Again, however, the information should be recorded in a manner that ensures that it is not disclosed to other persons or entities without the patient's consent.
- New legislation expands the scope of permissible disclosure, allowing an attending physician to reveal the results of a confirmed-positive HIV test without the consent of a patient under his/her care to a person reasonably believed to be the patient's spouse or sexual partner, a person with whom the patient has shared a hypodermic needle, or to county health officers.
- The new law allows the physician to do this with immunity from civil or criminal liability. The physician is not permitted to disclose any identifying information about the patient. (While the law does not expressly authorize the physician to transmit the identities of endangered third parties to the county health officer, such a disclosure would be necessary to enable the county to perform contact tracing.)
- This bill requires the physician, before such disclosure, to

discuss the test results with the patient, to offer the patient appropriate counseling, and to attempt to obtain the patient's consent for notification of endangered third persons. The physician must inform the patient that he/she intends to notify the patient's contacts before actually doing so.
- The physician may notify the patient's contacts only for purposes of diagnosis, care, and treatment or to arrest transmission of the disease. The physician must also refer those persons for appropriate care and counseling.
- The law specifically imposes no duty on a physician to notify his/her patient's contacts. However, a physician who intends to rely on the county health officer to perform this contact tracing should probably inquire whether the county health officer has or will in fact notify such contacts, as the county health officer has no mandatory duty to do so. If the county states that it does not intend to contact the endangered third parties, the physician may want to follow up personally.
- Under prior law, all insurance providers were prohibited from using the results of an HIV test in determining eligibility for life, disability, or health insurance. These prohibitions continue to apply to health insurance providers.
- Effective January 1, 1989, a life or disability insurer may refuse to grant a life or disability income policy on the basis of a positive ELISA test followed by a reactive Western Blot Assay performed on the same blood specimen, where the policy's issuance is otherwise contingent on medical review for other diseases or medical conditions. Such insurers may also decline to grant either of the above policies if the applicant has been diagnosed as having AIDS or ARC by a medical professional.
- An insurer that requires an applicant to undergo an HIV test must pay the cost of the test. Furthermore, if an insurer requests that an applicant take an HIV test, the insurer must obtain written informed consent for the test.
- The insurer must provide a wide range of information to the applicant, including a description of the test, its purpose, potential uses, limitations, and the meaning of, and confiden-

tiality protections for, its results; a description of HIV, its causes, symptoms, and methods of transmission, what a person can do, depending on the test's results, and a list of available counseling resources. Insurers may not communicate the results of a positive HIV test to other insurers.

My Comment: This article outlines the ridiculous and threatening positions the government and special-interest groups are placing practicing physicians in. After reading this piece of government "double talk," one should easily understand why physicians shy away from caring for AIDS patients. Who needs the aggravation or the risks?

The silence of the California Medical Association about this law shows that the CMA leaders have forgotten some of their main responsibilities – to insure the best interests of physician members and patients, to insure the delivery of quality medical care, and to insure the protection of the public. This law is a terrible piece of legislation, one which facilitates the spread of the AIDS disease and greatly increases the physicians' medico-legal liability. It is such confusing, irresponsible and discriminatory legislation which endangers the health of all AIDS-free people in California and the country.

From *Omni,* "The Dirty Truth About Toilets," pages 36-37, January 1989:

- Mom was right. You should wash your hands after using a toilet; in fact, it might be a good idea not to use public toilets any more than you have to. A recent study conducted by Charles Gerba, a microbiologist at the University of Arizona, found that toilet flushing spews germs all over the place.
- Knowing that feces contain various viruses and bacteria, Gerba was interested in seeing if toilets were being contaminated by the water sprayed upward during flushing action. He placed dye in a toilet bowl, stretched a lid-high sheet of paper over its top and then flushed. "We got a dye pattern reaching the toilet seat," he says. Then he did postflush time-lapse photog-

raphy and found that a cloud of spray shoots out of the toilet bowl after each flushing, "just like you see with a sneeze," he says.

- His research revealed that the contamination was not limited solely to the toilet seat but also flew outside the toilet, landing on among other things, the handle used to flush the toilet.
- "We saw quite a lot of contamination around the toilet rim where it will settle rather quickly," Gerba says. And when he placed caged mice in the room and flushed viruses, the mice got sick. "Flushing a toilet," concludes Gerba, "is a particularly good way of spreading viruses" such as the ones that cause hepatitis and diarrhea.
- Gerba and his colleagues have tested toilets across America by simply walking into a john, washing the toilet with a detergent, swishing the wash into the bowl, and taking a sample of the liquid. (Once a suspicious janitor saw Gerba with his head stuck in a toilet bowl and called the cops.) Back in the lab, the researchers ran tests to measure the amount of bacteria in each sample. Their results show that gas stations probably have the dirtiest commodes, "because most are not well maintained," says Gerba. The cleanest toilets are in hospitals, "probably," says Gerba, "because they're cleaned the most often." But libraries also have clean toilets. He has no idea why. As for which stall to go to: Avoid the middle one. "It's the most often used," he says.

My Comment: I have always felt that toilets, especially public ones, are excellent places where infectious organisms are found. This article proves such organisms are found in toilets and do cause infections. Since the AIDS virus is found in body fluids and in the rectum, it appears very probable that the AIDS virus could be found in some toilets. If so, can one get AIDS infected from a contaminated toilet? Personally, I believe so. Take great care when using a toilet, especially when away from home.

From *San Jose Mercury News,* "Report May Spur Prison AIDS Test," January 14, 1989:

- Sacramento – In a report that may spark new interest in mandatory testing of prison inmates, the State Department of Corrections estimates that it may be housing as many as 2,750 inmates with AIDS virus infections who have not been identified.
- The estimate, which is still being refined, was sent to the Legislature this week as part of a report on the prison system's AIDS management program.
- As of Thursday, state officials had identified 252 inmates with AIDS infections and had placed them in units apart form the main prison population. But there may be between 1,250 to 2,750 more who haven't been identified, they concluded.
- The figures "support mandatory testing of all prisoners for the reason of treatment, for the reason of staff protection, and for the reason of stopping the spread of the disease," Dr. Nadin Khoury, chief medical officer for the prison system said. "And we do not have the authority by law."
- The projections were based on some 6,000 anonymous tests of inmates who were entering the prison system. The preliminary estimates is that between 2 and 4 percent of those tested have some level of infection.
- Currently, a court order is required to administer an AIDS test to any of the state's 75,000 inmates. Under pressure from prison and AIDS activists, plus a number of health officials, the Legislature has been reluctant to approve measures for mandatory testing of any group.
- There's also been controversy over how the Corrections Department cares for known AIDS victims and where the money will come from to house and treat the state's burgeoning AIDS inmate population.

My Comment: Because of high costs and political pressure, this high risk group is being allowed to be inundated by the AIDS virus. I have heard rumors that prisoners with diagnosed AIDS are now being released from prison, due to the lack of funds and facilities to properly care for them and because of the fear of contracting the disease by the prison employees and inmates! True or not, if measures are not taken to diagnose and treat the AIDS infected prisoners and to protect the AIDS uninfected, our prisons will be overwhelmed by the AIDS virus, resulting in violence, riots, and, of course, death. Nearby communities will be frightened and demand protection, both from the violence and the AIDS plague. This problem will not go away by ignoring it; it will only continue to fester until it erupts into another national disaster.

From *American Medical News,* "Beaches studded with needles, bloody gauze," by Janice Somerville, January 6, 1989:

- As infectious medical waste closed beaches from Michigan to Massachusetts, the heat of public outrage rose with the summer's record-breaking temperatures.
- The debris – including HIV-infected vials of blood, hypodermic needles, gauze dressings, surgical gloves, colostomy bags, and dead rats with mysterious bald spots – highlighted a growing crisis in the nation's system of medical waste disposal, both on land and at sea.
- Acting with a speed rarely observed in the nation's capital, Congress passed sweeping legislation that would require the Environmental Protection Agency (EPA) to set up a 10-state system for tracking medical waste from point of origin to disposal, as urged in an Office of Technology (OTA) report released in early October.
- Passage of the act was preceded by a wave of local, state, and regional legislation, which began when infectious medical waste closed 50 miles of New Jersey beaches for three days in August, 1987.
- Debris continued to wash ashore during the summer of 1988, again closing East Coast beaches. This fall the problem spread to the West Coast, as vials of blood, gauze dressings, and other medical waste – believed to come from military hospital ships – were found on beaches in San Diego and Orange County, California.
- The OTA report pointed the finger at confusing and inconsis-

tent guidelines regulating infectious medical waste.
- Media coverage and the public outcry centered on the discovery that several illegally disposed syringes and vials of blood were contaminated with the human immunodeficiency virus.
- In an attempt to eliminate this risk to the public, and to monitor the disposal of medical residue, the act approved by President Reagan requires generators of medical waste to document their handling of blood, hypodermic needles, scalpels, and surgical and laboratory materials that have been in contact with infectious agents. Transport and disposal firms also would be required to provide similar evidence, creating a paper trail designed to catch violators.
- To the relief of many medical societies, the act exempted physician offices and other small facilities that generate less than 50 pounds of infectious waste per month but permits the EPA to lower that cut-off point. Several states also have enacted laws covering all generators. Many professional associations, such as the Connecticut State Medical Society, opposed including individual practitioners, charging it would burden them with licensing fees, stacks of unnecessary paperwork, and unwarranted governmental intrusion.
- The OTA report noted that "while hospitals and clinics may generate larger quantities of wastes, those generated by smaller facilities may be more susceptible to direct public exposure."
- Tighter regulations on the federal, state, and local levels will send the already spiraling cost of disposal to new heights, officials said. Costs already have doubled and tripled during the past few years, reaching $600 to $700 per ton of infectious waste, said officials from waste disposal firms and medical facilities.
- The federal act also set a new precedent by imposing fines of $25,000 per day for civil violations and $50,000 per day and two years in jail for criminal violations. If the public is endangered, the fine can reach $250,000 per day or up to $1 million for organizations.

My Comment: The most unfortunate truism noted in this article is that "public outrage" is usually the only impetus our government and medical leaders respond to when they must address and try to resolve unpleasant medical problems. Here, pollution of our land, water, and air with toxic and infectious medical waste and the failure of our leaders to lead are the problems. As a result, the public's health and safety are greatly endangered.

The "legislation" implemented by the government is riddled with loopholes. *Remember, there are enough AIDS viruses in a period at the end of a written sentence to infect every American.* Knowing this, what kind of chance do we have containing the spread of the AIDS plague with such poor legislation and such irresponsible leadership? *None!*

When I was being indoctrinated into the U.S. Air Force in the early 1960s, I and other physicians were required to take many orientation classes before assuming our duties. One class was about "germ warfare." The instructor entered from the back door and walked to the front of the classroom. More than 200 people were present. He put his satchel down on the floor and then placed a small opened vial on the podium. He looked at the audience and quietly said, "Please pull out your handkerchiefs and blow your noses." We did and, much to our astonishment, all of our handkerchiefs were stained blue.

The instructor said, "Ladies and gentlemen, if I used deadly lethal germs instead of safe germs in this opened vial, you would all now be dead in this demonstration." He went on to state that one airplane, flying from Maine to Florida, could easily kill all human life from the East Coast to near the Mississippi River by releasing various deadly germs. He finished his lecture by stating that the deaths and horrors caused by nuclear or any other kind of warfare were no match for that of germ warfare. Everyone in the class was stunned. Since that day, I have come to respect and fear what such contagious, lethal germs can do to human beings. Nuclear war is bad, but germ warfare is much worse, at least for humans it is.

I hope readers can appreciate my concern for the complacency of our people and leaders about the AIDS disease and deaths such germs can cause, the AIDS virus being but one of the worst of them. Such medical waste should be disposed of properly from all generators – no matter the cost.

From American Medical News, "Who knows AIDS status? Confidentiality varies by state," by Laurie Abraham, 1988 Top Stories, January 6, 1989:

- New York, Vermont, Washington, and Kansas were among the states that addressed confidentiality of HIV information last year. The State AIDS Policy Center at Washington, D.C. – based Georgetown U. – estimates that about half the states have some kind of confidentiality legislation on the books.
- Laws vary widely, but they generally allow members of the medical team to share a patient's HIV-status if necessary for care, and some permit physicians to notify sexual and needle-sharing partners of infected patients, if the patients themselves refuse to do so.
- The New York law sets forth the philosophy of confidentiality measures: "By providing additional protection for the confidentiality of HIV-related information, the Legislature intends to encourage the expansion of voluntary, confidential testing for HIV so that individuals may come forward, learn their health status, make decisions regarding the appropriate treatment, and change the behaviors that put them and others at risk of infection."
- Until new Legislation passed this fall, California had the strongest confidentiality protections in the country: M.D.s were required to get written consent before sharing a patient's HIV-status with health care personnel or entering it on the medical record. Only when a person was diagnosed with full-blown AIDS was written consent waived.
- The California Medical Association was pleased that the state Legislature amended state laws to allow physicians to share HIV test results on a need-to-know basis, said Mark Madsen, director of physician education. At the time of the initial law was passed, the test was still experimental, he said, so its use had to be more strictly regulated. Written consent "became too cumbersome when we realized the importance of the test

in everyday care and treatment."
- While 102 clearly deviated from the mainstream public health approach to fighting AIDS, other state confidentiality laws are harder to judge, said Mona Rowe, director of the State AIDS Policy Center.
- States such as Georgia have enacted confidentiality laws, but they allow such a wide range of disclosure that a hospital janitor could conceivably be told that a patient carries HIV. "Some states have up to 26 exceptions," Rowe said.
- This legislative unevenness prompted AIDS activists and medical groups, including the AMA, to push for a federal confidentiality law. Last year's effort failed, but American Civil Liberties Union attorney Chai Feldblum said the chances of passage were good in the upcoming congressional session.
- "We are seeing some positive (confidentiality) legislation on the state level," Feldblum said. "but the fact that states might retrench is one of the reasons we need the federal bill."
- But Illinois physicians are not alone in their opposition to state-mandated informed consent. M.D.s in Wisconsin, California, Oregon, and Massachusetts have begun to oppose rigid informed-consent statutes, which they say limit their ability to test. At its annual meeting in November, the Oregon Medical Association called for "routine" prenatal testing, which is likely to include loosening the informed consent procedures the state now requires.

My Comment: Another article explaining our country's misguided policy of protecting AIDS-infected people over the health and safety of AIDS-uninfected people. Our leaders continue to treat AIDS as a political disease and, as a result, we as a nation are unable to wage an effective war against the AIDS virus and the spread of the AIDS disease.

From *Smithsonian*, "America's deadly rendezvous with the 'Spanish Lady'," January 1989:

- In 1918, while the war in Europe still raged, we found ourselves

fighting a killer flu for which there was no cure.
- For millions of people fortunate enough to have escaped the horrors of World War I, the plague struck as the fighting neared its end and displaced war as the tragic centerpiece of everyday life. It was known as the Spanish flu and it spread worldwide. In just under a year, starting in the spring of 1918, it killed more than 22 million people, at least twice as many as died in the "war to end all wars." Some estimates, including people who died of complications, go as high as 30 million.
- In America, with curiously little fanfare, the flu brought to death a half-million souls, five times as many Americans as died in combat in France. How we tried to cope with the flu and its side effects became what historian Alfred Crosby calls the "greatest failure of medical science" ever. "Never before," an article in *Science* magazine stated in 1919, had there been "a catastrophe at once so sudden, so devastating and so universal." Describing 1918 here at home, a nurse from Milwaukee said that it was the "year men cried."
- But exactly what was communicated nobody knew. In fact, though flu shots are of some preventative help today, there is still no known cure for most of influenza's many forms.
- By fall, vomiting, dizziness, labored breathing, and profuse sweating were added to the previously mild symptoms. Sometimes purple blisters appeared on oxygen-starved skin. Projectile nosebleeds from pulmonary hemorrhages occurred, too. Victims often went into paroxysms of coughing, spitting out pints of yellow-green pus. Flu victims began dying in larger and larger numbers, some violently within a few days, their lungs, so doctors said, occasionally resembling "melted red currant jelly."
- From France this second wave of flu spread west to England and south to Spain where it killed eight million Spaniards, which is how it came to be known as Spanish flu, and even, ungallantly, "Spanish Lady."
- For the government and American medical authorities, it was crucial not only to find a cure and a preventative but to insure against possible public panic. Then, as it would now, the main

official responsibility lay with the Surgeon General of the United States, Rupert Blue.
- Today, the Public Health Service (PHS) is a far cry from what it was in 1918. Devastating infectious diseases like diphtheria, scarlet fever and smallpox have now all but been eliminated. The PHS now commands a yearly budget of $13 billion, a uniformed corps of 4,500 "shock troops" spread over all 50 states, and some 42,000 Civil Service doctors, scientists, technicians and administrators, not to mention such research installations as the National Institute of Allergy and Infectious Diseases, and the Centers for Disease Control in Atlanta, which have become so prominent lately in the struggle to control and cure AIDS. In 1918 Blue had only a relative handful of doctors and researchers to help him, and yearly budget – even then regarded as a pittance – of less than $3 million.
- Flu was not then a reportable disease anywhere in the United States, and many states did not even bother to file death statistics with the federal government – or to keep them at all.
- Alas, other dangerous infections were in the air – fatuity, folly, finger pointing, and wishful thinking. Cities as diverse as Santa Fe, San Francisco, Philadelphia, and Seattle bragged that they need not worry – the flu would be kept at bay by their ideal climates. People were presented with a welter of official commentary and patronizing reassurance, much of it nonsense. A community doctor in Arizona, perhaps trying to keep the lid on panic, reported 50 fresh cases as follows: "all mild, four deaths." Mild? An 8 percent death rate?
- The New York City Health Commissioner, Royal Copeland, seemed hell-bent on single-handedly jawboning the epidemic into remission by blaming it on unsanitary Europeans.
- It wasn't long before the nation's thin, blue line of surrogate health officers started fining public spitters as well as handkerchiefless sneezers and coughers, and issuing calls for mandatory face masks. Sales and production of masks exploded. Workers wore them in offices and in factories, and in some cities you couldn't climb on a bus or a trolley without one. But there was plenty of heated argument and plenty of

164 *Surviving the AIDS Plague*

backsliding from people who didn't believe masks helped; or didn't like being told what to do.
- As flu hopscotched around the county, the death toll mounted; from 2,899 in August to 10,481 in September to 195,876 in October, in the last four months of 1918, well over 300,000 died. Both sexes and all races were hit. Surprisingly, a general exodus failed to occur; the poor couldn't afford to run, and because the disease seemed so quixotic, the rich never knew where to go to avoid it.
- Historians still ask themselves how more than a half-million Americans could die in hardly more than ten months, in the most lethal internal convulsion since the Civil War (498,000 soldiers dead in four years), without laying a comparable mark on the country's psyche. But the astonishing truth is that during the epidemic, few people were in a position to see the big picture, and not one of the few was actively in charge overall, though the resulting chaos, assessed in retrospect, would result in an expanded Public Health Service with an unexcelled reporting system.
- Not that any of that would have mattered in the end. For nothing helped, really. Cause and cure – transmission and prevention – all remained mysteries. Transmission? Almost surely airborne by human breath, but what a Pandora's box of potentially ill winds that was. Phone booths were padlocked and streets sprinkled; cashiers were equipped with finger bowls of disinfectant. Public places from dance halls, pool rooms, and movie houses to libraries, schools, and ice cream parlors, even red-light districts, were buttoned up. Churches and saloons were shut tight, too, though not without spirited resistance.
- But controlling possible contagion on such a scale was virtually impossible. One sanitation officer counted 199 individual chances for exposure in any citizen's average day.
- Prevention? There were plenty of vaccines. Illinois alone tried 18 different kinds without success. Across the land, doctors rushed to create prophylactic solutions.
- Cure? Today we know there was none, so understandably in 1918 the medical profession was baffled.

- Cause? In some areas Pfeiffer's bacillus was detected almost daily in influenza victims, in other places it was absent altogether. Intrepid military volunteers were injected with 13 different strains of flu bacillus, had their throats swabbed with pulmonary secretions from the sick and allowed the inside of their noses to be painted with a broth of pure bacillus. Nothing happened. Indeed, in New York City an entire family of six was stricken, each member found to be infected with a different bacterium. It was chillingly ineluctable – as in the ditty recited on playgrounds everywhere:
  > I had a little bird
  > And its name was Enza.
  > I opened the window
  > And in-flew-Enza.
- "Hunt up your woodworkers and cabinetmakers and set them making coffins," one health department was morbidly advised. "Then take your street laborers and set them to digging graves." Devastated Pennsylvania had learned the wisdom of that counsel through grim experience. In one week a total of 5,000 people died in Pittsburg and Philadelphia. So overwhelmed was the latter city that 528 bodies piled up in a single day awaiting burial. More lay beside the gutters or in rooming houses.
- As fear spread, laws and law enforcement in some cities grew savage.
- Violence and vigilantism flourished.
- For every 1 who died in the United States, an estimated 50 had the disease.
- All that could really be done, it turned out, was to keep the patient quiet, warm, fed, and medicated against other life-threatening complications, but even that put a terrible burden on the people who were well, or though sick, still able to get about.
- With churches closed, people prayed elsewhere, sometimes using rude outdoor altars as they did in Main where a priest set up a table and a cross in a garage doorway, and worshipers knelt in the snow. Some deeply believed that the plague had

been visited on the world as divine punishment for human sinfulness. Acting Army Surgeon General Vaughan gave voice to a different, but statistically chilling, thought: "If the epidemic continues its mathematical rate of acceleration," he announced, "civilization could easily (disappear) from the face of the Earth."

- More than 25 million Americans were infected; perhaps a billion beings worldwide. Direct U.S. economic losses have been put at $3 billion, but an insurance industry expert calculated the influenza epidemic as an "actuarial nightmare," which would ultimately cost the United States alone ten million years in productive lives cut off in their prime. "Nothing else," writes Historian Alfred Crosby, "no infection, no war, no famine – has ever killed so many in as short a period."
- As for the mysterious Spanish flu virus, it seemed to vanish from the planet as if it had never been. Since then there have been plenty of milder flus, of course. Today we know that influenza viruses have a genius for assuming new forms when an old one has run its course.
- As evolutionary biologist Stephen Jay Gould recently told an AIDS-lecture audience: "We've had a couple of generations of great fortune: since the ... flu epidemic of 1918, there has not been a (lethal) pandemic disease that struck the human population. If you look through human history, a pandemic is everyday biology. With our usual hubris we felt that we'd learned through technological advances to be free of it forever. But we're not."

My Comment: The 1918 influenza plague was the worst plague this nation has had – thus far. We have had other smaller epidemics or plagues, such as smallpox in the early days and poliomyelitis in the mid 1900s; however, the 1918 influenza plague was more widespread and more deadly than these previous plagues. It was caused by a mutating virus which had no cure or effective vaccine – just like the AIDS virus. William H. McNeil (Plagues and People) wrote:

(a) Influenza has been around a long time and is remarkable

both for the rapidity of its spread, the brevity of its immunity it confers, and the instability of the virus that causes the disease. In 1918-19, the confluence of American with European and African troops in northern France provided the milieu for the emergence of an epidemic of unprecedented scope. New strains of virus were responsible, strains that proved unusually destructive to their human hosts. The disease spread throughout the earth, infecting almost the entire population of the globe, and killing twenty million or more. When the flu hit, medical personal and facilities were immediately overburdened and health services generally broke down; but the acute phase passed rapidly because of the very infectiousness of the virus, so that within a few weeks human routines resumed and the epidemic faded swiftly away.

A generation of research subsequent to 1918 established the existence of three distinct virus strains; and it is possible to create vaccines against all of them. The problem, however, is so complicated by the fact that the influenza virus itself is unstable and alters details of its chemical structure at frequent intervals. Any new and widespread epidemic is therefore almost sure to originate with a virus that has changed enough to escape the antibodies last year's vaccine can create in human bloodstreams.

(b) Changes in flu virus and mutations of other infectious organisms therefore remain a serious possibility. In 1957, for example, a new "Asian" strain of flu appeared in Hong Kong; but before it attained epidemic force in the United States, vaccine against the new variant had been produced in sufficient quantity to affect the incidence and intensity of the infection. This required, nonetheless, nimble footwork on the part of public health authorities and private entrepreneurs in recognizing the new influenza strain and starting vaccine manufacture on a large scale without delay.

Today, medicine has no real cures or vaccines for most diseases caused by viruses, such as influenza, the common cold, and AIDS.

The misery and deaths the 1918 influenza virus caused was great and well documented. The misery and death AIDS will cause mankind will be greater.

From *American Medical News,* "'AIDSism,' a New Form of Discrimination," Mary Ann Adler Cohen, M.D., Commentary, January 20, 1989:

- When a county board of a major hospital supports a policy that is discriminatory, unnecessary, unethical, and entirely without medical or epidemiological evidence to support it, other boards may be encouraged to follow suit.
- Acquired immune deficiency syndrome and other manifestations of HIV infection have created a multidimensional crisis with devastating biological, psychological, and social consequences. Among these are discrimination that we can call AIDSism.
- AIDSism is built on a foundation of homophobia, addictophobia, and fear of contagion and death. It has contributed toward comparisons of AIDS to leprosy and the plague. To violate the confidentiality of health care workers who are infected with HIV to prevent them from treating patients who choose not to accept their care makes no medical sense.
- The best weapons against AIDS are education and compassionate care. Through educational, research, and clinical activities, we can combat both AIDSism and the HIV epidemic. To discriminate against health care workers infected with an illness that cannot be transmitted through caring for patients is creating the worst kind of role model that the medical profession can provide.

My Comment: Another example which shows that many people feel the rights of the AIDS-infected people take precedence over those of the AIDS-free people. Until this kind of insane, irrational approach to the AIDS plague is abandoned, the AIDS virus will continue to decimate the populace.

From *The Wall Street Journal,* "Survey About AIDS Has Mixed Findings," People Patterns, February 7, 1989:

- For the past year, the National Center for Health Statistics has been surveying Americans on their knowledge of and attitudes toward acquired immune deficiency syndrome.
- The surveys found that most people are aware that AIDS can be transmitted by sex or sharing needles for intravenous drug use, and that pregnant women can pass the virus to their babies.
- But ignorance about other means of transmission persists. Over half of Americans think that you may be able to get AIDS by kissing someone who has the disease, which doctors say isn't true. A survey last fall found that 24% erroneously believe the virus is likely to be transmitted by mosquitoes or other insects. And 29% have the impression that AIDS can be contracted by being coughed on or sneezed on by someone who has the disease, which doctors say is impossible.
- Of those surveyed, 82% say they think there is no chance that they already carry the virus believed to cause AIDS, and 75% say there is no chance they will ever get it. Only 4% say they don't know what their chances are of getting AIDS. (Compiled by the staff of *American Demographics* magazine.)

My Comment: These findings, that 82% of people surveyed think there is no chance they carry the AIDS virus, and 75% of the people say there is no chance they will ever get the AIDS disease, is to be expected. Unfortunately, most people don't fear or react to danger until they are personally threatened. I also found disturbing the statement "how ignorant people are," about the transmission of AIDS, because most people polled think kissing spreads the AIDS disease and some think insect bites and being coughed/sneezed on spreads it, too. We are quickly informed by the reporter that "doctors say [this] isn't true." This unsubstantiated blanket statement is irresponsible and is obviously made to influence the reader.

I think people are always smart to use common sense, as well as any other proven method, to protect themselves from the AIDS virus. Remember, there are no "AIDS experts;" there are only some people who deal more with the AIDS problem than others. Since there is so little conclusive proof of anything concerning AIDS, the advice of these people should not be accepted without question. AIDS is not a recoverable disease and it results in certain death; therefore, it is better to be extra cautious than unnecessarily foolish when dealing with the AIDS virus.

From *San Jose Mercury News,* "'Gay Bashing' on the Upswing, Activists Say," December 5, 1988:

- From San Francisco to New York, reports of crimes targeted at homosexuals have increased dramatically in the last four years, up 300 percent by one estimate, in what gay leaders see as a violent reaction to the acquired immune deficiency syndrome crisis.
- Commonly called "gay bashing," the violations range from late-night beatings and slurs yelled in streets to more subtle acts.
- An audit by the National Gay and Lesbian Task Force in Washington shows reports of crimes against gays and harassment have more than tripled in three years, from 2,042 cases in 1985 to 7,008 cases last year.
- Gay bashers find both a motivation and a vindication in AIDS, activists say.
- "AIDS is perceived to be a gay disease. And as it moves out of the gay community into other communities, it has generated a lot of feelings of anger and hostility," said Laguna Beach Mayor-Pro Tem Robert Gentry, who is gay.

My Comment: As the AIDS plague worsens, people will become angry and turn to violence towards those they blame for the devastation of the AIDS plague. Unfortunately, this has been man's reaction in past plagues. Homosexuals, prostitutes, and drug addicts will most likely bear the brunt of this anger. I suggest these people keep a low profile, AIDS-infected or not, because I fear the public in the future will blame them for the AIDS plague and vent its anger/frustrations accordingly – right or wrong.

From *Spotlight,* "Kiss and Don't Tell, News You May Have Missed," January 30, 1989:

- When Dr. Robert Huse contracted AIDS, he tried to sell his pediatric practice near Houston. When word of his disease leaked out, the practice collapsed. Local medical authorities told parents that the doctor wasn't a threat to their children, but the parents weren't buying it. "Any risk is too great when you're dealing with my children," said one mother. Huse's advice to other doctors with AIDS: "Don't tell anyone."

My Comment: "Fear of AIDS" in action. Here, a physician's practice was destroyed when his patients learned he was AIDS infected, even after local "AIDS experts" had assured them there was no danger. In reality, both patients and health care workers fear the AIDS virus, because infection by it means certain death. The fact that the AIDS virus is still a mystery, with no cure, only compounds people's fear.

From *San Jose Mercury News,* "Soviet reports of AIDS are called 'understated'," Moscow, February 19, 1989:

- Reports of AIDS cases in the Soviet Union are "most likely understated and incomplete," the government newspaper *Izvestia* reported Friday as Soviet health officials puzzled over the case of 27 young children infected with the virus at a children's hospital in southern Russia.
- The Soviet Union only recently admitted that it had cases of acquired immune deficiency syndrome. Friday's new articles seemed to signal a growing attempt by the Soviet press to humanize and publicize the problem.
- Recently, an official of the Soviet Foreign Ministry announced that foreigners staying in the country for more than three months would be required to carry a certificate showing they were free of the virus or else be tested.

My Comment: This is more evidence the AIDS plague is

worldwide. Just a few months ago, we were being told AIDS is a disease of the Western World and that Communist bloc nations were AIDS free. *Absolute nonsense!* This contagious, 100% lethal disease is found worldwide and is spread by many routes; do not assume anything about the AIDS virus.

From the *New York Times,* "Latin Nations At High Risk For AIDS, Doctors Say," April 13, 1989:

- Some Latin American and Caribbean countries may be heading toward an epidemic of AIDS like that sweeping parts of Africa, a federal health expert said today.
- The expert, Dr. Thomas C. Quinn of the National Institute of Allergy and Infectious Diseases, and two colleagues estimated that 2.5 million people in the Western Hemisphere were already infected with the AIDS virus and that 500,000 were likely to be diagnosed with acquired immune deficiency syndrome by 1992.
- "We have great concern that we are starting to see a more heterosexual pattern of spread emerging in these countries," Dr. Quinn said. "Once it becomes an established heterosexual epidemic in those countries, it has a potential for rapidly increasing in sheer numbers, like in Africa."
- Dr. David D. Ho, who has studied the AIDS infection rate in Brazil, agreed with Dr. Quinn. Dr. Ho, an AIDS expert at Cedars-Sinai Medical Center in Los Angeles, was the senior author of a study directed by Dr. Eduardo Cortes of the Federal University of Rio de Janeiro.
- "If HIV-1 infection continues to penetrate the poor and less advantaged populations of Latin America and the Caribbean," the editorial said, "there is the potential for a massive epidemic in the Americas that may parallel the situation in Africa, where many cases remain unrecognized and unreported."
- In Africa, where the epidemic is most advanced, AIDS is spread primarily by heterosexual intercourse and affects men and women in almost equal numbers. But in the United States, victims are largely male homosexuals and drug users, and

men outnumber women about 10 to 1.
- Dr. Quinn noted that the epidemic in most Latin and Caribbean nations was far behind Africa's, but that there were signs it would follow a similar course. Among these are the relatively high proportion of female victims in some countries. The male-to-female ratio in French Guiana is 1.5 to 1; in Honduras, 1.7 to 1; in the Bahamas, 1.8 to 1; and in Trinidad, 4 to 1.

My Comment: More evidence which supports my fears: the AIDS plague is worsening by the day and the truth of the seriousness is minimized and withheld from the people. This article:
- Confirms the African AIDS epidemic is massive, with many AIDS cases being undiagnosed and/or unreported.
- Confirms AIDS in Africa is spread primarily by heterosexual intercourse.
- States millions of people are already infected in the Western Hemisphere.
- Confirms that women, as well as men, are susceptible to the AIDS virus.
- States there is a potential massive AIDS epidemic in the Western Hemisphere, much like that in Africa.
- If all people in our country (let alone the world) were tested for the AIDS infection and if all AIDS-infected people (in any of the three stages of the disease) were diagnosed and counted, the total number of AIDS cases would be unbelievable. The sooner this is done, the sooner we can determine the seriousness of the AIDS plague and begin effective counter measures.

From *Insight*, "Did Columbus Find Syphilis in America?" April 24, 1989, page 53:

- There is a good chance that, while in the Americas, Columbus and his crew contracted a nonvenereal form of syphilis and introduced it to Europe upon their return.
- Brenda J. Baker and George J. Armelagos believe the disease, which eventually became venereal, may have been responsible for a subsequent plague throughout Europe.

- There is no clear evidence that syphilis existed in the Old World before Columbus' return, the researchers say, and skeletal remains containing syphilitic lesions throughout North and South America provide overwhelming evidence that syphilis has existed in the Western Hemisphere since 3000 B.C.
- The researchers believe that some of the 1490s sailors contracted nonvenereal forms of the disease, all caused by the bacterium Treponema pallidum, through skin contact and then transported it to Europe, where it spread both sexually and nonsexually.

My Comment: Few, if any, countries have escaped the AIDS path, and it is now infecting human beings worldwide. Since accurate worldwide statistics are unavailable, we do not know how fast or where the AIDS virus is spreading or how many people it is infecting. As in Columbus' case with syphilis, our future history books will give us the answers to such questions, assuming the AIDS virus allows mankind to have a future.

From the *Los Angeles Times,* "No 'Capitalist' Disease, Soviets, At Last, Face up to AIDS," by Masha Hamilton, April 22, 1989:

- After years of officially dismissing AIDS as a disease of the corrupted West, the Soviet Union is now acknowledging its presence here and, with a palpable sense of urgency, has begun a massive education and treatment effort to try to make up for lost time.
- The Soviet health minister has likened the AIDS threat to that posed by nuclear weapons. Film makers are producing graphic and horrifying educational documentaries that break previous taboos in showing how the disease can be transmitted.
- And, in a striking admission of the problem, health officials in Leningrad opened a clinic just this month to conduct AIDS tests and provide physical and psychological treatment for AIDS patients. Clinic doctors, in their first interview with a Western journalist, said the hospital was needed because the number of AIDS cases in the country is vastly underestimated.

Potpourri of AIDS: Part II

- The decision to acknowledge the existence of AIDS, or acquired immune deficiency syndrome, in the Soviet Union has awakened a deep apprehension and even alarm among some in a population indoctrinated to believe the disease was a horror of capitalism that would pass them by.
- In Leningrad, hundreds wait in line each day for the anonymous blood tests offered at the new clinic.
- One frightened woman who visited the clinic confessed that she no longer takes the subway, where she believes the virus can travel like a wildfire.
- In another instance, a man rushed in one day, insisting on being tested because he was convinced he had contracted the disease during a fistfight that drew blood.
- "There is an epidemic of fear about the disease," Soviet AIDS expert Vadim Pokrovsky told the daily newspaper *Country Life* this week. "Hundreds and thousands of terrified people come to us saying they have diagnosed themselves as suffering from AIDS. Some stop visiting saunas and swimming pools and are afraid of foreigners."
- Assembling a team of doctors for the clinic was even a bit of a problem, because information about AIDS had been so suppressed that even some educated Soviets thought the disease could be transmitted through a sweaty handshake.
- "We're not afraid of panic – no, on the contrary, we are afraid of a lack of concern, of sloppiness in trying to prevent spread of the disease," Rachmanov said.
- The extent of Soviet medical concern over the disease might at first appear perplexing. Three Soviet citizens and three foreigners have died here from AIDS, according to official reports. A total of 192 Soviet citizens and 378 foreigners have been officially diagnosed here as carriers of the human immunodeficiency virus; the foreigners have all been deported.
- This compares to about 142,000 people who have contracted the deadly disease worldwide, according to the World Health Organization. The global figures are believed to be much lower than reality, however, because many countries under-report or fail to report cases. In the United States, about 90,990 AIDS

cases have been reported since the virus, which breaks down the body's immune system, was identified in June 1981.
- As a result, 100 times as many Soviets may have the disease as is officially acknowledged, doctors privately conceded in recent interviews at the Leningrad clinic.
- By the year 2000, according to a recent report in the Communist Party newspaper *Pravda,* some medical experts believe the country could have an astonishing 15 million carriers of the disease – a figure that, if accurate, would be 10 times the number estimated in the United States. About 200,000 people would have full-blown AIDS or already have died of the disease, according to the report, which has been seriously questioned by a number of authorities.
- "A long time ago, some noted epidemiologists reported with certainty that this new 20th Century plague would pass us by," the government daily *Izvestia* commented recently. "But the rapidly increasing number of Soviet cases shows AIDS is not somewhere 'over there, in their country.' It is here, among our population."
- "You write for a newspaper in Los Angeles? Then it is very important that you tell your readers something," said Dr. Andrei P. Kozlov, director of the AIDS clinic laboratory, leaning close to make his point.
- "Soviet scientists never supported the idea that this virus was created in the United States," Kozlov said. "It is necessary for the Americans to know we were not responsible for this stupidity."
- "I doubt Leningrad really had the first AIDS death. We were just brave enough to declare it," Kozlov said.
- Even with the best intentions, however, the Soviet Union still has some basic problems in trying to combat spread of the disease – severe shortage of both condoms and disposable needles.
- Soviets growing ever more concerned about AIDS have written to newspapers complaining about the lack of condoms. The Health Ministry newspaper *Medical Gazette* recently reported that some desperate couples had turned to using children's

balloons.
- At a city maternity hospital, 49 people, most of them children, contracted AIDS, apparently because ignorant reuse of an unsterilized needle. The case horrified many and apparently gave fresh impetus to plans to open the Leningrad clinic.
- "We used to be taught here in the Soviet Union that since we were decent people, we could not get AIDS," Kolmakov said. "Now we know the truth – anyone can get the disease, communist or capitalist, Soviet or American."

My Comment: As this article documents, AIDS is just as much of a problem in the communist world as it is in the Western world. The only difference between these two worlds is that the misdiagnosis, under-reporting, and the no reporting of AIDS cases is worse in the former than the latter.

It appalls me to see so many people trying to make AIDS a political disease or social disease, or a disease of homosexuals or anything but what it really is – a lethal, contagious disease of all peoples of the world. No person or nation is safe from the tentacles of the AIDS monster.

From *San Jose Mercury News,* "Financially strapped Mother's Milk Bank gets $30,000 reprieve," by Brandon Bailey, August 25, 1989:

- Santa Clara County supervisors agreed Friday to rescue a financially strapped organization that provides mother's milk for hundreds of babies who cannot survive on dairy milk or formula.
- At the urging of Valley Medical Center officials, the board of supervisors voted to give $30,000 to the Mother's Milk Bank, an independent, non-profit program that operates out of a trailer at the county hospital.
- Officials say the program, which started in 1974, is one of seven human milk banks in the nation and the only one in California. It collects milk from scores of donors in the Bay Area and distributes it to infants at public and private hospitals.

- Patients are charged $1.75 a bottle, but the program does not refuse families that cannot afford to pay, said Maria Teresa Asquith, who runs the bank.

My Comment: I included this article to show there are other body fluids besides blood that are housed in "banks." Milk and other such bodily fluids are fluids from which the AIDS virus can strike from and cause more horrendous problems. AIDS-contaminated breast milk from these banks can and do HIV-infect the babies drinking it. The milk is collected from lactating women, who sell/donate their breast milk. Our leaders and the established media are so concerned about blood used for transfusions being safe (particularly AIDS-free), that they overlook the other lesser used (but just as important) bodily fluids.

All people donating or selling any bodily fluid (as well as any body organ) should be HIV tested, because if they are HIV-infected, their donated body fluids or organs can AIDS infect the AIDS-free recipients. People should be assured everything possible has been done to insure the body fluids/organs they receive are HIV-free – sperm from sperm banks, organs from organ banks, milk from milk banks, etc. The lethal AIDS virus can be transmitted just as well from these bodily fluids/organs as from blood.

From *The Cutting Edge,* "Interview From London" (John Seale, M.D.), Vol. 3, No. 7, July 1989:

- CE: Will civil liberties have to be curtailed to meet the threat of the AIDS epidemic?
- Seale: "The public must be fully informed of the true nature of the threat of AIDS. Once they are informed, the mass of the population will accept measures essential to halt the spread of the virus, even though they will inevitably require severe curtailment of the liberty and civil rights of everybody, just as happens in wartime."
- "And, incidentally, the longer the truth is obscured from the public, and the greater the multitude of innocent people who die most horribly as a result, the more ferocious will be the

explosion of hatred and revenge against those scientists and government officials guilty of perpetrating the deception."
- CE: Are Doctors Douglass and Strecker exaggerating when they claim that this plague could wipe out most of Western civilization?
- Seale: "The virus has the properties of a skilled, devious hidden and implacable invader with the capacity and willingness to kill every man, woman and child in our country. It may now be spreading amongst us precisely because it has this capacity. It is unwise to assume that such a force cannot be vanquished without taking actions which the people accepted as entirely appropriate to fight two World Wars; particularly dissemination of the virus is being actively encouraged by some who wish to destroy our society."
- CE: The government is spending tens of millions of dollars in viral vaccine research. Is this a promising avenue for solution to the AIDS epidemic?
- Seale: "The outlook for a successful vaccine is bleak. None is available for the lente virus diseases of animals. A search for a vaccine against infectious anemia of horses for 80 years, and against maedi-visna sheep for 40 years, has proved futile. Indeed, when antibodies to a lente virus are produced artificially by vaccination, the vaccinated animals die after subsequent infection more rapidly than those which are not."
- CE: Could AIDS be a kissing disease?
- "Cell-free (infectious) virus particles were detected easily in saliva over two years ago, but quantitative studies have still not been published. It is certainly possible that AIDS could be a 'kissing disease.'
- "The scale of the deceptions and misinformation perpetrated by virologists, clinicians, and editors of scientific and medical journals about the infectivity of genital secretions compared with that of blood, serum and saliva, has been astonishing. In the presence of a new, lethal virus spreading amongst people, for which no vaccine or cure is in sight, every sane person would assume that scientists have been working flat-out to verify precisely how it is transmitted. This is not true, and

certainly kissing as a mode of transmission cannot be ruled out at this time."
- "Having assumed for a variety of motives, that AIDS is a sexually-transmitted disease, like syphilis or gonorrhea, a negligible research effort has gone into the critical matter of transmission. A few preliminary papers were published, and their findings have been repeatedly quoted as showing the opposite to what they actually showed. When this was pointed out in letters to the editors of the major medical and scientific journals, publication has been refused."
- "As far as it goes, the tiny research effort into infectivity of bodily fluids indicates that saliva is more infectious than genital secretions."
- CE: Will condoms help prevent AIDS?
- "As the small amount of research that has been done indicates that saliva is more infectious than genital secretions, the idea that condoms can have any significant effect on the spread of AIDS is utterly preposterous. Governments all over the world are spending millions of dollars advising their citizens to prevent AIDS by using condoms on the basis of manifestly fraudulent misrepresentation of scientific evidence presented by scientists themselves.'
- "It must be remembered that the AIDS virus is unusually stable outside the human body. It retains almost all its infectivity after seven days in water at room temperature, and some, after being kept dry, for over a week. A virus with this degree of stability which persists in saliva, cannot possibly fail to be transmitted in many ways apart from sex."
- CE: Could one catch AIDS from coughing or sneezing?
- "If an AIDS viron is inhaled into the lung it is engulfed by an amoebe-like macrophage from the lining of the alveoli (air sacs). It has been shown repeatedly in the laboratory that the AIDS virus readily infects macrophages, and the virus replicates within them, thereby enabling infection of people initiated by this route.
- "Understandably, and wisely, the government has advised dental surgeons in Britain always to wear masks to avoid

AIDS virus infection when using high-speed drills. These drills make aerosols of saliva similar to those produced by sneezing."
- "Chronic lymphoid interstitial pneumonitis is a well-recognized variety of pneumonia caused directly by infection of the lungs with the AIDS virus. When associated with pulmonary tuberculosis, a very common complication of AIDS, it is inevitable that coughing will produce some aerosols containing tubercle bacilli and the AIDS virus. After the fluid in the aerosols evaporates, the minute dry flakes containing tubercle bacilli and AIDS virus float in the air indefinitely, and both remain infectious for days."
- CE: Then it would seem that you are saying that AIDS is not basically a sexually-transmitted disease?
- Seale: "That is correct. You must remember that the animal retroviruses, from which AIDS was probably derived, are not sexually-transmitted diseases. The maedi-visna virus of sheep is transmitted by respiratory aerosols, and the infectious anemia of horses is transmitted by large biting insects. I have no doubt that AIDS can be transmitted by both of these methods. AIDS is definitely not a classic sexually-transmitted disease, but is only incidentally transmitted by the fact that sex is an intimate type of contact."
- CE: How is medical science responding overall to the AIDS epidemic?
- Seale: "In general, not well, I'm afraid. An epidemic slow virus disease is new to medical science and its significance largely incomprehensible to doctors, because it is outside both their practical experience and theoretical training. Epidemics were supposed to have been abolished, and it is difficult to change cherished beliefs. Many doctors are profoundly shocked to be confronted with the disease in young people for which they have no treatment. Many of them have developed profoundly neurotic attitudes toward the disease and fiercely defend the right of AIDS patients to confidentiality and freedom of association, totally ignoring public health responsibilities to insure that others are not infected."
- (From *The Cutting Edge,* January 1989, interview continued.)

CE: How does AIDS compare with other epidemics in history?
- Seale: "The AIDS virus is the most lethal virus which has ever spread world-wide amongst people in recorded history. It is already known that 50 percent of people will die within ten years of being infected; the ultimate mortality twenty years after infection may be close to 100 percent. The previous record holder, the smallpox virus, killed only 25 percent of people infected by it – the remainder recovered and were never troubled by the virus again."
- CE: What about prolonged exposure of family members and normal intercourse with an infected spouse?
- Seale: "The probability is very small of transmission of HIV-I during a single, biologically normal, interaction between an infected and uninfected person."
- CE: Is it possible that practically everyone, in your country and ours, will eventually be infected with the virus? How can we stop it?
- Seale: "Because infected people remain infectious for life, and usually live for eight or more years, it would be expected that, within a few decades of its first arrival, almost the entire population of a nation would become infected with the virus. This catastrophe may be prevented if active measures are taken to test people for the virus, and ensure that those infected do not transmit it to others, in the early stages of the epidemic."
- "The speed with which saturation of the population with HIV-I will be reached will be accelerated by poverty, overcrowding, re-use of medical hypodermics, intravenous drug abuse, frequent contact with the rectal mucosa of different people, frequent changing of sexual partners, inability or failure to screen populations for the virus regularly, maintenance of secrecy for those known to be infected, and dysinformation about transmission."

My Comment: The information in this interview is controversial but logical, and probably true. I believe the people who listen to and heed Dr. Seale's comments, recommendations, and warnings have a better chance of avoiding the HIV infection than those who don't. I commend *The Cutting Edge* for having the courage to print Dr. Seale's comments.

From *Santa Barbara News-Press,* Ann Landers, "Wedding Guest With AIDS No Threat," September 13, 1989.

- Dear Ann Landers: I am engaged to be married next February. My fiance and I are having a serious disagreement that comes up every time we discuss our wedding plans. It's about a friend he insists on inviting. The man has AIDS.

 I have made it plain that I do not want "R" at the wedding, even though I realize that the virus cannot be transmitted by just being in the same room with a person who is infected.

 What if someone should accidently use R's fork, or drink out of the same glass? What if he should sneeze across the table or, heaven forbid, give me a kiss of congratulations? Very few people know about R's condition, but if the news should leak out between now and then, I'm sure many of the guests would be afraid to attend. Also, is it fair of us not to tell people about the risks they may be taking?

 It makes me angry that this man is putting a crimp in our wedding plans and causing so much trouble between my fiance and me. A word from you would be a great help – Westchester Dilemma.

- Dear Dil: Good grief, girl, where have you been these last two years? On the moon? Don't you read the papers? How does it happen that you are not aware that the AIDS virus cannot be transmitted by using the same fork, drinking out of a cup, sneezing over the table or giving someone a kiss? You need to educate yourself. Start with your public library.

My Comment: Dear Angry Dilemma: You are not alone. Such concern and fear of AIDS is very real and justified. The people who have no such fears or concerns are either AIDS-uninformed or AIDS-ignorant. Remember, if you follow the advice of a "supposed AIDS expert" and unnecessarily become HIV infected, they will be proven wrong and you will die. These self-proclaimed AIDS experts are very free with their AIDS advice because it is literally "no skin off their nose." When all is said and done, it's you and everyone else who will have to make such decisions for themselves, because there are no real answers for the AIDS disease and its problems today. *Remember, there is no room for error or mistakes with the HIV – infection by it means death!*

CHAPTER VIII
POTPOURRI OF AIDS: PART III

*He who corrects a scoffer gets himself abuse;
do not reprove a scoffer, or he will hate you;
reprove a wise man, and he will love you.
Give instruction to a wise man, and he will be still wiser.*

Proverbs 9:7

AIDS: 10 percent of cases hit elderly, *San Jose Mercury News,* April 10, 1991:

Aids generally is considered to have little effect on the older population. In fact, 10 percent of diagnosed AIDS cases are among people over age 50, and many elderly people provide care to children, grandchildren or friends with AIDS.

In most cases of AIDS in the older population, the disease was transmitted sexually or by blood transfusion.

Older people inadvertently may be exposed to the AIDS virus because they are the most frequent recipients of blood transfusions.

Another problem in diagnosing AIDS in older people is that some symptoms of AIDS resemble those of other diseases of old age. Like Alzheimer's and related dementias, AIDS can cause changes in memory, personality and behavior. An important difference is that AIDS changes are more rapid and inevitably involve physical symptoms as well.

AIDS also can affect the elderly population through their family and friends. In early 1988, a case-management and homemaker-service agency in Philadelphia found that more than half of the care-givers for their AIDS patients were over 60.

Of course, older adults should have no fear of contracting AIDS if they have never had a blood transfusion, never used drugs intravenously and have maintained a longstanding monogamous relationship with someone who also has the same history.

My Comment: Like I said, the HIV can infect and kill anybody, anytime, anyplace – including elderly people. Through the years, the established media and "AIDS experts" have had to eat their words time and time again, about how and who the AIDS virus infects and kills. Originally they said AIDS was a disease of homosexuals, then heterosexuals; then primarily a disease of men, now a disease of both men and women; then a disease of only young people, now elderly people, etc etc. The main points of the article are AIDS infects the elderly (as well as anybody else) and it is more virulent in older people than in younger people. I find the last paragraph disturbing because it is not true. Whenever a new finding about the AIDS disease surfaces that might help us understand what we are dealing with and shed some light on what we should do, the established media tries to minimize it and tries to channel our thoughts into believing what they want us to believe. It has been shown elderly people can and do infect each other with the HIV, even if they have not had intercourse for years. The reasoning here is that the HIV-infected person probably infects the AIDS-free person via casual or social contact, but of course more research is needed on these modes of HIV transmission. In the near future, the established media will probably have to admit this is true also and then have to eat its words again. I hope eating so many words doesn't make them sick, it sure would me.

AIDS through the AIR, *The Spotlight,* March 18, 1991:

The Centers for Disease Control (CDC) in Atlanta is going to have to fund a study after Dr. Donald Jewitt, professor of orthopedic surgery at the University of California at San Francisco, conducted a study showing that aerosols containing HIV-infected blood were produced during orthopedic surgery when bone cutting tools were used. He found that these particles were small enough to penetrate a surgical mask. The finding would also implicate high-speed dental drills, apparently. Previously the CDC said it was impossible for AIDS to spread through the air.

My Comment: Here we go again. The CDC and other "AIDS experts," who have been telling us emphatically not to worry about AIDS-contaminated aerosols (because AIDS cannot become airborne in aerosols), may now have to eat their words again. For years, a few people (like myself) have been warning people about the HIV's ability to become airborne in aerosols – from people's coughs or sneezes, high speed dental and bone drills etc. Once airborne the HIV does have the ability to infect people, *if the conditions are right*. This is *probably* the way some dentists and physicians are getting infected. Of course more research on this mode of transmission has to be done, before we know if the HIV can truly infect people this way; but since some pretty knowledgeable people highly suspect it does, it is better to protect yourself from AIDS-contaminated aerosols than not. Remember, there is no room for error or mistakes with this disease, *so play it safe and always take AIDS precautions*. Try not to breath any aerosols, which you think may be AIDS-contaminated. I know this is almost impossible, but at least wear glasses and a mask, if you think there is any chance of this happening at any time.

U.S. to lift entry ban on AIDS, VD patients, *San Jose Mercury News,* January 27, 1991:

Washington (AP) – The Bush administration served notice Friday that it intends to lift rules prohibiting foreigners with AIDS, leprosy or any of five venereal diseases – including gonorrhea and syphilis – from entering the United States.

The new policy, said Health Secretary Louis Sullivan, will "bring us in line with the best medical thinking, here and abroad."

After consulting with medical experts, administration officials concluded the new policy will not pose an additional AIDS risk to Americans because the human immunodeficiency virus which cause AIDS, is not spread by casual contact. The same reasoning applied to the other diseases being removed from the disqualification list for visitors and immigrants.

"The risk of...HIV infection comes not from the nationality of the infected person, but from the specific behaviors that are practiced," said a draft regulation of Sullivan's Department of Health and Human Services. A final version will be drawn after a 30-day period for public comment and could be implemented in June.

HIV infection and the six other disease have been on a regulatory list used to bar foreign visitors, workers, refugees and immigrants from entering the country. Infectious tuberculosis would be the only one to remain, because it can be spread more easily.

HIV has been the only listing that has provoked much controversy.

Congress put HIV on the list of contagious diseases in 1987. But Congress and the administration came under increasing pressure from AIDS activists, medical experts and international groups last year to remove it.

Shortly before an international AIDS conference in San Francisco last summer, the administration relaxed the restriction by offering a special visa to people with AIDS, formally called acquired immune deficiency syndrome.

But the action was not enough to quell the protests, and dozens of countries and organizations boycotted the meeting because of the U.S. immigration policy.

Last fall, Congress passed the Immigration ACT of 1990, which instructed the health and human services secretary to develop a new list, based on scientific and medical considerations.

My Comment: In my opinion, this is an insane policy to recommend, let alone, implement. Countries like Korea, China, Thailand, Japan, Taiwan, and Cuba won't let HIV positive people enter their domains, hoping this would help contain the AIDS plague. Meanwhile, America opens its doors to all the HIV positive peoples of the world. – *Why?*

This is another exercise in self-destruction. Abolishing the bans on the contagious diseases mentioned is because these diseases are thought to pose no threat to the general public – there are now cures and/or vaccines for all of them, *except AIDS!* As you know by now, anybody who is HIV positive has the contagious AIDS disease – a disease with no cure or vaccine. To purposely allow people infected with such a lethal disease, to enter the country and endanger the populace, is unforgivable. This will be a "rerun" of the conquistador disaster I wrote about earlier in the book – when adventurers looking for riches brought various communicable disease from the Old World, because these people had no immunity to these contagious diseases. Equally important, this policy will only worsen the socio/economic AIDS problems we have already have and further burden the already overburdened American taxpayer. I guess that old saying is true – "we are destined to repeat our mistakes of the past." *Again, I say why?*

AIDS Transmitted From Injury During Contact Sports, *National Health Alert,* The AIDS Epidemic & Health Care Workers Safety, Volume 1, No. 3, May 1990:

A 25 year old Italian soccer player contracted the AIDS virus after an injury caused by a collision with another player during a soccer game. The Infectious Disease physician reported that the virus was apparently transmitted through severe cuts of the forehead sustained by both players.

Two months after the accident the player was found to be HIV positive. One year before, he had tested negative and had no other risk factors.

The other man involved in the accident was a member of a soccer team composed of residents of a drug rehabilitation center and had previously tested positive for HIV. (Lancet, May 5, 1990, pg. 1105)

My Comment: Here is more proof of the HIV infecting a person by entering his body from a break in the skin, in this case, during a contact sport. "AIDS alarmists" like me have been saying this mode of HIV transmitted is possible and probable for years, now articles like this confirms and proves it. Now over a year has passed since this documented proof came to light, and to my knowledge, nothing has happened. No people, male or female, participating in contact sports are HIV tested – before or after they play. Why? I believe it most important that anybody participating in contact sports be HIV tested before they play for obvious reasons – if anyone is HIV infected, their HIV contamination blood can infect other participants (if it gets on any surface of their bodies). The rougher the contact sport (football, boxing, basketball etc.), the more likely blood contamination of the participants will occur and thus the more important HIV testing is. The obvious question now is, what does a participant who tests HIV positive do? In my opinion, the answer is equally obvious – *he/she does not participate*. Yes, it is a cruel world we live in.

HIV In Saliva: Only Infectious in the Dental Office? *National Health Alert* newsletter, Volume 1, No. 2, February 1990.

Even though HIV is known to be present in saliva, the CDC says it is unnecessary to follow universal precautions in regard to saliva exposure except for dentists. For example, according to present CDC guidelines, a nurse or technician handling sputum specimens is not required to use gloves. (Federal Register Dept. of Labor, OSHA, May 30 1989, pg 23112)

The surgeon General has said that AIDS cannot be transmitted by saliva, yet the American Heart Association concerned about exposure via saliva, has issued guidelines allowing rescue workers performing cardiopulmonary resuscitation to avoid direct mouth-to-mouth contact with unconscious victims. Mouthpieces, resuscitation bags and ventilation devices should be made available.

It is impossible to reconcile these different standards. Either saliva is potentially infectious or it is not. Several cases of transmission by saliva have already been reported. Therefore, the correct approach should be clear. (JAMA, Oct. 27, 1989, pg 2231 and Lancet, Sept. 20, 1986, pg 694).

My Comment: Why aren't the "AIDS experts" or authorities informing the general public, as well as health care workers, that HIV contaminated saliva is infectious? Sooner or later they will have to, but when? How many people have to needlessly become

HIV infected before the warning flags go up?

AIDS Virus Remains Alive and Infective For 7 Days, *Health Alert* newsletter, Volume 1, No. 1, November 1989:

A 1985 report from the Pasteur Institute in Paris, France, revealed that concentrated AIDS virus in saliva remains alive and infective on a dry surface at room temperature for 7 days. (Lancet, Sept. 28, 1985, pg. 721)
These studies were performed by allowing the virus to dry on a surface and then collecting a small specimen every few days and placing it in a test tube with human lymphocytes. Specimens collected after 7 days were able to infect the lymphocytes with AIDS.

My Comment: This is only one of other articles that discusses the HIV's frightening ability to still be infectious, when in a dry state. Again, more research has to be done before all the ramifications of this fact are known; but until then, I caution everybody to be careful of HIV contaminated bodily fluids – *wet or dry!*

AIDS Virus Not Killed By Many Disinfectants, *Health Alert* newsletter, Volume 1, No. 1, November 1989:

The AIDS virus has been reported to be easily inactivated by many disinfectants as well as by household detergents. However, recent studies have shown that 70% alcohol fails to inactivate HIV that is dried on a surface. 2% glutaraldehyde (Cidex, Surgikos) was effective, but 1% glutaraldehyde did not inactivate HIV within 15 minutes. (Peter Hanson et al: London, St. Stephen's Hospital. Presented at Montreal AIDS Conference June 1989)
The previous reports showing that HIV is susceptible to many disinfectants were based on suspension tests – with the virus wet, not dried – iIn hospitals and other clinical settings, in which form it will be resistant to inactivation by many disinfectants.

My Comment: This is an important article because it brings up a most important point – the effectiveness of various soaps, detergents and disinfectants to kill the HIV, wet or dry. Cleanliness is certainly one of the best defenses in preventing HIV infection, but it must be *effective cleanliness*. Just saying to use soap and water or bleach or hydrogen peroxide etc. is not enough. We must know the particulars – what strength, how long the application, which agent, etc. If I could, I would bet right now some people have been and many others will be HIV infected by the use of HIV contaminated instruments and other such medical equipment – because of failure to kill the HIV during the cleaning process. I know I sound like a broken record, but much research is yet to be done on soaps, detergents and disinfectants, which will tell us the most effective HIV killing agents to use and how they should be used. Once this information is known, it should be readily available. The research that yet has to be done on the HIV and the disease it causes boggles the mind – at least it does mine.

Italian Doctors Cite HIV Hazard In Kissing, *Health Alert* newsletter, Vol. 1, No. 1, November 1989:

Researchers analyzed the saliva of 45 couples for blood, cells of which can transmit the AIDS virus. They found 55% had traces of blood after eating, 80% after brushing their teeth and 91% after passionate kissing. (Journal of the American Medical Assoc., Vol. 261, pg.244, Jan 13, 1989)

My Comment: Great Article! The point here is that saliva often has small amounts of blood in it. So, when somebody gets somebody else's saliva on/in their body, they usually get two bodily fluids, not one – the saliva with the small amount of blood in it. What do you think are the chances of somebody you kiss having some amount of blood in their saliva? Just guessing, I would say somewhere between 50 and 100%, with the answer being closer to the latter than the former figure. Knowing this, can somebody get HIV infected when coming in contact with HIV contaminated saliva from French Kissing, oral sex, intercourse, or social kissing? Good question! Be my guest, you answer first this time; however, if you guess wrong, you better go to the beginning of the book and start rereading again...

AIDS Patients Should Be Cared For in "Centers". *Health Alert* newsletter, Volume 1 No.1, November 1989:

AIDS patients with pneumocystis carinii pneumonia are more than three times likely to die in hospitals that have limited experience in treating AIDS than in those with more experience, according to a Rand Corporation study. (American Medical News, June 16, 1989)

Regional AIDS treatment centers should be established to offer the most up-to-date diagnosis and treatment.

My Comment: There are many reasons why HIV infected people should be treated in such facilities, but the most important one is that they have a very complicated, serious, contagious, infectious, fatal, medical disease. Very few facilities or physicians are capable or qualified to treat people with this disease. The public, HIV infected and HIV free alike, must understand that treating people with this disease is a *specialty in itself.* We already have some facilities and health care workers treating only patients with the AIDS disease; but in the near future, we must and will have such officially recognized "centers," because here is where AIDS patients will get the best medical care and will have the best chance to survive. Being an AIDS specialist will be as accepted and respected as is being an obstetrician, a surgeon, a pediatrician or any medical specialist. I am talking about good medical care here – not politics, civil rights, discrimination or anything else! Whoever cannot understand this has a problem; *a real problem.*

Study Wary Of AIDS-Only Hospitals, *San Francisco Chronicle* newspaper, September 13, 1990:

BOSTON – Separate hospitals for AIDS patients could lead to a decline in care and increase the chance of discrimination, the 22-member New York City Task Force on Single-Disease Hospitals said in a study published in today's New England Journal of Medicine.

The creation of such hospitals "would promote negative stereotyping and bias against those with the disease, particularly as the disease comes to affect black and Hispanic persons disproportionately," the group said. "The creation of AIDS hospitals would interfere unduly with the freedom of choice of these patients" and result in poorer quality care because such hospitals often have trouble attracting funds and staff.

My Comment: More nonsense, will it never end? In America we have many health facilities and health care professionals who specialize in various diseases and specialties. I don't hear anybody yelling "foul" here. We have children and women hospitals, cancer centers, pediatricians, surgeons, obstetricians, gynecologists, etc. etc. The treatment, research and prevention of AIDS is a specialty in itself; and as time goes on and more people become AIDS infected or AIDS dead, the more obvious this fact will be and the more people will accept it. A person with AIDS is sick, real sick – even more so than a person with cancer. At least the person with cancer has some chance to survive, but a person with AIDS has *none*. He/she started dying theday the HIV infection began. This is why we need health care workers and facilities that specialize in the treatment of AIDS-infected people. AIDS is a lethal, complicated, contagious, medical disease – a disease that requires much knowledge and experience to treat. By having such AIDS specialists and facilities, the AIDS infected people can be offered longer and more comfortable lives, as well as increased hope for a permanent cure in the future. AIDS treatment centers are coming, whether we want them or not. Why? *Because they will be needed and they will offer better AIDS medical care than anywhere else, that's why!*

AIDS Warning Sought For Lambskin Condoms, *San Jose Mercury News,* May 4, 1991:

SANTA BARBARA (AP) – Businesses selling condoms may have to post warnings advising customers that those made of natural membranes are less effective than the latex variety in preventing the transmission of AIDS.

As proposed, the warnings would read "Tests have shown that latex condoms can prevent the passage of AIDS, hepatitis and herpes viruses, but that natural lambskins condoms may not do this."

The proposal for the warnings came through the actions of Santa Barbara businessman Jim Nissley, who said he contracted the AIDS virus while using a lambskin condom.

Nissley said he wrote a letter to the federal Food and Drug Administration asking them to post warnings on condom packages.

Studies show that latex condoms are 99.6 percent effective in stopping the spread of the virus, but lambskins condoms are only 95 percent effective, Chovil said.

"If lambskin condoms don't provide protection, I'm concerned about these state and federal education programs that imply using them is safe sex," Stoker said.

My Comment: America continues to promote the myth that condom use during sex protects the sex participants from the HIV. America is obsessed with this myth. Believe me, "Condomizing America" will not contain, let alone eradicate, the AIDS plague. If a person (with no immunity) has sex with another person who has the flu or smallpox or chicken pox or AIDS, he/she will most likely get the disease in question – *whether there was condom use or not.* Why? Because these are *all contagious infectious viral diseases,* spread by contaminated bodily fluids – *including AIDS!* Even if condoms could prevent the HIV from passing through them (*which they cannot*), they certainly do not prevent the exchange of other HIV contaminated bodily fluids (sputum, saliva, vaginal secretions, sweat, and blood) exchanged between the two partners having sex. I often recommend condom use during sex for many reasons, but to prevent an HIV infection is at the bottom of the list. If I believe this way, why do I recommend condom use at all? Because maybe, just maybe, I am wrong and condom use does somehow protect the sex participants from the HIV (by a way I am not yet aware of) – *but I sincerely doubt it.* Also let me add here that surveys have been done (and well documented) where sex partners have passed the HIV infection to each other *with and without condom use* and where elderly couples (who haven't had intercourse for many years) have passed the HIV infection to each other, as well. So you see, there are many reasons why "Condomizing America" for protection from the HIV is a myth, a myth which I think should be discarded and forgotten.

Incidence of AIDS Rising in People Over Age 50, *San Francisco Chronicle* newspaper, April 1991:

NEW YORK – Hidden for years by secrecy, shame and in some cases the assumption that their symptoms were simply those of aging, a growing number of older people are emerging as victims of AIDS.

AIDS now occurs far more frequently in people over the age of 50 that among children under the age if 13.

According to the most recent data from the national Centers for Disease Control in Atlanta, there have been 15,696 cases reported in people over 50 compared with 2,686 in children under 13. Older people account for 10 percent of the more than 150,000 AIDS cases reported to the government.

"This topic is one that a year ago no one was talking about, and now it has come of age," said Len McNally, program officer for the New York Community Trust, which finances AIDS programs, and former director of the Village Nursing Home program in Greenwich Village.

Although little research has been done on AIDS among older people, experts say the prevalence of the disease among them raises a number of challenges, both medically and socially.

From a medical standpoint there are signs that the disease progresses through an older body faster and that it causes more severe afflictions.

There is also the risk of delayed diagnosis because many of the initial symptoms of acquired immune deficiency syndrome, like muscle weakness or forgetfulness, are hallmarks of aging.

My Comment: As the mystery of the AIDS disease unfolds, many surprising and ominous findings continue to surface. Worse yet, things we thought were true about AIDS yesterday, have been proven false today, and visa versa. The future will be no different.

It is this trait which makes this disease so deadly and why I say there are no "AIDS experts." How can there be, when we really don't know where the HIV came from, the way the HIV is transmitted, the cure to eradicate the AIDS disease or the vaccine to prevent the HIV infection.. In fact, we don't even know half the answers, let alone all of them, to the AIDS puzzle. Just a short while ago, the elderly were thought to be safe from HIV. Now we find out they too are not safe from the HIV. In fact, AIDS is worse for the elderly than for the younger people. Again, I repeat, one must be very careful what one believes and whose advice one follows, concerning this disease. If I said it once, I've said it a million times, there is no room for error or mistakes with the HIV, because an HIV infection today means certain death.

1 in 5 Infected by AIDS in Some Parts of Africa, *San Francisco Chronicle* newspaper, September 17, 1990:

EPIDEMIC HAS REACHED ASTONISHING LEVELS :
NAIROBI, KENYA – The AIDS epidemic continues to course through Africa, outracing the prevention campaigns that have now been started by every government.

In many cities the spread of the AIDS virus among young adults, the parents and breadwinners, has reached astonishing levels.

In several – including Lusaka, Zambia and Kampala, Uganda – More than 20 percent of adults are infected.

In many other cities where 5 percent of adults now carry the virus, as in Nairobi, or 10 percent as in Abidjan, the Ivory Coast, the numbers are still rising steadily.

Once thought to be largely confined to urban areas of central and eastern Africa, AIDS spread rapidly in the late 1980s to huge new parts of the continent and, ominously, from city to countryside, where most people live.

It is striking men and women alike, the rich and the poor, portending social effects on a scale unmatched anywhere else.

In Africa, the growing misery was evident during weeks of reporting in seven countries.

Perhaps no scene in Africa today is sadder than the elderly in the unnatural activity of burying their grown sons and daughters.

Because so many people were infected so recently and the virus often takes years to kill, the worst lies ahead. With more than 5 million adults carrying the virus, and hundreds of thousands of infants, disease rates will soar.

Dismayed leaders are beginning to ask what the loss of large numbers of people in their prime years will do to society – economically, politically, spiritually.

A "very conservative" estimate of infected African adults as of 1989 is 5 million, said Dr. James Chin, chief of AIDS surveillance at the World Health Organization.

My Comment: This article supports what I have been saying AIDS is doing in Africa – it is decimating the human species. Over 75 million Africans are now believed to be HIV infected, and the numbers are mounting by the day. The work forces of Zaire and Zambia copper mines have almost been destroyed by the HIV, thus adversely affecting their main export – copper. This, plus the great drop of tourism (because of the "Fear of AIDS"), has ruined their economies. Twenty-five percent of the people in Tanzania are HIV-infected, and in some places, it is over forty percent. Well over 100,000 South Africans are believed to be HIV infected. Zimbabwe reports over 400,000 people (4.2% of the population) are HIV infected. Country after country in Africa is slowly admitting/reporting similar numbers. The AIDS plague is now raging in Africa and I'm afraid the future for the people there is bleak. The human species is thought to have first started in Africa, I wonder if it will first disappear there as well. "What goes around, comes around."

Women Fears She Got AIDS From Pap Test, *USA Today* newspaper, April 24, 1991:

A Chicago woman fears she may have contracted the virus that causes AIDS after undergoing a Pap test with a swab used on another patient.

The fears were raised by doctor's recommendations after the examination that she begin taking AZT, a drug used to combat

AIDS.

Corboy said the woman had not been tested for the virus because it was too soon for the virus to show up in a test.

Corboy said the woman, in her early 30s, was tested by a resident physician last week. He said the resident came back to her shortly after the test and said: "something terrible has happened. I used a swab on you that has been used on an infected person."

James Curran, of the Centers for Disease Control in Atlanta, said he had not heard of anyone contracting the AIDS virus through used swabs.

"It would be very unusual," he said. "If there was the absence of the inoculation of blood, the risk would be zero or very low."

But the waiting is wrenching. "she is very optimistic, very prayerful, very concerned – and she's scared."

My Comment: Is this woman's fear of contracting the HIV infection justified? *No – not unless you are that woman!* It is generally accepted that the HIV is spread from contact with HIV contaminated bodily fluids. *Cervical* (mouth of the uterus or womb) *mucous is a bodily fluid;* therefore an HIV infection from contact with this bodily fluid is possible, *if the HIV is in the cervical mucous!* The question is, what is the probability. This, only time well tell; meanwhile this poor woman has to hope and pray she does not get the HIV infection.

Surgeon's Risk of Getting HIV, *San Francisco Chronicle* newspaper, March 27, 1991:

CHICAGO – Surgeons often get splashed, soaked, or accidentally injected with patient's blood in ways that increase risk of becoming infected with the AIDS virus, a federal study says.

The survey by the national Centers for Disease Control found that surgeons came into contact with patient blood in almost one of five operations involved an incision.

Other operating room workers came into contact with blood less frequently, according to the study of 206 operations during six months at Grady Memorial Hospital in Atlanta.

Contact was defined as getting stuck with a needle or cut with a sharp object that had touched patient blood; getting splashed with blood in the eyes, nose or mouth; or having one's skin touched or garments soaked with blood.

My Comment: I am a surgeon and let me tell you right now, this article is "full of beans!" Surgeons come in contact with their patients' blood about 50% of the time, *not* 20% (one of five operations) as started. For starters, our surgical gloves leak (for one reason or another) in about 50% of the time. Also, bodily fluids (primarily blood, but also such fluids as vomitus, amniotic fluid and saliva) often get into our eyes, nose and mouth and on our skin, shoes and clothes in either the liquid or dry state. Many a time have I had to change my undergarments and/or socks and shower (often in then middle of the night), because they were accidently soiled by various bodily fluids of the patient I was delivering or operating on. Why and how does this happen? Because getting accidently soiled by patients' bodily fluids comes "with the job" and because we health care workers often have inadequate protective equipment/apparel (such as defective gloves and non water repellent operating gowns, shoe covers and drapes) to work with – that's why and how! The statement that "operating room workers come into contact with blood less frequently" is *hogwash*. All one has to do is watch the nurses and housekeepers clean up a room after a surgical procedure or obstetrical delivery is finished, to realize the HIV danger they are in. Often, the surgical/obstetrical rooms look like a disaster hit them after being used – bodily fluids everywhere. These hospital employees *often* get soiled/contaminated with various bodily fluids of previous patients – *especially the housekeepers, the most AIDS uninformed and AIDS vulnerable group of people in the hospital*. This article angers me because it is articles like this (that minimize the risk of the HIV infection to health care workers) which are misleading and false, and which are responsible for hospitals across the country not protecting their health care workers adequately with proper AIDS information, AIDS education and AIDS protective gear. *If nothing changes, the HIV will decimate America's health care workers* – just like smallpox decimated the peoples of the New World in the 16th Century.

America cannot afford to let this happen. I again repeat, *America's HIV-free health care workers must be protected, as much as possible, from the HIV in their workplace* – I cannot emphasize this enough!

Mysterious HIV Case – Gay Basher Infected, *San Francisco Chronicle* newspaper, April 1991:

NEW YORK – Doctors say it is possible that a man was infected with the AIDS virus through cuts on his hands when he beat up gay men.

The scientist said the patient, who was not identified, denied having sex with anyone but his wife since he married 25 years ago. He said he had been impotent for about 10 years; his wife was not infected. He said he had never received a blood transfusion, but acknowledged having used intravenous drugs with a sterile needle.

The man later recounted that he and co-workers had sought out and beat gay men in the New York area, where he worked as a truck driver from 1982 to 1988.

"He told me he did this too many times to remember," Carson said, "in the neighborhood of several times a week during that period."

The patient said he often got small cuts on his hands and large amounts of victims' blood on himself during those beatings, the doctors reported. The AIDS virus is most often transmitted through sexual intercourse with an infected partner or through exchanges of the blood.

The national Center for Disease Control in Atlanta has confirmed six cases of health care workers who contracted the AIDS virus through exposure to infected blood in ways unrelated to needles.

My Comment: More documentation confirming that AIDS contaminated blood on one's body surfaces can and does cause an HIV infection. How much proof do we as a nation need to admit that the HIV infection spreads from one person to another by contact with HIV contaminated bodily fluids – *most bodily fluids, not just blood?* Does it have to be when millions of Americans areHIV infected and AIDS dead? I certainly hope not.

AIDS Cases In Prison Increasing Fast, Doctor Testifies, *San Jose Mercury News* newspaper, April 24, 1991:

SACRAMENTO (AP) – AIDS is rising dramatically in California's prisons at the rate of more than 3 percent per month, the prisons' top heath officer said Tuesday.

Dr. Nadim Khoury, testifying before the legislature's joint prison committee, said the number of AIDS cases were increasing "at between 3 percent and 4 percent per month." Overall, California's prison population – currently just over 100,000 – is increasing at a rate of less than 1 percent per month and is expected to reach more than 200,000 by the end of the decade.

Currently, system – wide, AIDS patients may be part of the general prison population until their disease reaches a critical stage, at which point they are assigned to a hospital ward, Kindel said.

Prison officials say the increase of Aids is partly attributable to improved diagnosing, but they stopped short of urging mandatory AIDS testing of inmates, a politically sensitive issue in the Capitol. "That's something the next Corrections Department director may want to do, but we are certainly not going to be doing that," Corrections Department Director James Gomez said.

"Maybe somebody ought to question the attorney general for an opinion, what happens if we do that (AIDS) test along with all the other incoming tests," suggested Assemblyman Richard Floyd, D-Carson, a member of the committee. "It's an explosive situation."

My Comment: About 4 % of America's prisoners are believed to be HIV positive. This article shows that the AIDS problem in California prisons is worsening and creating havoc. I'm sure the AIDS prison problem is as bad, if not worse, in the rest of the states of America. What should we do? *Address the problem – now!* Everybody seems to be waiting for "somebody" to do something and, as expected, nothing is done by anybody.

Rural Nurses Fears Helping AIDS Patients, *Insight Magazine,* March 4, 1991:

In an 18 month study of almost 1,000 nurses working in several rural counties of Pennsylvania and New York, more than 22 percent responded that they would not be willing to care for AIDS patients, and 90 percent were anxious about any form of casual contact with someone infected with the human immunodeficiency virus. While some nurses surveyed did not say they would refuse to treat an AIDS patient, they were worried about doing so and said they would be afraid of contracting the disease from the patient.

Eighty percent of the nurses said their spouse would be upset if they were exposed to an AIDS patient, and 82 percent said their children would react the same way.

Researchers found that nurses who participated in a three-month workshop to learn more about the disease developed more positive attitudes toward AIDS patients. (Dina Van Pelt)

My Comment: This article states what I see everyday, a mounting fear of the HIV and the AIDS disease by patients and health care workers alike. The politicians, researchers, social, workers, etc. all try to rationalize away or minimize the dangers of the of the HIV, but I think most health care workers on the front lines and in the trenches (the ones who have direct contact with patient)s know the ominous consequences of an AIDS infection and trying to convince them otherwise is fruitless, let alone irresponsible. What angers me is that so many of the "expert advice givers" are people who have no medical training at all and who don't know what they are talking about – they are simply regurgitating, word for word, what some other similar "expert advice giver" has told them . These people I can forgive because they are really trying to help people. However, the people who really irk me are the "AIDS experts" or physicians (with no or little direct patient contact) who eagerly advise physicians on the front lines, about what to do or not to do for proper AIDS treatment and prevention. They follow the principle of "do as I say, not as I do," and continue lessening their own chances of exposing themselves to the HIV.

The New Red Plague, *The Cutting Edge* newsletter, Vol.4, No. 8, August 1990:

Politics aside, we have a new red plague – the red-staining tuberculosis organism. It is the most frightening of the diseases we face in this New Age of Pestilence, one that we thought we had conquered. Not only is formally drug-sensitive tuberculosis now drug-resistant, but we now have a new form, mycobacterium avium intracellulari, which has *never* been sensitive to any antibiotic. The Centers for Disease Control, in a report on HIV and tuberculosis said, "Persons who share air with an infectious person through a common ventilation system are at highest risk of contracting tuberculosis infection." Avoiding the "Q" word, the CDC goes on to say: "Because TB is transmitted by the airborne (coughing, sneezing) route, persons at highest risk for acquiring infections are 'close contacts,' e.g. persons who sleep, live, work or otherwise share air with an infectious person through a common ventilation system. Persons with suspected or confirmed TB who have pulmonary involvement, cough and/or positive sputum smear, *should be immediately placed in respiratory isolation...*" The dreaded "Q" word not used by the CDC is *quarantine.*

Do we have a problem with TB? Consider this from the Centers for Disease Control: *"Only one percent of the estimated ten million persons in the U.S. who are infected with TB are identified and being treated."*

Dr. John Mills of the University of California, San Francisco, warns that once TB is reactivated, it is highly contagious *and can be be spread easily by casual contact or through the air, by simply passing an infected person.*

"People are obsessed by the possibility of casual transmission of the AIDS virus," Dr. Mills said. "I think there should be real concern about a far more likely possibility: the casual transmission of TB."

Consider this:
1. A high percentage of AIDS patients harbor undiagnosed tuberculosis.
2. "You can't catch AIDS through casual contact," (say government experts) therefore you must work in close proximity to AIDS patients of suffer the penalties of a discrimination suit and possible jail sentence (where you will catch AIDS

and tuberculosis).
3. The experts agree that *you can catch TB* (including the incurable kind) *by casual contact* (see above).
4. The obvious corollary: *the government is promoting tuberculosis.*
5. Which confirms the Douglas Rule of Inverse Government Action (DRIGA): The more government tries to solve a problem, the worse it gets.

Our friend and colleague, Dr. John Seale of London, warns of the lethal combinations of tuberculosis and pulmonary AIDS. Testifying before the British House of Commons he said, "When pulmonary AIDS is combined with pulmonary tuberculosis, a very common complication of AIDS, it is inevitable that coughing will produce some aerosols containing tubercular bacilli and the AIDS virus. After the liquid in the aerosols evaporates, the minute dry flakes containing tubercular bacilli and AIDS virus float in the air indefinitely and both remain infectious for days."

The unvarnished truth is that we are facing a grim situation with untreatable tuberculosis in our schools and crowded work places. Only a hermit can be said to be truly immune to the possibility of infection with the new, deadly tuberculosis.

My Comment: I only include this excellent article to emphasis the fact that AIDS-infected people can/do spread more than the HIV to other people – in this case, tuberculosis. Aids-infected people are reservoirs of other contagious infectious disease – tuberculosis, various intestinal parasites, cytomegalic disease, syphilis and gonorrhea, to name a few. In America, the incidence of tuberculosis has been on the decline for the past 35 years, but not for the past few years. Now the tuberculosis disease is on the rise and worse yet, it is difficult to treat. The deadly HIV is felt by many to be the main responsible culprit for the recent increase of tuberculosis, as well as other infectious diseases – time will tell.

AIDS Violence, *The Cutting Edge* newsletter, Vol 4, No. 8, August 1990:

The AIDS-infected are swallowing poison, plunging out of windows, smashing their cars and shooting themselves at a prodigious rate.

"You have no control over this illness at all, so it gives me some kind of control when I can say I can end my life any time I want to," Said Chuck Sporeman, a 43-year old nurse who has AIDS. Sporeman tried to kill himself twice in 1988, after his male companion of 13 years died of AIDS.

Andrew Weisser, a spokesman for the Los Angeles AIDS Project, says the the relatively small number of AIDS-related suicides reported publicly "is just the tip of the iceberg" (Malcom Forbes for example).

Dr. Peter Marzuk of Cornell University says that AIDS patients face the greatest risk of suicide just after they are diagnosed, and again when AIDS effects on the brain cause depression, delirium "or other treatable psychiatric disorders." (AP Hemet News, February 21, 1990)

My Comment: An increasing number of suicides is another unpleasant offshoot of the AIDS plague. I believe we will see more and more AIDS infected people committing suicide as the AIDS plague worsens. The reasons will be many, but the cause will namely be one – *AIDS!*

AIDS In China, *The Cutting Edge* newsletter, Vol. 4, No. 8, August 1990:

China representatives have reported that AIDS is "spreading fast" and for the first time has been detected in remote areas and among drug users. "AIDS in China is no longer a myth. The spread of this disease is in fact very serious," a Chinese radio quoted a senior health ministry official as saying. "Our abilities to control this disease are limited," he added. The government reported 153 Chinese have been diagnosed thus far with AIDS.

My Comment: As time goes on, more and more countries are starting to finally admit, they too have an AIDS problem. If anybody really believes China (a nation of almost a trillion people) has only 153 AIDS-infected Chinese, then they will believe anything. As I've said throughout the book, *the HIV infects and kills anybody, anyplace and anytime, and AIDS is a disease of all peoples of the planet earth – no country is immune!*

Should AIDS Stop Care Givers?, *San Jose Mercury News,* February 21 1991:

Since the AIDS epidemic began, doctors, nurses and other health care workers have been on the front line of the battle against the disease – including some infected with the HIV virus themselves.

Many health care employees who tested positive have continued to work for years, without any documented transmission to patients.

On one side, the powerful American Medical Association states that infected physicians should stop performing their job if their work poses "an identifiable risk" to patients or inform patients of their status. Doctors have an ethical obligation to do no harm that is almost as old as the medical practice itself, the AMA argues.

Then, there are those infected by the HIV virus, who say such policies would force them to sacrifice a career and livelihood because of exaggerated public fears.

Hacib Aoun, a physician who contracted AIDS from a patient at Johns Hopkins Hospital in Baltimore, has called such restrictions "an awful message to send to the health care worker."

"We ask you to be in the front lines, but if something happens to you, we will not stand behind you; you will be abandoned and will be deprived of the privilege of practicing medicine," he said in a speech at an international AIDS conference last year.

Opponents of restrictions for HIV-positive health care workers say the risk of transmission pales when compared with other dangers in a hospital setting. How many drinks did the surgeon have recently? How alert is the doctor at the end of a 36-hour shift? What unsafe practices have resulted in infection or death from other causes in a hospital setting? asks Ben Schatz, who heads a San Francisco information group for HIV-positive doctors.

To Lorraine Day, the former chief of orthopedic surgery at San

Francisco General, even a remote chance that a patient might be infected is too much. She resigned from her post last year because she felt that she couldn't protect herself from AIDS on her job.

"The uninfected must be protected," she said. "Surgeons do pose a risk, and the risk if a patient gets it is a 100 percent chance of dying."

"I don't have the right to put a patients life at risk. If surgeons don't want to get tested, its because they are selfish and they don't want to worry about the rights of someone else."

But many other health care workers, who don't know whether patients themselves are infected, resent any demands that they disclose their own HIV status.

So far, health care workers are more vulnerable to being infected by their patients than the other way around.

"I personally have a strong feeling I need to take care of people no matter what their condition," said Maria Allo, chief of surgery at Santa Clara Valley Medical Center. "Society is being very unfair if everyone's rights are protected except the rights of the health care worker."

My Comment: There are many interesting issues here, but they all come down to the same thing – who should be HIV tested, who should know the results of the HIV test and what does a positive HIV test mean for either the patient or the health care worker? These issues could be debated endlessly; but if we look at what we are dealing with (a disease that is infectious, contagious, 100% fatal and had no cure or vaccine), the only *responsible* solutions are:

1. Both patients and health care workers should be HIV tested (and *the rest of the public as well,* but this is another issue I answer elsewhere in the book).
2. If a patient tests HIV positive, he/she has AIDS and should be treated/counselled for AIDS. All health care workers have the right (at least, in America they do) to participate or not to participate in the treatment of this AIDS patient or any other patient.
3. If the health care worker tests HIV positive, he/she has AIDS and should be treated/counselled for AIDS. This health care

worker should not have any direct patient contact, unless that patient also has AIDS.

4. HIV-free patients have the right to request treatment from health care workers who are HIV-free and/or who do not participate in the treatment of HIV positive patients.

These solutions are "truisms" which we cannot hide from – they protect patients and the health care workers alike from the killer HIV, which is the goal of preventative medicine. I know the pain, suffering, unpleasantries etc. implementing these "truisms" will cause, but there are no other alternatives. Would we be *"responsible"* if we did less and thus sentence many innocent people needlessly to their deaths by the killer HIV? I for one, hope not.

AIDS international: Suppressing AIDS Information in the Middle East, *The Cutting Edge* newsletter, Vol. 4, No.9, September 1990:

A number of countries in the Middle East with soaring rates of AIDS infection are keeping their doors closed to W.H.O. officials and other AIDS organizations. Infection rates among prostitutes and drug addicts are increasing dramatically in the Middle East.

Two Middle Eastern countries, Saudi Arabia and the United Arab Emirates, refuse to report any statistics on AIDS. This reticence can be attributed to cultural taboos concerning homosexuality (which is condemned and widely practiced), drug abuse and prostitution. Many believe that the AIDS epidemic in the Middle East may be as bad as or even worse than that among upper classes in Africa, but no one can really tell. (U.S. Military please note)* Medical Tribune, April 5, 1990.

My Comment: More documentation proving AIDS is a global plague and that no country is immune from it, whether they admit it or not. As I have often said, the world figures of AIDS cases (how many people have the HIV infection and how many people have died from AIDS) are far from accurate because too many countries are not AIDS testing, reporting or counting – for one reason or another. But as the AIDS numbers trickle in, we are beginning to realize the AIDS plague is truly man's greatest threat.

The CDC Issues a Stunning Report, *The Cutting Edge* newsletter, Vol. 4, No. 9, September 1990:

After two years of anonymous testing for AIDS in 26 hospitals across the country, the CDC has issued a stunning finding. In New York City – New Jersey area, 25% of men age 25-44 are seropositive for AIDS.

The above statistic is not only the highest in the U.S. but it is also higher than reports from Central Africa. In three hospitals in the New York – New Jersey area, the overall rate for AIDS was 8%.

Although some studies have suggested that the U.S. incidence of new sero-positive and actual AIDS cases is declining, Dr. Dondero, a CDC epidemiologist, challenges this data asserting that the recent survey shows a steady increase nation wide for all the demographic groups tested. Another astounding study was a New York survey showing that 3% of all new-born babies in the Bronx are now HIV-positive. *Medical Tribune, May 3, 1990.

My Comment: The important thing to note here is that the AIDS plague continues to worsen, no matter who says what. Keep your eyes on the trends of AIDS. If they are up (which they are), the plague is worsening.

Royal College of Surgeons Supports Mandatory AIDS Testing, *The International Healthwatch Report,* Vol.IV, No. 7, January 1991:

LONDON, JANUARY 10 (REUTER) – In a report which has AIDS activists up in arms, the Royal College of Surgeons has issued a policy statement saying that British surgeons who may be contaminated with AIDS infected blood during operations have a right to test patients for AIDS without their consent.

The statement by the surgeons' group is a topic of heated debate within the medical profession.

The British Medical Association, representing doctors generally, said anyone who tested a patient without consent might be committing "an assault."

The surgeons also want high-risk patients to be tested for infection with the deadly AIDS virus with consent before an operation.

ANALYSIS: Scores, perhaps hundreds, of medical workers in the United States have been infected with HIV through treating AIDS patients. It is absolutely imperative that surgeons have the right to test patients before performing invasive surgical procedures. Nurses and physicians have a right to know which patients are infected with HIV.

Pregnant nurses should never be required to work with AIDS patients because of their risk of contracting cytomegalovirus (CMV) which can cause severe birth defects and even death to a developing baby.

Usually it is the surgeons, who are on the front lines working with razor sharp instruments and needles while up to their elbows in potentially infective blood, who start clamoring for routine HIV testing of patients.

My Comment: I couldn't have said it better. This is a fine newsletter edited by Gene Antonio ("The AIDS Cover Up") and I commend it for this informative article and analysis. It is this kind of AIDS information which must reach the public, as well as our politicians and medical profession, if we are ever to contain and eventually eradicate the AIDS plague. *What worries me, however, will our leaders learn and act on such good information? So far, I doubt it!*

AIDSWEEK, Signs of an Accelerating Epidemic, *San Francisco Examiner* newspaper, Bruce Hilton, January 27, 1991:

It was a week of milestones and assessments in the HIV epidemic. The federal Centers for Disease Control said the number of deaths related to AIDS has passed 100,000. The CDC also said:
- As the rate of deaths grew over nearly 10 years, half were in the last two years. There were 24,264 in 1989 and 31,196 last

year.
- Twice as many – 215,000 – could die in the next three years.
- AIDS has become the second-leading killer of young men 24-44 years old. "Unintentional injuries" including homicide, is still No. 1.
- By the end of 1991, it will be the No. 5 killer of U.S. women that age.
- Gay or bisexual men and drug abusers of both sexes still account for more than 86 percent of HIV deaths.

My Comment: What can I say, this article speaks for itself. The trends of the AIDS plague (more people getting infected, more people have terminal AIDS, more people dying of AIDS, worsening socio/economic/political AIDS problems) are all *up*. Yes, the AIDS plague in America is here and worsening by the day.

Florida AIDS bill focuses on doctors, *USA Today,* April 18 1991:

Florida Gov. Lawton Chiles is pushing for a law – the first of its kind in any state – to require HIV infected health care professionals to report their condition to a medical board.

"We feel like this is kind of the first steps you ought to take. It's prudent," Chiles said, adding that the professional boards should "see that the disease is not transmitted. I think we've got to go this far."

West Palm Beach orthodontist Robert Engel, who said he was diagnosed with AIDS last week, closed his 750-patient practice Tuesday.

"I feel that is my ethical responsibility as a health care professional," Engel wrote.

"No matter what the CDC decides, this will probably hit the floor of Congress." says Carissa Cunningham of the AIDS Action Council. "We need to take people's fears very, very seriously. But there's no way to guarantee a risk-free environment. If people feel they're being protected (by legislation) they're wrong."

"It will inevitably lead to mandatory testing – that's the slippery slope we're on," says Cunningham. "People with HIV will be driven out of the health professions."

Patients are Upset

"I feel sad that (Engel) is sick, but I feel anyone dealing with patients and having that disease is a danger," said Shirley Citers whose child was Engel's patient.

My Comment: The problem with this article is it only addresses one side of the issue – the patients' side. Who is addressing the other side – the side of the health care workers? Don't they deserve to be protected from the HIV also? Don't they have any civil or human rights? It is true, patients can and do get HIV infected by HIV-infected health care workers, but *visa-versa is more so true!* How do most healthcare workers get infected? Are they all homosexuals or drug addicts or prostitutes etc.? *Of course not.* They are getting infected by patients and in their workplace (hospitals,offices etc.). The point is both parties should be HIV tested and each has the right to know if the other has AIDS, *before a patient/health care worker relationship is established.* It appears to me the politicians in Florida are doing what they do best – *playing politics.* I guess they feel it would cost them too many votes, and maybe even their offices, come election time if they did what was right – *mandate all patients and health care workers, as well as the rest of the general public, be HIV tested.* If you mandate one group of people to be HIV tested, *you must mandate the same for all people* – you can't have your cake and eat it too, *it's all or none!*

Women are awakening to the trauma of AIDS, *USA Today,* November 27, 1990:

Nurse practitioner Risa Denenberg hears about a woman who'd been coming to Bronx Lebanon Hospital in New York for two years to interpret for her Spanish-speaking husband with AIDS.

Denenberg, new to the staff, asked the woman if she'd considered getting tested for the AIDS virus herself.

"She says, 'Do you think I really have to?'"

Unfortunately, Risa Denenberg says, the incident was typical:

Even women at the highest risk for the HIV infection still don't realize they could have AIDS and need treatment.

"It's painfully obvious, but women who get care do better," she says.

Health care providers don't tend to suspect AIDS in women, either – and don't recognize it when they see it, say Denenberg and others seeking more attention for growing numbers of women with AIDS.

Denenberg, who contributed a chapter on complications in women, says women with advanced HIV infection often suffer gynecological problems before other complications such as pneumonia, They Include:

- Recurring, resistant vaginal yeast infections.
- Pelvic inflammatory disease – infection of reproductive organs, often caused by sexually transmitted microorganisms.
- Abnormal Pap smears which are early warning signs for cervical cancer.

These problems can occur in women without HIV infection, but they are both more common and more severe in women whose immune systems have been destroyed by the virus, the activists say.

The CDC says changing the AIDS case definition to include such conditions – not usually life-threatening in and of themselves – could obscure AIDS trends and hamper forecasting. They say their definition of full-blown AIDS is designed for statistical purposes; physicians and other agencies are free to devise their own definitions.

A few studies have looked at the effect of pregnancy on HIV-infected women. The consensus so far: It doesn't speed up AIDS in the mother, except in the latter stages of disease.

Other research indicates women die faster after diagnosis than men – but most experts suspect that's because women are diagnosed later.

One small study done at the Walter Reed Army Institute of Research, Washington D.C., suggests AIDS kills women over 30 faster than younger women – just as it kills older men faster than younger ones.

My Comment: No truer words have been spoken! AIDS is a disease of people, all people – males and females alike. It is true that men are affected by the AIDS disease 10 to 1, *but only early in the epidemic*. However, once the AIDS epidemic is in full swing, the ratio evens out one to one. This happened in Africa, Haiti and Brazil, where the AIDS plague first broke out and where now the AIDS virus is infecting both sexes equally. Here in the United States, the AIDS ratio today is 6 males to 4 females but evening out rapidly. Unfortunately, most people in America still believe AIDS is a disease of homosexuals, prostitutes and drug addicts and mainly males. In reality, women are just as susceptible to the HIV infection as are men and worse yet, the AIDS disease is more virulent in women – they are sicker and die earlier. This is why I strongly believe all males and females should be AIDS tested, especially pregnant women. In pregnancy, the AIDS disease is bad for the pregnant woman, the fetus she is carrying and the people around her. In any event, America's females are in more danger from the HIV than are men because women are HIV tested less, women are diagnosed later in the AIDS disease and women are sicker and die faster from the HIV infection. In my opinion, the most neglected people in this war with HIV are women and health care workers, in that order. As the AIDS plague matures, this observation will prove to be correct.

AIDS screening advised for some pregnant women, *San Jose Mercury News,* January 16, 1991:

PANEL SUPPORTS TESTING IN HIGH-INCIDENCE AREAS
WASHINGTON – The AIDS antibody test should be offered to all pregnant women who live in areas where there is a high prevalence of the deadly disease, an expert committee of the Institute of Medicine recommended Tuesday.

But such screening for infection with the human immunodeficiency virus should be strictly voluntary and should occur only with written informed consent, said the committee, a part of the prestigious National Academy of Sciences.

More that 80 percent of the children with AIDS acquired the infection during gestation or at the time of delivery, the panel said.

AIDS is expected to become one of the five leading causes of death among women of reproductive age if current trends continue, the CDC has said.

Because diagnosis of HIV infection "can have powerful psychological and social consequences," the committee emphasized that women should have the right to refuse to be tested.

"Prenatal HIV screening should not be mandatory because of the multitude of costs involved," Said Dr. Marie C. McCormick, committee chair and associate professor at the Harvard Medical School. "There are great psychological and social costs to women who test positive for HIV, including the threat of discrimination in health care, employment, and access to housing."

The panel recommended against routine testing of newborns, saying that such screening "cannot be justified at present" because it is not meaningful. All babies carry antibodies obtained from their mothers; thus, a positive test does not necessarily mean that an infant is truly infected.

Further, there are risks in treating infants for HIV infection, the panel said.

My Comment: I said it before and I'll say it again, all pregnant women should be tested for the AIDS disease – at least once, but more likely in each of the three trimesters of their pregnancy. Just recently, the State of California mandated that all pregnant women be tested for Hepatitis B, and guess what – there was no human outcry of discrimination, breech of confidentiality, violation of civil rights etc. The same goes for the other diseases we are mandated to test for in pregnancy – syphilis, gonorrhea, German measles, Alpha fetal protein (for spinal cord anomalies) to name a few. Why is AIDS any different – *especially since it has no cure or vaccine?* I include this article because it exemplifies the mainstream thinking – it says a lot about nothing, it rationalizes why we aren't HIV testing all pregnant women, it minimizes the importance of HIV testing pregnant women and omits the other side of the argument (why we should HIV test all pregnant women). I guess the fact that it is good medicine to diagnose AIDS early in pregnancy and offer treatment and counselling to the unfortunate pregnant HIV-infected woman just doesn't seem as important to most people as are these other reasons – *not unless you are the pregnant woman that is HIV infected!* No matter, I believe time will force us to not only HIV test all pregnant women, but everybody as well – whether we like it or not.

Fear of AIDS Changes Behavior of Women, *San Jose Mercury News,* May 15, 1991:

Nearly one-third of all sexually experienced single women in the United States have changed their sexual behavior because they are worried about AIDS, federal officials reported Tuesday. "It is encouraging that a substantial number of unmarried women at higher risk recognize the dangers of HIV infection and have taken positive steps to lessen that risk," said Dr. William Roper, director of the Centers for Disease Control in Atlanta.

My Comment: More evidence that the sexual behavior of Americans is changing. I believe that if accurate polls were taken today, they would show Americans practice *less* "singles bar/pickup" activity, *less* blind dates, *less* promiscuity, *less* premarital and extramarital sex, *less* prostitution and *less* bisexual activity. Also, I do believe Americans are practicing more monogamous sex and getting married earlier. All this change because of a little (0.1 micron) virus *with a knockout punch.* Yes, the "fear of AIDS" will change a lot of other things in our society, including our sexual behavior.

AIDS in the USA, *USA Today* newspaper, May 17, 1991:

As of March 31, 171,876 people had been diagnosed with AIDS. How did they get it:

- Got it from mother	2,963
- Blood disorder/transfusion	5,323
- Undetermined	6,215
- Heterosexual contact	9,191
- Homosexual/Bisexual male contact & drug abuse	11,153
- Homosexual/Bisexual male contact	99,941
- I.V. drug abuse	37,090
Total	171,876

My Comment: If only this many Americans have AIDS, what is the problem in the USA – a country with 250 million people? The problem is, these are only the people in the third stage of AIDS, and only those that are diagnosed and reported. If we tested all Americans *(instead of the very small percentage we are presently testing)* for the HIV infection and counted everybody diagnosed with the AIDS disease (people in the first, second and third stages of AIDS disease, as well as those people with AIDS dementia), the number of HIV-infected (AIDS) people would be in the *millions*. This is why the people in the "know" are concerned – *super concerned!!!*

AIDS in the USA: The infected health-care workers, *USA Today* newspaper, May 17, 1991:

As of March 31, 6,436 health care workers had been diagnosed with AIDS. What their jobs are:

- Physicians	703
- Therapists	319
- Dentists	171
- Paramedics	116
- Surgeons	47
- Technicians	941
- Medical Aides	1,101
- Nurses	1,358
- Others	1,680
Total	6,436

My Comment: These are only the health care workers that have been diagnosed and reported with third stage AIDS. How many are undiagnosed or have been diagnosed with third stage AIDS but are unreported? How many have the first or second stage of AIDS or AIDS dementia? How many of the six and one-half million health care workers in America have been AIDS tested – if it is over 1-2%, I will be greatly surprised. If all health care workers were AIDS tested and all testing positive were counted, the number would be shocking. Since I have realized America's health care workers are in a dangerous AIDS environment and can/are getting HIV infected, I have been crusading for the most effective HIV protective equipment money can buy to protect them. Presently, the majority of our health care workers are not taking proper AIDS precautions and the majority of our health care facilities do not have any HIV protective equipment/gear/policies. This must change as soon as possible, or our health care workers will go the way of the dinosaur. Lastly, let me correct one important misconception. We health care workers wear caps, glasses, gowns and gloves to primarily protect *us* from germs from patients, not visa versa. It is we health care workers who are more likely to get HIV-infected from patients, not visa-versa; therefore, if you want us around in the near future, please demand our leaders protects us – *NOW!!!*

AIDS Groups May Try To Block Boston Meeting, *San Francisco Chronicle* newspaper, May 27, 1991:

A movement to cancel or boycott an international AIDS conference scheduled in Boston next year surfaced during the weekend because of indications that the federal government will continue to bar immigrants infected with the virus from entering the United States.

Bowing to pressure from conservatives, the Bush administration has reportedly shelved new regulations that would have removed a ban on immigrants and foreign travelers infected with HIV. The move has renewed the hostility of those opposed to the ban.

The Department of Health and Human Services has not formally announced that it is backing off from proposed regulations lifting the ban, but Washington sources have said that the department is holding the matter in abeyance. The draft regulations were expected to go into effect Saturday, June 1.

Last June, major AIDS organizations around the world boycotted the same gathering in San Francisco, the key scientific meeting on the disease in the world. Many scientists and others who chose to attend the San Francisco conference wore armbands with U.S. immigration policies, while noisy protestors made their feelings known outside.

No Medical Grounds
Most leading health authorities, including Health Secretary Louis Sullivan, have said there is no medical basis for excluding people infected with the human immunodeficiency virus because it cannot be transmitted casually. The dispute now centers on whether immigrants infected with the virus will become a financial burden on the nation's public health system if they become ill and have no health insurance or assets to pay for their care.

My Comment: Thank goodness this insane proposed immigration bill of 1991 has been shelved, even if it might be temporary. Now, the special interests groups and many "AIDS experts" will apply fierce political pressure on the politicians to reverse this decision and pass the bill. They will do or say anything to achieve their goal – even if it is at the expense of the health of the public and country. To them, reason or facts or common sense does not "compute" – *only imposing their beliefs, right or wrong, on others is what counts!* However, it appears the "silent majority" and organized medicine are finally starting to wake up, so maybe all is not lost yet. Now is the time to speak up and drown out the AIDS-uninformed/AIDS-ignorant people. This article proves the politicians are listening to your cries and reading your letters and responding responsibly thereafter. It was the many letters (over 40,000) and the multiple objections (by many organizations, both medical and nonmedical) that finally convinced our legislators to shelve this terrible immigration bill. So hereafter, *let your voice be heard on all important AIDS social/economic/political issues*. More people than you think are listening. The battle is on – not just people vs. the HIV, but AIDS informed/AIDS concerned people vs. AIDS uninformed/AIDS ignorant people too. *It is about time!*

Lastly, I must comment on the last paragraph of the article, because it is very misleading. I doubt if any "leading authorities" (whoever they are) would bet their reputations and life savings on the statement that "the HIV cannot be transmitted casually." If any do, they either do not know that the HIV can *probably* be transmitted casually or they are lying for personal reasons. Also, to state the dispute now centers on whether or not immigrants (ill with contagious diseases) have enough money to pay for their own health care is another stupid statement. Nobody should be allowed to enter the USA with a contagious disease (especially one with no cure or vaccine), whether they have millions of dollars or none. The only issue is *keeping our HIV-free people HIV free – PERIOD!*

"Nurse has a right to know," Ann Landers, *San Francisco Chronicle* newspaper, May 22, 1991:

Dear Ann Landers: I am a registered nurse working in an intensive care unit. I love my job and I want to be a nurse for the rest of my life. This letter is a plea for my safety as well as that of my husband and family.

Yesterday, while handling blood and other secretions, I accidentally stuck myself with a dirty needle. I was being cautious and wearing rubber gloves. The hub of the needle stuck to the glove, then turned and stuck deeply into my index finger.

The next hour and a half was spent getting the doctor to come into the hospital and obtain consent from the patient's family to do an HIV test on him. This family consented. They could have refused. The results are confidential, which means they will not reveal them to me even if it is positive.

No consent is necessary for the hepatitis screen, for which I have already been immunized, nor is consent necessary for any other lab test. I do not want to hear about gay rights because AIDS is no longer a gay disease. It is a fatal infection spreading throughout the general population. I have no fear of caring for AIDS patients. I do feel I have a right to know if a patient I'm looking after has AIDS. Am I unreasonable? My supervisor thinks so. I'm plenty upset. – R.N. in Iowa

Dear Iowa R.N.: I have said this in the column before and I have no hesitation about saying it again. I believe health professionals who serve patients have the right to know if those patients have AIDS. Their instructions are to take precautions and assume every patient is infected, but in instances where the patient knows he is infected, he should have the decency to tell the nurses, doctors, dentists and others who take care of him. Since you had direct contact with this patient's bodily fluids, you certainly are entitled to know if he is HIV positive. *Los Angeles Times Syndicate and Creators Syndicate*

My Comment: The concerns and fears of this R.N. are typical of those of health care workers on the front lines of medicine – those that have direct patient contact. If things do not change and America continues to treat AIDS as a political disease, the public better expect one of the following scenarios:
1. The health care workers will be decimated by the HIV.
2. Health care workers by the droves will retire early from medicine or quit the profession.

Either scenario will result in a terrible shortage of health care workers. Health care workers are human beings, just like you. *They too, want to live and they too, have loved ones and friends, who want them around.* If anybody thinks differently, they are either too dumb to understand this or just plain crazy. I think Ms. Landers' response is the typical one, when this issue is addressed. A lot of well meaning sympathy and consoling, *but no action!* In this case, R.N. is just as concerned and just as frightened now as before Ms. Landers' advice. *Nothing has changed!* This R.N., and other health care workers like her, are screaming for help, *NOW!* They know an HIV infection means certain death, it is their business to know. They don't want to hear about their moral or ethical obligations, *they want to hear that someone is going to help them not get infected by the HIV in their workplace – it is as simple as that!*

Bottom line – America, protect you health care workers from the HIV *TODAY,* or don't expect very many of them *TOMORROW!*

CHAPTER IX

REFLECTIONS, COMMENTS AND OPINIONS

OF AN OBSTETRICIAN & GYNECOLOGIST

Again, I considered all travail, and every right work, that for this a man is envied of his neighbor. This is also vanity and vexation of spirit.
Ecclesiastes 4:4

PLAGUE

Plague – What is it?
Pestilence means any affliction or calamity, any deadly epidemic disease. **Epidemic** means spreading rapidly among many people in a community, as a disease. **Pandemic** means an epidemic over a large region. Put all these words together – Pestilence, Epidemic, and Pandemic – and you have PLAGUE.

AIDS qualifies as a plague, just as did the Black Death. Calling AIDS what it truly is – a plague – alerts most people immediately as to how contagious and lethal the disease really is. Even though the bubonic plagues happened many years ago, the many millions of people they killed are still remembered by people today. Today, we are at war with a world-wide disease – AIDS – which will ultimately kill more people than the Black Death (if not *all* people).

I think AIDS will prove far worse than the bubonic plague. The bubonic disease kills its victims within hours to days, while AIDS kills within months to years. Therefore, bubonic plague victims can infect only a limited number of other people since they die so rapidly. In contrast, AIDS-infected victims can live for many years, infecting countless other people. Finally, a cure is now available for the bubonic plague, but not for AIDS.

When all of the characteristics of the two diseases are compared, one can understand why I think AIDS is much more dangerous to mankind and why I think AIDS will ultimately prove to be the "Plague of Plagues." AIDS is the most formidable foe man has ever had to face. I only hope he has the wisdom and strength to ultimately prevail.

"AIDS POLICY"

I have repeatedly referred to the term "AIDS Policy." It simply means a plan of precautions to slow or prevent the spread of the AIDS disease amongst human beings. Unfortunately, there is no such adopted federal, universal "AIDS Policy" of minimum precautions which all states in the union must follow to help protect the AIDS-uninfected public. As a result, states now do nothing or very little with regards to AIDS precautions.

Self-interest and special interest groups are the most powerful and effective political forces in state policy. In California, for example, multiple such groups have been very successful in interfering or stopping the legislature from passing effective precautionary laws to help slow or prevent the spread of the AIDS virus.

As an example, the legislators were in early 1988 unable to pass legislation which would have made it a felony (instead of a misdemeanor) for an AIDS-infected person to purposely have sex with an unsuspecting, uninfected person. In addition, a California proposition which would have allowed physicians to test any patient for AIDS (among other things) was defeated by a two-to-one margin in November 1988. It's unfortunate that the real danger of the AIDS disease is unknown by most people, minimized by many, and misrepresented by others.

A federal, universal "AIDS Policy" is desperately needed for all states to follow. The sooner such an effective "AIDS Policy is formulated and adopted at the federal level, the better. The states must then follow and continually improve it as we learn more about the disease. The public will then become much better informed and able to protect itself from the AIDS virus. Such a policy will lessen the confusion, fear and misunderstanding that now exists.

As a practicing physician, it saddens and angers me to see so many people, especially many of my own colleagues, resisting such a plan – a plan which will surely save many lives. Because of their never-ending opposition of such a plan, many innocent people will unnecessarily die from AIDS. I urge everyone I can to write or call their U.S. representative and insist they support and help pass such a mandatory "AIDS Policy" as soon as possible.

HUMAN RIGHTS

The issue of human rights for AIDS-infected people arises again and again. The healthy public is continually bombarded with pleas to not "discriminate" against these unfortunate victims, because it's immoral, unjust, unfair, inhuman and heartless. Hogwash! The public has been purposely led to consider the AIDS disease as a political/human rights disease instead of what it really is – *a contagious, infectious, lethal, medical disease!*

Human or civil rights have nothing to do with the AIDS disease or the war against AIDS. While originally primarily a "homosexual" disease, AIDS is now infecting all of us: young or old, male or female, homosexual or heterosexual.

The healthy public must be protected at all costs. It's they who will work to keep the country going. It's they who will work to pay the taxes to keep America strong, and to take care of the sick, including the dying AIDS-infected people. If the public isn't protected from the AIDS virus, everyone will eventually become AIDS-infected. Then what? Who will run the country then? One doesn't have to be a genius to see the consequences if this is allowed to happen.

My position has always been to protect healthy people from disease – any disease. Here is where our medical and political leaders are letting the healthy public down: For their own personal and special-interest group reasons, they are jeopardizing the health of the nation by neglecting their responsibility to protect the ENTIRE PUBLIC.

As a result, the AIDS virus continues to relentlessly infect, spread and kill – faster and faster. Unless nations begin to wage an "all out war" against the AIDS virus, man will disappear from earth.

POGO, a popular comic strip character, states it best: "We have met the enemy, and the enemy is us." AIDS needs no help to do its dirty work; it is unfortunately doing quite nicely on its own! Let us all fight the AIDS virus now. Our very survival depends on it.

I treat sick people – human and civil rights have never had anything to do with my responsibility for making them well. Interference by government, business, and medical bureaucrats is the very reason private medicine and high quality medical care in America are being rapidly destroyed. Wake up, America!

GOVERNMENT

Is our government telling us the truth about AIDS? Yes and no. It tells us that there is an AIDS disease, it is caused by a virus, it is contagious, it does kill, and it is a problem. But government does not tell us how fast it is spreading, how it spreads, accurate statistics of how many people are HIV-infected, how to best protect ourselves, and what it is doing to our economy, nation, and world.

Why isn't it telling the whole truth? I believe it is because the truth is too frightening, too dismal, and too controversial. The government is trying to avert a panic which would, in turn, adversely affect the country's function and future. However, as time goes on, the magnitude of the AIDS problem will become evident to most people.

How soon? When? *When enough people – especially family members, relatives and friends – begin showing signs and symptoms of AIDS, and especially when they begin dying in larger and larger numbers from the disease.* Then, and only then, will the real war on AIDS begin and the first effective counter-attack by man be launched.

Most distressing are the leaders in government and medicine who are purposely misleading the public and obstructing any real progress in this fight with AIDS. Because of these "AIDS experts," our populace and nation have been lulled into a state of complacency and false sense of security. AIDS is still a mystery to all of us. By claiming they "know" the answers to this mystery, many innocent people will believe them and become good candidates for the AIDS infection.

We must not assume anything about AIDS if we are to survive. To defeat AIDS, we must find a cure. To find a cure, we must stay alive and healthy, work together, work hard, allocate the necessary resources, and continue unraveling the mystery of AIDS. By so doing, I believe a cure for AIDS will eventually be found.

ORGANIZED MEDICINE

Organized medicine's leaders are presently not representing the best overall interests of most physicians, the public, and the nation. When I started private practice in 1964, I joined the American Medical Association (national), California Medical Association (state), and Santa Clara County Medical Association (county), because I wanted to be a part of organized medicine. Back then, those organizations helped maintain and improve the high quality of medical care delivered by its members, and protected the rights of both patients and physicians.

Since then, however, these organizations have deteriorated to the point that now they are essentially ineffective and do not represent the majority of America's physicians. Why is this? Simple: Organized medicine's leaders have failed to keep the profession up with the march of time and are representing only part of their membership. As a result, the health needs of the nation are not being properly addressed or met.

More and more Americans are not receiving adequate medical care (37 million as of January 29, 1989 – *San Francisco Chronicle*) and the quality of medical care continues to deteriorate because of poor leadership, lack of funds, and bureaucratic interference. Many of organized medicine's leaders appear to be more concerned with medical politics and money than health care.

Other reasons for this breakdown include the wide diversity of societies and physicians in the organization (many of which have deferring and conflicting interests), its policy of backing down in most confrontations with its adversaries, and its own enormous cost of doing business.

Organized medicine's embarrassing silence on AIDS (what it is, how it spreads, how contagious and lethal it is, etc.) is the most current example of how organized medicine is being irresponsible and neglecting its obligation to protect the people.

When the AIDS plague accelerates its spread and our nation is consumed with suffering and death, organized medicine's failure to lead an effective attack will be one of the main reasons. This will indeed be a sad chapter in the history of medicine and of this nation.

HOSPITALS

Today, the hospital is one of the most likely places to come into contact with the AIDS virus. Hospitals definitely belong on the list of "high risk" places where the AIDS virus can be found.

Why is this? For many reasons, most of which aren't known by the general public. One main reason is the lack of a universal, federal "AIDS policy" which would include mandatory testing, isolation techniques, appropriate education, etc. Presently, hospitals around the country do what they want concerning the AIDS disease.

Some test all patients coming into the hospital for AIDS and others don't. Some have strict precautionary measures for protecting both their work force and AIDS-free patients, and others don't. Some don't "discriminate" against AIDS-infected patients (that is, they treat them exactly like the AIDS-free patients), and some do (they try to protect them from each other). Some have strict confidentiality rules to protect the identity of the AIDS-infected patients, and others don't.

Hospitals should be where sick people go to get well – not places where the treacherous AIDS virus is present and chances of accidentally becoming infected by it are increased. Therefore, the chance of becoming infected by the AIDS virus in a hospital increases or decreases depending on the effectiveness of each hospital's "AIDS policy." The better the policy, the less chance of

HIV infection and vice versa.

In many hospitals, the "AIDS policies" are inadequate or even non-existent. Considering the above, I thus recommend that everyone avoid hospitals unless absolutely necessary. In addition, patients should pick their hospitals very carefully, taking into consideration not only its quality of health care and cost, but the kind of "AIDS policy" it has. What a tragedy to go into the hospital to have a baby or hernia repair and come out with a 100% lethal disease like AIDS.

Everyone – health care workers and patients, alike – should insist that our hospitals recognize the dangers of AIDS and take appropriate precautions to protect us. Hospitals are run by people and people do respond to pressure; therefore, overwhelming demands from the public for AIDS protection will force effective "AIDS policy" implementation by all hospitals.

Insist on such protection. *Your life and your loved ones lives are too important to gamble.*

PHYSICIANS

Today, the majority of physicians do not understand or want to understand the AIDS virus or disease, because they fear it. They fear it more than the general public, because their training as physicians taught them what infectious and contagious organisms are and what damage they can do to the human body. Their profession exposes them to the realities of sickness and death from such organisms on a daily basis. When confronting a disease like AIDS (a mystery, contagious, incurable and usually lethal), their fear is multiplied many times.

Many physicians are so concerned about AIDS that they don't want anything to do with the AIDS virus or disease. They fear they may get infected and take it home and infect their family, relatives, and friends. They fear they will have to quit practicing medicine if they become infected, thus losing their livelihood. They fear losing their AIDS-free patients if they treat AIDS patients and the "word gets out."

Physicians fear being unknowingly exposed to the AIDS virus

when treating patients (who have not been HIV tested) in high risk areas such as the hospital emergency, surgical, and obstetrical departments. They fear they are unable to treat AIDS-infected patients properly because they know they haven't been trained how to treat them. Their fear is very real and increasing with time. Many physicians are now retiring early to avoid the problem, changing their practice habits to minimize their exposure to the AIDS virus, and refusing to treat AIDS-infected patients.

One of my obstetrician colleagues is so fearful of becoming infected that he actually made and wore a gown out of a plastic garbage bag to deliver one of his patient's baby. No "AIDS safe" gowns for the medical personnel were available. After this news circulated about the hospital, the embarrassed hospital officials immediately made water repellent gowns available throughout the hospital.

Also, a pediatrician came to me and asked me never to call him to take care of any baby from an AIDS-infected mother. He said he didn't want to take any chances of getting HIV infected, which would result in ruining his career and family life.

I see and hear these fears every day. Make no mistake about it, physicians on the front lines of medicine are the most exposed and most likely to be infected by the AIDS virus, and we know it! The same applies to the other health care workers who help treat the sick. The end result is apprehension, caution and fear.

Physicians who minimize the risk of AIDS are usually not the physicians on the front lines. Most of them make a practice not to frequent anyplace where the AIDS virus is likely to be present.

Recently, a professor at a very large teaching institution was talking to a group of physicians about how active his obstetrical-gynecologic service is. I asked him if his institution sees or treats any AIDS patients. He said, "Yes, more and more all the time, but I make sure I don't go near those people." Then I asked, "Well, who does treat them?" "The residents and interns, of course, who do you think!" he replied.

I was horrified.

Then, in a recent hospital Infectious Control Committee meeting, everything and anything was eagerly discussed – except AIDS.

When I broached the subject of AIDS, the physicians and other health care professionals didn't know anything about it and did not want to even discuss it. I asked if any AIDS cases were admitted to the hospital and how many HIV tests were done during the previous month. I was told that none of this information was gathered or available and the subject was dropped. I guess people believe if we ignore this disease, it will just go away.

Today, too many of such "AIDS-ignorant" physicians don't hesitate to manipulate the reins of leadership of our faltering medical organizations and, as a result and as expected, organized medicine is now far behind in the war against AIDS. Why is it that our own worst enemy is usually ourselves?

HIPPOCRATES OATH

The Hippocratic Oath is an oath physicians take and promise to abide by. This oath sets forth an ethical code for them to follow in the practice of medicine. Through time, this code has served the medical profession well, though some physicians seem to completely ignore it. Worse, this oath is often used by various people (politicians, journalists, medicrats, etc.) and entities (insurance companies, hospitals, and medical societies) to manipulate or try to force physicians into doing things they do not want to do, such as practice medicine according to the whims of insurance companies or government (not to the standards of good medical care), or treat patients they do not feel qualified to treat.

Because I work on the front lines of medicine, I see and understand the growing fear of AIDS that the public and knowledgeable physicians have. I understand why a physician is reluctant to care for a patient with AIDS, especially if he or she has little experience treating them. I understand his concern/fear of becoming HIV infected himself if he treats AIDS patients. I understand why he doesn't want an HIV-infected patient being mixed with his other AIDS-free patients. The physician knows that becoming AIDS infected means sure death.

I don't think any physician should be forced to treat any person or vice versa. The physician himself is the best judge whether he/

she can or should treat a patient, no one else. If a physician does not want to treat an AIDS-infected patient – whatever his reasons – I don't think anybody has the right to question or belittle him, or try to coerce him to do differently.

The decision of whether or not to treat AIDS patients is a very difficult and important decision for a physician to make. It is, most of all, a personal decision, and no one should inappropriately use the Hippocratic Oath or any other tactic to sway the physician's decision.

BUSINESS & SOCIETY

With the onslaught of the AIDS plague, like all plagues, will come tremendous changes in the way we do things, including changes in our economy and society. These changes will be economically advantageous for a few people, but disastrous for most.

Drug companies researching and selling potentially helpful AIDS drugs and stock brokers selling stocks of these companies will benefit. Others who will benefit economically include health facilities (hospitals, laboratories, X-ray facilities, etc.), health providers, and suppliers.

However, most will probably not benefit economically. Insurance companies, housing and apartment markets. and facilities serving the general public (restaurants, hotels, motels, theaters, etc.) will definitely suffer. The AIDS virus and disease will be responsible for changes in people's personal habits, attitudes, and behavior, thus changing our society. More fear, apprehension, greed, precaution, violence, anger, hostility, and confusion will be some of the major changes in our society's makeup. Civil rights, human rights, and discrimination of AIDS-infected people (so important to many people today) will become less important in the near future. Protection from the AIDS virus for the healthy people will be the primary concern by all governments and most people. AIDS then will be treated as the medical disease it truly is.

SAFE SEX

AIDS "experts" recommend "safe sex" as a means of preventing the spread of AIDS. They, as well as the public, all have their own definitions and interpretations of what "safe sex" is, most of which is different, vague and confusing. In reality, there are only five kinds of "safe sex":

(1) No sex at all – complete abstinence.
(2) Masturbation.
(3) "Test tube sex" – the AIDS-free male partner puts his semen (sperm) in a test tube and another person (usually a physician) injects part or all of it into his sexual female partner with a sterile needle and syringe apparatus. In this type of sex, there is absolutely no contact between the sexual partners, except for the passage of semen from one to the other.
(4) Sex between two "AIDS-free" participants.
(5) A huge condom over each of the sexual partners – what I call a "full body condom." I must admit that having sex in this manner would be uncomfortable, difficult, and no fun at all, but I can guarantee no contact between these two sexual partners.

Our AIDS "experts" fail to consider or admit that sex involves more than the passage of sperm from one to the other partner. Since I know that the sex act (intercourse) can involve other associated actions, such as biting scratching, kissing. and sucking, I doubt that a small piece of rubber (which, by the way, is occasionally penetrable by the AIDS virus) on the male's penis would constitute "safe sex" and keep an HIV-infected partner from infecting the other.

If anybody really believes the "AIDS experts" that "condomizing America" is the answer to control the spread of the AIDS disease, I'm afraid that person has his/her head in the sand. This is just another example of how our AIDS "experts" are deceiving the public, as well as themselves. into a false sense of security.

CASUAL CONTACT

"Casual contact," another euphemism our "AIDS experts" use to allay people's fear of AIDS. Again, the definition is vague and means different things to different people, but it does exactly what the government and AIDS "experts" want to prevent the public from facing the reality of AIDS. Since it has been shown the AIDS virus can survive up to 10-14 days in a dry or liquid state, it certainly appears possible (and/or probable) for one to become infected with the AIDS virus if he/she comes into contact with the virus in such a state under the right conditions.

For this reason, I feel it is *irresponsible* for anyone to state categorically and without proof that no one can or has ever been infected by the AIDS virus by simply coming into contact with it from a glass or plate. How do they know?

If such a mode of transmission is impossible, why did the Pasteur Institute burn all the clothes and bedding and thoroughly disinfect the hospital room of Rock Hudson, the movie star who was treated there for AIDS? Why is the disease spreading like a prairie fire around the world, infecting both high- and low-risk people, male and female? The only reason that makes sense to me is that the disease is spreading by many modes of transmission.

I believe the spread of the AIDS disease by casual contact is possible and probable – only time will tell. I know many physicians and other health care workers who are terrified of becoming infected by the AIDS virus from such contact.

In any event, AIDS is literally changing our country's health care system. Today, medical and dental schools are having trouble filling their quotas; physicians are altering their practices (less surgery, less obstetrics, etc.) to minimize their AIDS risk; some are retiring early or refusing to care for high risk patients.

The fear of AIDS has much to do with the present growing shortage of nurses, nursing aids, X-ray/laboratory technicians, and other such health care workers. These workers are concerned about "casual contact" with AIDS-infected people. When the AIDS disease reaches plague dimensions, everybody will be afraid of everything and everybody, especially "casual contact" with the AIDS virus.

AIDS CHILDREN

Recently, there has been much disturbance created by several AIDS-infected children going to school. The concern by many vociferous parents of the AIDS-free children was that their children might get infected with the AIDS virus if these AIDS-infected children were allowed to attend school.

Much ado was made by the parents, school officials, and media concerning this issue, but in each case, I feel the real issue was completely overlooked.

Their fear was that the AIDS-infected children would spread their disease to others; of course, a very real possibility. However, what was completely overlooked was that the AIDS-infected children were being placed into a very dangerous environment (school) when allowed to attend school. There they would be subjected to many other commonly found infectious organisms – organisms which could easily infect them and shorten their already shortened lives, due to their impaired immune systems.

This situation illustrates that most well-meaning people really don't know the first thing about protecting anybody – the AIDS-uninfected from the AIDS virus and the AIDS-infected from opportunistic organisms. Everyone seemed to dwell on the *rights* of the AIDS-infected children to attend school, rather than the safety of any of the children involved.

Unfortunately, AIDS-infected children are no better off than AIDS-infected adults – all are dying. They must all be treated as appropriately and as humanly as possible, but not at the expense of the AIDS-uninfected public. With proper vigilance and education, and great effort, I'm confident we can overcome this plague. Our survival as a nation depends on it.

WHAT HIV INFECTION MEANS

Accurate tests to detect exposure to AIDS are available through most medical laboratories and offices. The most commonly used test today is a screen for antibodies in blood to the HIV virus. Other tests include an antigen detection test now available for research use only and the Western blot test.

ANTIBODY TEST

The human body produces antibodies to fight infections. Within a few weeks or months after infection with HIV, the body forms antibodies in the blood which can be detected by a simple medical test. This test, called the enzyme-linked immunosorbent assay (ELISA), is widely available through hospitals, medical centers, and public health clinics.

A laboratory performing the test for HIV antibodies goes through several steps to ensure accuracy. If the initial result is positive, the test is repeated and confirmed by a different method, usually the Western blot test.

Because antibodies are not formed for a few weeks or months after the initial infection with HIV, there is a period of time when an infected individual may test negative for antibodies. An AIDS infected individual could, therefore, be tested immediately after exposure and produce a negative result.

Symptoms associated with the infection may appear shortly after infection or much later.

Your physician may recommend additional testing to ensure the correct results. The ELISA antibody test may be repeated in two to three months. In the future, an antigen test may also be given.

ANTIGEN TEST

While the ELISA test detects antibodies the patient forms against HIV, the antigen test, which is currently available for research use only, directly detects a portion of the actual virus.

This new test can detect the presence of HIV even before antibodies are produced. When commercially available, this test will permit doctors to detect the presence of infection much earlier than the antibody test.

Positive antigen test results are confirmed by a process that used HIV antibody to neutralize the AIDS virus if present. This process is used to verify antigen test results.

WESTERN BLOT TEST

The Western blot test is more technical and difficult to perform than the other methods. Results, used to confirm antibody test results, must be interpreted by a skilled technician to ensure accuracy.

The Western blot can take several days to perform and may require an additional sample or special handling. Because it is more labor-intensive and expensive than the other tests, the Western blot is not used for initial screening of blood samples.

What do the results mean?

When properly confirmed, a positive test result indicates that an individual is infected by HIV. Infected individuals can transmit it to others through blood or sexual contact. For this reason, it is important for those providing testing to offer counseling, as well.

While HIV antibody test results do not predict which infected individuals have AIDS or may develop AIDS in the future, the antigen test, when available, may be able to do so. Individuals infected with HIV may remain outwardly healthy for a long period before developing an illness related to the HIV infection.

Because it generally takes years for AIDS to develop in infected individuals, today it is difficult to determine exactly what proportion of those infected will ultimated develop AIDS. Current estimated indicate 30 to 50 percent will develop AIDS, but some scientists now believe that an even higher percentage (up to 100%) of those infected will eventually die of AIDS-related complications.

Where can a person get tested?

Testing is available in public health clinics, hospitals, and doctors' offices. In addition, most city and state health departments have set up programs to provide AIDS information and counseling. Your city, county, or state medical society can often provide additional information about testing.

Are results confidential?

Test results may be either confidential or anonymous, depending on the particular clinic or office. In a confidential test, the patient's name and test results are known only to the physician and immediate staff. It becomes part of the patient's private medical file.

Tests performed by many public clinics are anonymous – they do not keep records by name. Each patient is assigned a number when blood is taken. Patients must return to the clinic in person and provide the assigned number to receive their test results.

In most states, results are released only to the patient. In a few others, positive results must be reported to the state health department. Ask your doctor or clinic how results will be recorded and reported.

What if my test is positive?

Has anyone ever stopped to really consider what an HIV-positive test really means for the individual tested? *It means the person testing "HIV positive" has the AIDS disease.* It's amazing that the consequences of such a test haven't really been openly or honestly addressed.

It literally means a complete change of lifestyle, both for the AIDS-infected person and his family. The HIV-infected person's lifespan is immediately shortened and his association with his fellow men immediately and adversely affected. Since such an HIV-infected person can infect others, at any time during the rest of his life, he/she must constantly be on guard not to do so.

At the present time, the AIDS-infected person starts dying from the moment he/she becomes AIDS-infected. Many people become severely depressed and even suicidal. For these reasons, most people are reluctant to be tested and are content to rationalize the threats of the AIDS problem.

INFORMED CONSENT

One of the most important agreements in medicine is the "informed consent." This is a legally enforced written agreement between a patient and the health care providers. If properly executed, it means the patient fully understands the what, how, when, and where of a medical procedure to be performed.

It also means all the people signing the consent fully understand the treatment procedure, as well as all of its risks and advantages. Through the years, this contract has become more and more important. Now it is one of the most important legal documents in medicine. It rightfully protects both parties of the contract. If improperly done, it could lead to disastrous results for the health providers and/or patient.

The above is true – except in the case of the AIDS disease. Depending on which state one is in, this informed consent protection is primarily only for the benefit of the AIDS-infected patient. Since there is no universal federal "AIDS policy," each state does what it wants. Here in California, the rights of the AIDS-infected patients take precedent over those of the health care providers.

Because of powerful, vocal, self-interest and special interest groups, vote-seeking California politicians and irresponsible medical leaders, AIDS is treated more as a political disease instead of what it really is – *a deadly contagious medical disease*. Physicians have to obtain a patient's informed consent to order an HIV test or to tell anybody, including relatives, the results. The HIV test report can't even be put in the patient's chart; it must be placed in a sealed envelope marked "confidential" and only opened if the patient agrees in writing. Also, this sealed envelope must not be kept in the patient's chart.

Once a physician diagnoses a patient as AIDS-infected, he cannot stop treatment unless he transfers the patient to another physician or health facility, both of which have to agree in writing. Also, the physician can tell no one his patient is infected with the AIDS virus; if he does, he is breaking the law.

When an AIDS-infected patient is in the hospital, no one can be told about his ailment because, if disclosed, it would violate his civil rights. In late 1988, the California Legislature passed legislation to help alleviate some of the above "red tape." I fear it will be too little too late.

Because of these misguided policies, many innocent people have been unnecessarily exposed to the AIDS virus. Patients going to doctors' or dentists' offices, relatives of AIDS-infected patients, and health care providers in hospitals are just a few.

It is these kind of ridiculous and irresponsible rules and regulations which interfere with the prevention, as well as the proper diagnosis and treatment, of the AIDS disease. An effective, federal, universal "AIDS policy" is desperately needed, which will force all states to take the same effective, appropriate action, both for treatment and prevention of the AIDS disease.

CHAPTER X
RADIO TALK SHOW QUESTIONS/COMMENTS

*A soft answer turneth away wrath; but a harsh word stirs anger.
The tongue of the wise dispenses knowledge,
but the mouth of fools poureth out folly .*
Proverbs 15:1-2

Since mid 1990, I have been a guest on many radio talk shows through out America. Of course the topic of all these shows was the AIDS disease and my goal for being there was to inform and educate the general public about both the HIV and AIDS. In doing these shows, I came to some very important conclusions. The majority of the public:

1. Is misinformed, dysinformed or uninformed about the HIV and AIDS disease.
2. Is concerned and fearful of the HIV and the AIDS disease.
3. Is not comfortable with the established media's reporting of the AIDS disease and AIDS plague.
4. Is concerned why the politicians (they elect to represent them at all levels of government) fail to recognize/treat AIDS as a lethal contagious medical disease, fail to propose and pass laws that can reasonably protect people from the AIDS virus and fail to realize that the AIDS virus threatens the very survival of mankind.
5. Is resentful of being "kept in the dark" about the AIDS plague.
6. Wants to know more than only the establishment's explanations about the HIV and AIDS disease (that is the other side of the AIDS coin) *and the sooner the better.*
7. Wants to practice effective precautions against the AIDS virus, if they know what they are.

8. Wants our government and medical organizations to quit playing politics with the AIDS disease, to quit favoring special interest groups and to face the fact *now,* that the AIDS plague is worsening every day and that serious efforts to control and eradicate it must begin immediately.

Now let me proceed to tell you some of the more interesting questions people have asked me on these radio talk shows, as well as my comments. There is much repetition and duplication of material from the book in my comments, because much of the book's information was completely new to the media listeners and had to be presented. However, I feel this is a plus for the reader because repeating much of the book's material serves as a good review of the more important information. The more often the book's information is reviewed, the better the reader should understand the HIV, the AIDS disease and the socio/economic/political problems of AIDS.

Is AIDS a homosexual disease?

Comment: No. AIDS is a disease of all people – *all people.* The AIDS virus, (which only attacks the human species) infects anybody, anytime and anyplace – man, woman, or child. No continent, subcontinent or island chain on this planet has escaped the wrath of AIDS. The media has not adequately informed the American public what AIDS has done and is doing worldwide (hundreds of millions of people infected and dying – men, women, children, babies and elderly); therefore, many Americans now believe AIDS is primarily a problem in the U.S. and primarily a venereal disease of homosexual people. Nothing could be further from the truth. Here in America, homosexuals (as well as other high risk people like drug addicts, prostitutes, and bisexuals) are only the first group of people to have the unfortunate pleasure of being the AIDS virus' first victims. Now, *all* Americans (Homosexuals and Heterosexuals alike) are at risk for the AIDS infection; and as time goes on, and the AIDS virus becomes more aggressive and more virulent, this risk will surely increase *for everybody.*

Can I get Aids from a swimming pool?

Comment: Possible, and I think probable. As already stated, the AIDS virus (HIV) can stay alive up to 14 days in a dry state, and *even longer in liquids*. It has been shown, that under the right circumstances, the AIDS virus can be activated and infectious in these two states; therefore, we must conclude infection from these two states is possible and probable. So far, there has been no known reported cases of AIDS contracted from any swimming pool. More research has to be done on such potential infection modes of transmission before we know the true answers. However, until such answer are known, it is better for one to be cautious than foolhardy – because infection by the AIDS virus is certain death. The water in swimming pools is usually treated with chemicals and often contaminated with dirt, bugs, various human body fluids (saliva, sputum, sweat, urine, etc.) and who knows what else: therefore, swimmers can come in contact with such contaminates (if present) and thus expose themselves to various infectious organisms, including the AIDS virus. I don't recommend swimming in any pool (public or private) which is dirty, where the AIDS status of the swimmers is unknown and where the possibility of coming in contact with the AIDS virus exists. Swimming in swimming pools, where only known AIDS-free people swim, is certainly safe from the AIDS virus. Realistically, it isn't possible to know the AIDS-status of people swimming in swimming pools; *but* your chances of swimming in an AIDS-free pool are better when you swim in a private pool (where you know who the swimmers are) than in a public pool (where you don't know any of the swimmers). In short, it is always more prudent to be cautious than sorry; therefore, I recommend people use good common sense when swimming. *Don't swim in just any pool, only in pools which you think are clean and AIDS-free.*

Should physicians (or other health care workers) who are AIDS-infected treat AIDS-free people?

Comment: There is no simple yes or no answer to this question because there are two sides to it, like a double edged sword. I have always been of the opinion that anybody testing positive for the AIDS virus (HIV) has the AIDS disease and is thus, contagious to other people. This being the case, not only can AIDS-infected health care workers infect AIDS-free patients, but AIDS-infected patients can infect AIDS-free health care workers. Recently, the media has reported cases where each has infected the other. These reports have confirmed my fears; thus I now believe AIDS-infected health care workers should not treat/care for AIDS-free patients. In all fairness, however, health care workers should have the right to choose, whether they want to treat/care for AIDS-infected patients or not. Our constitution guarantees this right for everybody. Remember, there is no room for error with AIDS – infection by the AIDS virus is literally *a death sentence*. In the near future, I see AIDS-infected people being treated in AIDS-only hospitals, hospices and clinics – operated by AIDS-infected and volunteer health professionals. Medical care for both the health care professionals and patients infected by the AIDS virus will be separate from that of the AIDS-free public, for two reasons. One is to protect the AIDS-free patients from the AIDS virus and the other is to provide better medical care for the AIDS-infected patients. Aids patients require specialized medical care because their disease is very complicated and dangerous; thus, I feel only AIDS specialists in AIDS specialized facilities should treat these patients. Harsh and unfair as this may seem, it is but one of the many unpleasant tactics which must eventually be done, in hope of controlling the spread of this killer plague.

Can someone get AIDS from a public drinking fountain?

Comment: Possible, and I believe probable, under the right circumstances. When possible, don't drink water from any public drinking fountain, wait until you find known clean water. If you cannot wait and you must drink, follow the following precautions:
1. Make sure the drinking fountain is clean; if it doesn't look clean, don't drink from it.
2. Make sure the water flow or stream is well above the drink-

ing fountain nozzle or spigot.
3. Let the water run for awhile, so the water stream can clean the drinking fountain spigot; thus insuring cleaner water to drink.
4. When drinking the water, make sure your mouth does not touch any part of the fountain spigot. Only water from the water stream should touch your lips and mouth.

Until it is 100% proven, that a person cannot get AIDS from a public drinking fountain, I would follow the above precautions.

Don't you think your message will make people panic, causing more harm than good?

Comment: No. My job as a physician is to make sick people well and keep well people well. My main tool for doing this is to tell my patients the truth, because if they know what they and I are both dealing with, we can do my job better. Unfortunately, the truth is not always pleasant and often difficult to accept. Everyday I tell patients many things, most of which usually makes them feel better or happy. Sometimes, however, my news is bad and makes them feel sad or depressed or helpless or unlucky or desperate, etc. Yes, even panicky sometimes. Thru experience, however, I have learned it is better to tell patients what they are dealing with, than not. I am now trying to tell people the truth about AIDS, at least what I believe to be the truth. I have complete faith in the American people to act accordingly, once they are told the truth about the dangers of AIDS they face. They will roll up their sleeves and battle the AIDS plague head on. It is this instinct of survival, to face danger and fight in the American people, which has made and kept this country free and strong. *It is not panic of people from truth I fear, it is the people's complacency and ignorance of AIDS from lack of truth which frightens me.*

Should AIDS-infected people feel discriminated against or that their civil rights are being violated if other people avoid them?

Comment: No, not at all. It is man's nature and human behavior to avoid something he doesn't understand or fears. Since AIDS is a disease with no known cure or vaccine and which is very little understood, it is only natural for people to fear it. Avoiding AIDS-infected people has nothing to do with anything (civil rights, discrimination, legal rights, etc.) *except fear*. People fear AIDS for the same reason they feared the Black Death in the past, *because it can kill them*. Since no one knows all the ways AIDS spreads or kills and since the AIDS virus is infecting more and more people everyday, more and more people will avoid AIDS-infected people – not because they are inhumane, or uncaring or bigots, etc., but because they are afraid. Whether this is right or wrong is academic, *it is reality*. To try to legislate fear away, is like trying to empty the oceans with a teaspoon.

What does it mean when a person tests positive for the human immuno deficiency virus (HIV)?

Comment: *It means that person has AIDS*. It means that person is a carrier and is contagious to others for the AIDS virus (HIV). It unfortunately means that person's life will be shortened and his lifestyle changed forever. For some strange reason (strange?), the established media continues to perpetrate the myth that a person who is HIV positive does not mean he/she has AIDS – it only means that he/she will probably get it sometime in the future. This is a terrible deception and a great injustice to the American people. What the media should do is tell the people the truth, in plain simple English –

1. AIDS has three stages – the asymptomatic first stage, the second "ARC" stage (when symptoms of AIDS begin to show themselves) and the third terminal stage (when the victims have 6-18 months to live).
2. The HIV test is positive in all three stages of the AIDS disease.
3. *A person who tests positive for HIV (the AIDS virus) has AIDS!*
4. A person who tests HIV positive and who is in any of the

three stages of AIDS is contagious and classified as a carrier of the HIV. He/she can infect other people at anytime and anyplace, depending on the circumstances.
5. A person who tests HIV positive has an incurable fatal, contagious disease and *is a sick* person. He/she is not like other people. The sooner he/she knows and understands this, the better for them and the people around them.

Is a person with the AIDS disease like anybody else?

Comment: *Absolutely not.* A person with AIDS has a fatal, contagious, incurable disease. He/she is a sick person and is a threat to himself/herself as well as to others. It really upsets me that the person with AIDS thinks (until he is obviously AIDS-sick) he/she is like everybody else. Why not, he/she is constantly being told this by special interests groups, the government, the legal profession, and yes – even the medical profession. It is hard for me as a physician to sit back and see sick people misled into believing their illness won't/shouldn't interfere with their lifestyles. Nothing could be farther from the truth for AIDS-infected people. Not only are these people a threat to others, but to themselves – *especially if they believe they are not sick, "only HIV positive."* AIDS-infected people must be made to realize they are sick, real sick – *no matter what stage of the disease they are in.* Their immune systems are methodically being destroyed by the AIDS virus; thus, their ability to fight off opportunistic disease and infections steadily decreases as times goes on. Therefore, these people must protect themselves at all times from infectious organisms, which may shorten their already shortened lives. It is insane for AIDS-infected people to put themselves in environments, where they expose themselves to opportunistic diseases/infections – such as crowded theaters, coliseums, restaurants, schools, colleges etc. The point here is people that are healthy or ill with other diseases can and do carry literally hundreds of infectious organisms, many of which are a danger to AIDS-infected people. *Physicians must speak out and warn the AIDS-infected – "protect others from the AIDS virus and yourselves from opportunistic disease/organisms.* You are sick people but with proper treatment and counseling, you can live constructive and safer lives."

Are AIDS-free patients mixed with AIDS-infected in hospitals?

Comment: Yes they are, at least in California they are. I am vehemently opposed to this practice. We health professionals are told to treat every patient in the hospital as if they have AIDS and to use "universal precautions," that is glasses, gloves, caps and gowns. This protocol is to decrease the chance of accidental infection by the AIDS virus from hospital patients. However, there is *no such protocol, as superficial as it is, for protecting the patients in the hospital from the AIDS virus.* Since both the health professionals and patients are not routinely tested for the AIDS virus, no one knows who has or who has not AIDS. Patients are all mixed together with no regard to whether they have AIDS or not. In fact, AIDS-free patients are mixed with AIDS-infected patients without their knowledge or permission. This is pure insanity. Here we have a lethal contagious disease, just waiting for the opportunity to claim another victim, and we in medicine just can't seem to wait to accommodate it. The sooner both AIDS-infected health care workers and patients in hospitals are diagnosed and separated from the others, the more common sense it makes. What a travesty if a person goes into the hospital to have a tonsillectomy or a baby and comes out with AIDS – and all because both the legal and medical professions give the AIDS-infected victims and the AIDS virus "civil rights."

Do you think the AIDS-infected and AIDS-free patients should share the same hospital room?

Comment: No. Why? Because I feel the AIDS free-patients can accidently get infected by the AIDS virus from their AIDS-infected roommates. How is this? If the AIDS virus can somehow reach the blood stream of the AIDS-free patient, whether from a dry or liquid state, infection is possible. When patients share a hospital room, they also share the room air and furnishings, as well as a bathroom; therefore, they in one way or another, do usually come in contact with each others body fluids – aerosols (coughs and sneezes), blood (rugs, floors, bathrooms), saliva or sputum (bathrooms), urine or feces (bathrooms) etc. Presently when patients in hospitals have contagious or infectious diseases, they are isolated from other patients; and for good reason – *to protect the other patients from these conditions.* To treat AIDS any differently is wrong and, I think, criminal. I believe all patients entering the hospital should be tested for AIDS and those testing positive, should be separated from the AIDS-free patients. The quicker we treat AIDS as the lethal, contagious disease it is, the more people will ultimately survive.

How safe is U.S. bank blood and when should it be used?

Comment: This question is one of the most frequent, as well as important, questions I am asked on radio talk shows. Blood banks began testing blood for AIDS in 1985. Whenever any antibodies against the AIDS virus are found in any unit of blood, that blood is not used. The problem is that occasionally, some blood test negative for AIDS when it really should test positive (called a false negative test), and some blood test negative because the antibodies against the AIDS virus are not yet developed in the blood (indicating AIDS contamination). When people become infected by the AIDS virus, they "seroconvert" and test positive for AIDS – 90+% of the time in three months and over 95+% of the time in six months. However a few people don't test positive for AIDS for *three years and and even longer*. Unfortunately, when and if such AIDS-contaminated blood is accidently used for transfusions, the recipients can and do get AIDS. Today the risk of getting AIDS from a single unit of blood is one in 40,000; however, the average patient needing blood receives 5.4 units of blood. This increases this patient's risk to one in 7,400 (*Insight* magazine, August 20, 1990). It is reported that 1,000 people get AIDS (and 16,000 people get one of five different strains of hepatitis) from blood transfusions per year. (*Omni* magazine, Sept. 90). Because of this risk of AIDS

(as well as hepatitis) from blood transfusions, I recommend the following:
1. If you are going to have elective surgery, donate your own blood for your own use in advance. This can easily be done, and because it is your own blood, it is 100% safe for you. This blood is called autologous blood and if it is not used, it can be frozen up to 10 years for your future. The cost for this service today is $10/unit of blood /month.
2. If #1 is not possible, have a few of your close friends or relatives (who you feel are AIDS-free and healthy) donate their blood in advance for your use.
3. If #1 and #2 are not possible, then use blood from the blood banks, if a blood transfusion is necessary.

Today physicians use blood transfusions very sparingly, because of the AIDS and hepatitis risks. Blood transfusions are life saving, so the risk of blood transfusions must certainly be accepted if blood is needed. The main thing for you, the reader, is to remember the above risks and recommendations of blood transfusions and to accept a blood transfusion only when it is absolutely necessary.

Can I get AIDS by using a public toilet ?

Comment: Interesting and increasingly worrisome question. The transmission of the AIDS infection has to do with the contact of AIDS virus (HIV) contaminated bodily fluids of human beings. Everybody, in one way or another, often comes in contact with other people's bodily fluids (dry or wet) when using a toilet – whether they want to or not, or wether they think they do or not. The dirtier the toilet, the more chance of such contact. Since the AIDS virus is found in the bodily fluids of a person who has AIDS, it is possible for people using toilets to come in contact with the virus, if an AIDS-infected person used the toilet beforehand. Remember the AIDS virus can be activated from a dry or liquid state, under the right conditions; therefore, it is theoretically possible, under the right conditions, for a person to get AIDS-infected from using an AIDS-contaminated toilet. No cases, of a person getting AIDS-infected from a toilet, have been reported – *so far!* A recent survey has shown that hospital toilets are the cleanest and gas station toilets are the dirtiest, with the rest somewhere in between. When using a public restroom be very careful, because you don't know if the AIDS virus is around or not. Also, *many* people using public restrooms *do not wash their hands,* before or after using the toilet. This certainly increases the possibility of the AIDS virus being present. In any event, I recommend the following precautions when using a public restrooms:

1. Wash your hands before using the toilet.
2. With a paper towel, flush the toilet, and step way back, well away from the aerosol of the toilet flush.
3. Wipe off the toilet seat and handle with a paper towel.
4. Put a disposable paper cover or toilet paper on the toilet seat, before using the toilet.
5. When finished, flush the toilet with a paper towel and then wash your hands again; but this time, turn the faucet water off with a paper towel on the faucet handle – *because the person before you may not have washed their hands.*
6. If you cannot leave the restroom through an open doorway or by pushing the door open with your foot (again, the person before you may have opened the door with unwashed hands), grab the door handle with a paper towel and open it. Then hold the door open with your foot, throw the used paper towel in the waste basket and then leave through the open doorway.

I know the above is involved, requires a lot of paper and is maybe unnecessary; but until it is 100% proven that people cannot get AIDS-infected in restrooms, I recommend these precautions. There is no room for error with this disease.

Also, I highly recommend the local health departments make it mandatory for all public restrooms to be "super clean," and that they monitor and strictly enforce this requirement.

Is it true that it is very difficult to get infected by the AIDS Virus?

Comment: Anybody who believes this myth probably believes in the tooth fairy as well and is just begging to be the HIV's next victim. It is beyond me why and how some knowledgeable people can honestly make such irresponsible, unsubstantiated statements. The burden of proof, that it is difficult to get infected by the AIDS virus (HIV), is on the people who make such statements, *not on you or me*. Until they have this proof, *which I know they usually do not*, one should always protect themselves as much as possible from the AIDS Virus. Common sense tells us this statement cannot possibly be true, not when the AIDS virus has already infected millions of people worldwide and now threatens the very survival of the human species itself. Because the AIDS virus has already infected so many people so fast, common sense again tells us the virus must be easily spread from person to person by many ways. Until we prove and know these ways, don't assume anything about the AIDS virus. It is better to be careful and cautious with this disease than complacent or careless, because there is no room for error – infection by the HIV means certain death. Respect the HIV at all times and remember, it is a mutating killer virus, without cure or vaccine, and can infect you anytime in any place – *if you give it the chance.*

Why aren't the health professionals, as a group, more concerned about the AIDS plague?

> **Comment:** *They are,* but unfortunately, not openly.
> They are concerned about:
> (1) The lack of available, unbiased, truthful AIDS information and education, both for the public and themselves.
> (2) The lack of available AIDS-protective gear for them in their work place (hospitals, offices etc.).
> (3) The fact that the nation is treating AIDS as a political, venereal disease with "civil rights", instead of what it really is – a lethal, fatal, contagious medical disease of plague proportions.
> (4) The "authorities" are forcing them to fight the AIDS plague with their hands handcuffed-by legal, coercive, and punitive methods.
> (5) The "authorities" are more concerned about the health care

of the AIDS – infected people and the protection of AIDS – free patients from the AIDS virus than they are about the legal rights and health of the care workers.

(6) The possibility of becoming infected themselves by the AIDS virus, which would shorten and change their lives forever.

Because of these concerns and fears, many health professionals are retiring early, quitting medicine or changing their practice modes, so they don't come in contact with patients. If some of our health professionals (and I include nurses, laboratory and x-ray technicians in this group) would have the courage to speak out and tell the American people the truth about the present inadequate and dangerous AIDS situation, many of their concerns/fears would be addressed and corrected. Why? Because the AIDS-informed American people would then become outraged and demand it! It is high time we health professionals put our fears of political or "special interest group" repercussions aside and speak out – *the American people are desperate for someone to tell them the truth about the AIDS plague.*

Do you think AIDS is a venereal disease?

Comment: No. An organism that causes a venereal disease (syphilis, gonorrhea, various types of vaginal infections, etc.) must adhere to some basic criteria. These are:

(1) It attacks primarily the reproductive tracts of human beings.
(2) It breeds primarily in the reproductive tracts of the human beings.
(3) It is found in the highest concentrations (numbers) in the reproductive tracts of human beings.
(4) It spreads from human being to human being primarily by sexual contact between human beings.
(5) It can live outside the human body for only minutes to hours.

The AIDS virus adheres to none of these basic criteria. *It has its own set of criteria, which are far more numerous, broad and deadly.* In short, the HIV attacks and infects the entire human body by many ways, until its host succumbs. A venereal disease – *AIDS is not!!!* A Lethal, 100% fatal, Contagious disease – *AIDS is!!!*

What are the human body fluids and in which ones are the AIDS virus found?

Comment: The body fluids are:
(1) Blood (blood cell and liquid)
(2) Serum (liquid part of blood)
(3) Saliva
(4) Sputum
(5) Breast milk
(6) Vaginal secretions
(7) Sperm (semen)
(8) Spinal fluid (the fluid bathing the brain and spinal cord)
(9) Amniotic fluid (the fluid bathing the fetus in the womb of a pregnant woman)
(10) Urine
(11) Sweat
(12) Tears

When the HIV invades and infects the human body, it infects the entire human body – *including all the bodily fluids.* Therefore, the AIDS virus is found in all bodily fluids, *but not in the same concentration or numbers per unit value.* The highest concentration of HIV per unit value is in blood and the least in tears and sweat. The real question now is "are all these bodily fluids infectious, since they are AIDS contaminated?" I think the best way to answer this question is by this quote: "Anyone who tells you categorically that AIDS is not contracted by saliva is not telling you the truth. AIDS may, in fact, be transmissible by tears, saliva, bodily fluids, and mosquito bites" – Dr. William Haseltine, prominent Harvard AIDS researcher (*New Dimensions* magazine, April 1990)The important point to remember is if a person comes in contact with an AIDS (HIV)-contaminated bodily fluid, that person could get infected by the AIDS virus. *It is the bodily fluids of people which are the vectors for the virus*, and which carry the HIV from person to person. Therefore, it is the AIDS-contaminated bodily fluids of AIDS-infected people which we must protect AIDS-free people from, if we are to control the spread of the AIDS disease.

What are the recommendations of the CDC (Center for Disease Control) for the control of the spread of AIDS?

Comment: The CDC is unfortunately using a double standard for their recommendations – one set is for the health care providers and the other is for the general public. The nation's health care providers are told to consider everybody coming to hospitals as if they all have AIDS. Also, they are told to use "Universal Precautions" (masks, gloves, gowns, and goggles) if any patients test HIV positive, (which means, of course, they have AIDS). These "universal precautions" are to hopefully protect the health care workers from any contact with AIDS-contaminated bodily fluids. Meanwhile, the general public is told (for their protection from the AIDS virus) to practice "safe sex," which is to either abstain from sexual relations or wear a condom, when having sex with any sexual partner. So, one group of people (health care workers), the CDC recommends protection from all bodily fluids and for the other group (the general public), the CDC recommends protection from only semen and/or vaginal secretions of the many bodily fluids. *What insane, discriminatory, bad, ridiculous recommendations these are*. When a person is AIDS-infected, *all of his/her bodily fluids contain the AIDS virus;* therefore, AIDS-free people must protect themselves from all AIDS-contaminated bodily fluids, to avoid any chance of becoming infected by the AIDS virus. I think this double standard of the CDC is deplorable and must be stopped immediately. The CDC must equally protect all the people from the AIDS virus, *immediately*. This policy is nondiscriminatory and gives everybody the same chance to protect themselves and survive the AIDS plague.

How do you think the AIDS disease spreads from person to person?

Comment: No one knows all the ways the AIDS virus spreads, only some of the ways. If we knew all the ways of HIV transmission, we would have a much better chance of containing the AIDS plague. Unfortunately, our government is presently more concerned about people's human/civil rights with AIDS than *the loss of human lives* from AIDS.

I think the AIDS virus is spread by more than one way – in fact, by many ways. The most important thing to remember is when a person is AIDS-infected, his/her whole body in infected – *including all their bodily fluids.* These bodily fluids contain the AIDS virus and if any person is contaminated by any of these fluids, an AIDS infection is possible and probable. However, some AIDS-contaminated bodily fluids contain many more AIDS viruses per unit value than others and are thus more infectious – blood being the most virus laden and sweat/urine being the least, with the rest somewhere in between. This being a truism, the possibility of an AIDS-infection is thus far greater if a person comes in contact with AIDS-contaminated blood than with AIDS contaminated urine or sweat.

Now, back to the question. I now believe there are three main categories *(most effective, effective, and controversial ways)* from which the AIDS virus spreads from person to person. These are:

Most Effective Ways (coming in contact with AIDS-contaminated blood)

(a) Contaminated needles
(b) Contaminated blood transfusions
(c) Contaminated blood splashed in eyes, mouth, skin (broken or intact)
(d) Etc.

Effective Ways (coming in contact with AIDS-contaminated saliva, sputum, breast milk, semen, vaginal secretions)

(a) French kissing (saliva, sputum, blood)
(b) Oral sex (saliva, sputum, semen, vaginal secretions, and even blood)
(c) Sexual intercourse (semen, vaginal secretions, sweat, saliva, sputum, blood)
(d) Breast feeding (breast milk)
(e) Aerosols from coughing, sneezing, high speed orthopedic/dental drills, spitting (saliva, sputum, blood)
(f) Etc.

Controversial Ways (Possible/probable – coming in contact with any AIDS-contaminated bodily fluid – *any bodily fluid*)

(a) Blood sucking insects – mosquitos, ticks, bedbugs, etc. (blood)
(b) Social kissing (saliva, blood)
(c) Casual contact (dry AIDS virus on plates, glasses, eating utensils, handshakes, furniture, fomites, etc.)
(d) Contact sports – football, sports, wrestling, etc. (blood, sweat, sputum, saliva)
(e) Etc.

Much research has yet to be done before we know if some or all of the transmission ways or modes mentioned above are ways the vicious AIDS virus spreads from person to person. As the AIDS virus infects more and more people, it will probably become more virulent and finally reach the critical mass stage, at which point it will increase its modes of spreading/transmission and then proceed to infect far more people than it did or now does. If or when that time comes, and I hope it never does, the AIDS plague will literally explode – infecting and killing unbelievable numbers of people worldwide. Lastly, and most important, the AIDS virus' ability to spread, infect, and kill people is now grossly underestimated in America. No matter how the HIV spreads, this arrogant, foundless assumption has lulled most Americans into a false sense of security, self denial and complacency – attitudes which will greatly assist the AIDS virus in its war with man.

Will "safe sex" protect people from the HIV infection (AIDS)?

Comment: No, and for many reasons. First of all, the term "safe sex" is a ridiculous term. If ten people were asked to define it, there would be ten different definitions. What the CDC (Center for Disease Control) and most "AIDS experts" mean by "safe sex" is either abstinence from sex or partners having vaginal or anal intercourse with the male sex organ (penis) covered with a condom. Secondly, in the act of love making, there is contact with more bodily fluids than just semen and/or vaginal secretions. To be specific, they are saliva, sputum, sweat, semen, vaginal secretions, and even blood. It is ridiculous to assume that partners making love (wearing condoms and who are super careful) do not come in contact with any of each others bodily fluids (mentioned above). *What nonsense!* In my opinion, if the sex partners are that careful and that successful in not coming in contact with any of each others bodily fluids when making love, then they may as well quit wasting their time and forget the whole process. Thirdly, the AIDS virus (HIV) is very small (.1 micron to be specific) – a fact which greatly assists the virus' ability to spread. To give you some idea of how small the HIV is, it is 1 million (1,000,000) times smaller than the infectious organism (a parasite) that causes malaria. If a condom is placed under an electron microscope, one would see the pores (the spaces between the weave of the condom's rubber threads) measure 1.5 microns in diameter; therefore, this means the much smaller AIDS virus can and does pass thru a condom at will – like water thru a colander. This being a truism, one can easily understand why condom use offers no help in protecting either partner from the AIDS virus during love making. However, the CDC and persons claiming to be "AIDS experts" still insist that condom use is a protection against the AIDS virus and continue to encourage condom use. *This advice is wrong and dangerous.* It fosters a false sense of security and leads some people to inappropriate action and behavior, which is sometimes dangerous to themselves and even to others. Lastly, and most important, we must all remember *there is no such thing as AIDS "safe sex"* (unless it is between two people who are HIV free or who are HIV positive) *and the HIV infects by many ways.* As far as I'm concerned however, there is no such thing as "safe sex" – it is a ridiculous term. People who believe and practice "safe sex" are only fooling themselves – certainly not the AIDS virus, me and now, *you!*

What does the CDC consider "unsafe sex?"

Comment: For many years, the CDC has said sex between two partners without condom use is unsafe sex. Recently, the CDC has been forced to add "French kissing" and "oral sex" to its list of "unsafe sex." As we learn more about the AIDS virus and its modes of transmission, I feel this list will grow many times over. In the near future, I foresee people having to show proof they are HIV free before they do many things, especially when indulging in any sexual activity with each other.

Do you think pregnant women should be tested for AIDS?

Comment: I think *all* pregnant women should be tested for HIV every three months of their pregnancy. The AIDS plague will prove to be the worst medical disaster this country has ever had, especially in my specialty of medicine – obstetrics. In the 1980s, the HIV decimated the homosexual community and other such high risk groups, but the 1990s will prove to be the decade the AIDS virus attacks both men and women equally and indiscriminately. Presently, the HIV infects twice as many men as it does women, but this two to one ratio is rapidly changing to one to one. Another important, little known fact is that the AIDS disease is worse (more virulent) in women than in men, especially when women are pregnant. Unfortunately, AIDS- infected pregnant women have babies which are AIDS-infected in over 50% of the time and which have a higher evidence of congenital anomalies. The longer the fetus is exposed to the AIDS virus, the more likely the fetus will be AIDS-infected and/or have a congenital anomaly when it is born. In summary, not only is the fetus in danger, when the mother is AIDS-infected, but so is the mother herself (because the AIDS disease often worsens during pregnancy). Most important, it must be remembered that all AIDS-infected people are carriers of the HIV and are contagious, *including AIDS-infected pregnant women and babies*. Therefore, anybody near AIDS-infected pregnant women must be careful not to come in contact with their bodily fluids, if any chance of the HIV infection is to be avoided.

The sooner all pregnant women are tested for AIDS, the sooner AID-infected pregnant women can be diagnosed. When diagnosed these women should be counseled and treated in high risk obstetrical centers by obstetricians and perinatologists specializing in AIDS obstetrical and neonatal care. With proper counselling and treatment, these unfortunate pregnant women and their newborns have a better chance of survival. If I didn't know any better, I would think the AIDS virus could think and plan strategy, before it attacked in its war with man. Not only does it attack man's immune system and brain, but his ability to reproduce – *his main means* to increase his numbers and thus insure the survival of his species. AIDS is testing man's ability to survive, so we all better get serious about preventing the spread of the disease as well as finding a cure and/or vaccine for it. *"Time is of the essence."*

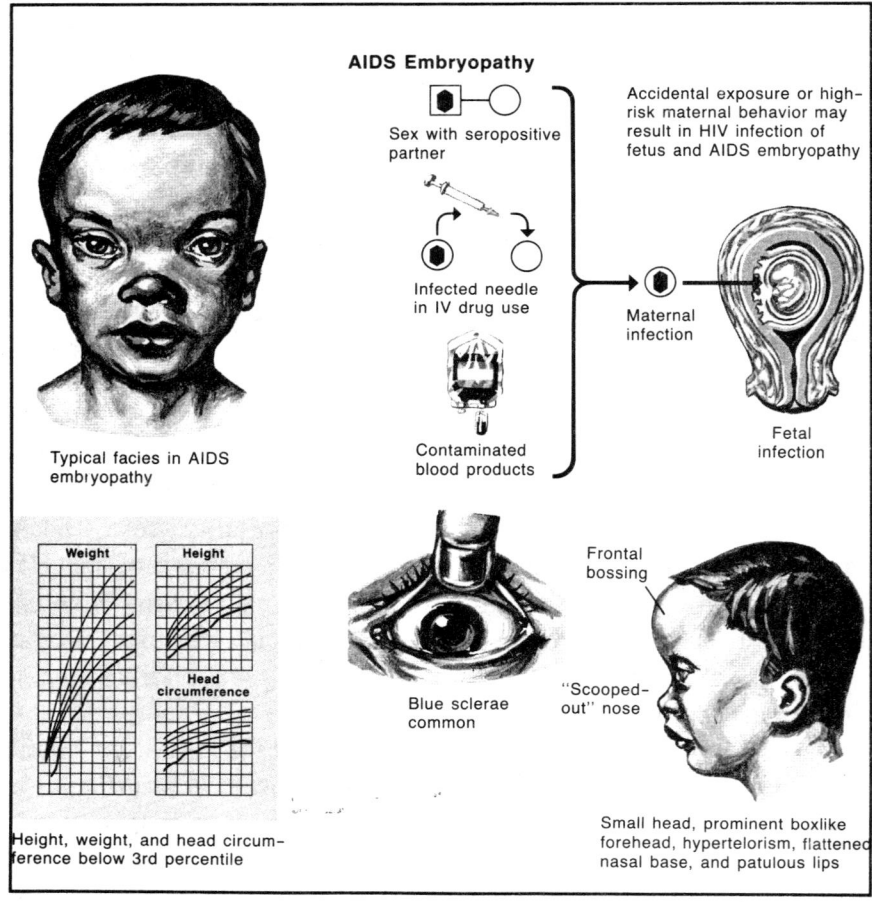

Figure 4

"AIDS Embryopathy," Clinical Symposia, Volume 42, November 1990

The fetal rubella syndrome, characterized by deafness, mental retardation, cataracts, and congenital heart disease, made it very clear that viral infections could produce substantial effects on the developing human fetus. It is now clear that the human immunodeficiency virus (HIV), the causative agent in acquired immunodeficiency syndrome (AIDS), causes a malformation syndrome when the fetus acquires the infection from the mother early in gestation (Figure 4).

Many babies with AIDS have similar dysmorphic features, including shortness of stature and growth retardation that may begin in utero. In a series of 20 patients, 70% had microcephaly – the head circumference was below the third percentile for chronologic age. Craniofacial abnormalities include a prominent, square, or boxlike forehead in the frontal view; lateral bossing; hypertelorism; a flat nasal bridge, giving the forehead a scooped-out appearance in profile; long palpebral fissures and blue sclerae; a short nose with a flattened columella and a well-formed triangular philtrum; full, patulous lips with a particularly prominent upper vermillion border, and mild slanting of the eyes. Although the above facial features occur in 50% to 75% of the patients, there is a variation in facial appearance, which is characteristic enough so that these patients can easily be identified. The children with clinical symptoms of immunodeficiency at an early age were those who had the most striking dysmorphic features. The timing of fetal viremia seems to influence the type and severity of abnormal morphogenesis. Prospective date on fetal rubella syndrome showed that when the fetuses were exposed to infection after the first trimester, only 15% developed the classic syndrome. The earlier the infection occurred, the more severe were the abnormalities. Infection with the HIV virus may be difficult to diagnose definitely in the first 5 months after birth. Recognizing the syndrome as AIDS related prompts a more vigorous search for the infection organism.

Comment: If there is any article to support my position, that all pregnant women should be HIV tested at least once during their pregnancy, this article is it. Seeing pictures of the deformities AIDS babies might have are worth a thousand words and enough to weaken the strongest of hearts. Also, this article should convince any "doubting Thomases" why HIV testing in pregnancy is *important* (and a *must*) and why all pregnant women (and their obstetricians) should insist it be done. *The longer the fetus (the unborn child) is exposed to the AIDS virus in utero, the more chance the baby will have AIDS or a congenital anomaly when born!* The "nightmare of nightmares" (AIDS in pregnancy) has started and we must start diagnosing, treating and counseling all of our pregnant women with the AIDS disease, *NOW!* Not to do so, in my opinion, is irresponsible, negligent and literally a death wish for the human species.

Can anybody get AIDS-infected when eating in a restaurant? If so, should people stop eating in restaurants?

Comment: In my opinion, yes – a person can get an HIV infection by eating in a restaurant, if that restaurant is AIDS-contaminated. My opinion is not just off the wall and without substantiation. Believing the AIDS virus can live up to two weeks in a dry state (and even longer in liquids) and believing the AIDS virus is infectious in this state (if activated under the right circumstances), then common sense dictates I must believe HIV infection is possible when contact with it is made. The extraordinary reproductive and mutating capacity of the AIDS virus (when bodily invasion with even a minute amount of the virus) is a matter of grave concern. According to Dr. John Seale:

"It is probable that, as with so many viremic diseases, a single viron (virus) introduced directly into the blood will regularly transmit infection" (The AIDS Cover-Up – page 7).

Therefore, if a person gets the AIDS virus on his/her hands (from restaurant plates, forks, cups, food, etc.) or in his/her eyes/mouth/lungs/skin (from a sneeze/cough by a restaurant AIDS-infected customer or employee), an HIV infection is possible.

Now, believing the above, do I believe nobody should eat in

restaurants or other public facilities? *Absolutely not.* However, I do believe we all must follow a few basic precautions, to minimize any chance of coming into contact with the AIDS virus, when eating away from home. Most important, make sure the eating facility (private or public) you eat in is clean – cleanliness is one of the best indicators of an AIDS-free environment. Also, if you think an eating facility has an AIDS-environment (a place where the AIDS virus is most likely to be found in or a place where there are AIDS-infected employees or a place where there are customers who are high risk to be harboring the AIDS virus), I would not eat there. Instead, I would patronize another eating facility, where I felt safer and could thus enjoy my meal. My advice, when eating in restaurants, is to keep your ears and eyes open. When entering an eating facility, check everything for cleanliness before eating (tables, forks, plates, glasses, waiters, waitresses, cooks, food, etc.). If *anything* is dirty or sounds/appears dirty (employees, customers, utensils, salad bars, kitchens, etc.), I would cross that eating facility off my list of places to eat in.

As the plague worsens and finally becomes obvious to everybody, the public will insist the government ensure all public eating facilities are super clean and are as HIV-free as possible. I foresee all public eating facilities being government inspected, approved and labeled "AIDS-safe" before they are allowed to serve the public. Violators will probably be severely fined and/or punished. Also, such things as disposable eating utensils (plates, forks, glasses, etc.), individually wrapped tooth picks, waitresses/waiters wearing disposable gloves (for each table) etc. will be the *expected* instead of the *exception*. Yes, we will still eat in public eating facilities, but, only if they have a proven "AIDS-free" environment.

What is AIDS Dementia?

Comment: *AIDS Dementia is AIDS,* another form of AIDS. Basically, there are two types of HIV infection (AIDS). The more common type attacks the immune system (70% of the time) and is called AIDS. The less common type attacks the brain (30% of the time) and is called AIDS Dementia. Both types of AIDS eventually kill their victims – the former by destroying the immune system which allows others diseases to kill the victim secondarily and the latter, by actually destroying the brain and thus killing the victim directly. Unfortunately, the CDC does not include the AIDS Dementia victims in its tally of AIDS-infected people in the United States – another reason the AIDS statistics are ridiculously low.

The symptoms and signs of AIDS Dementia are anxiety, depression, forgetfulness, memory loss, cognitive loss, neurosis, psychosis, and eventually sensory and motor loss. In short, when the victim's brain is finally destroyed, the victim dies. As time goes on, we are finding that more and more AIDS-infected people have some form of both types of the HIV infection.

As the mystery of AIDS continues to unravel, I'm sure we have many such surprises ahead of us. I only hope not all are as horrific as AIDS Dementia.

Both tuberculosis and HIV infections are on the rise, is there any relationship between the two?

Comment : Yes. Worldwide, tuberculosis infects over 8 million people and kills over 3 million people every year. Interestingly and unfortunately, over three million people are not only infected with the tuberculosis organism, but with the AIDS virus (HIV) as well. Why is this? As the HIV destroys the immune system of its victims, they become more and more susceptible to other infectious organisms, such as tuberculosis and histo-plasmosis. Also important, is the fact that 1.7 billion of the earth's 6+ billion people carry the tuberculosis organism in a "dormant or sleeping" state and the fact that AIDS-infected people are reservoirs for many other infectious diseases/organisms (such as tuberculosis, cytomegalovirus, toxoplasmosis, histoplasmosis, salmonella, herpes and various intestinal parasites). Because of these reasons, the tuberculosis disease is on the rise, with and without the accompanying HIV infection. The 32 year, five percent per year progressively downward trend in tuberculosis statistics has been halted and recently reversed. Now in the United States, 9.5/100,000 people are infected each year, which is 5% higher than last year. (*San Jose Mercury* newspaper,

October 16, 1990)

What can one do to survive the AIDS Plague? What are your recommendations?

Comment: First of all, remember that a good defense is better than a good offense – *take great caution not to get infected by the AIDS virus*. Secondly, if you are HIV infected, *Stay alive* – until a cure is found and you can be cured. I feel certain a cure for AIDS is out there someplace and, in time, we will find it. I only hope we find it sooner than later.

Presently, I think the following precautions should be followed:

(1) Learn all you can about the AIDS virus (HIV) and the disease (AIDS) it causes. Discard the information/advice which you think is incorrect/bad and only follow the advice which you think is correct, to avoid the HIV infection. Always remember, there is *no room for error with this disease* – an HIV infection is certain death.

(2) Always consider the AIDS disease as a lethal, fatal, contagious medical disease – not a political/venereal disease or a disease with human/civil rights.

(3) Respect the AIDS virus at all times. Remember, it can infect anybody, anytime and in any place, and there is no cure or vaccine for/against it.

(4) Know when you are in an "AIDS environment" and when you are in one, be careful not to come in contact with any other person's bodily fluids (which might be AIDS-contaminated). What I mean by "AIDS environment" is a place where the HIV might be in or with people who may be harboring the AIDS virus.

(5) Don't inject/use drugs. This is good advise whether you are worried about AIDS or not.

(6) Don't practice or indulge in prostitution.

(7) Use soap and water, detergents and disinfectants liberally – cleanliness is one of the best protections against the HIV.

(8) When having elective surgery, donate your own blood before your surgery. Then, your own blood (autogenous blood)

is available if you should happen to need it during your surgery. If there is no time to donate your own blood for your surgery, then try to get a few close friends or relatives (who you feel are AIDS-free and healthy) to donate blood for your surgery. If none of these options are available, then I certainly recommend using blood bank blood if necessary. Please keep in mind, most doctors don't transfuse their patients unless it is absolutely necessary. Also, it is better to have a blood transfusion (when necessary) than not, because that could mean the difference between life and death.

(9) Practice "safe sex." I hate this term because it is so vague; however, what I mean by it is:
  (a) Don't be promiscuous.
  (b) Don't patronize prostitutes.
  (c) Practice monogomous sex.
  (d) Know the HIV status of your partner. If he/she is HIV negative, you have no problem. If he/she is HIV positive, make sure your partner gets treatment and counselling as should you. Both you and your partner has to know how not to infect each other – your partner infecting you (and others) with the HIV and you infecting your partner with an opportunistic disease.

(10) Contact your legislators at the local, state and federal levels. *Demand* they recognize AIDS for what it is – a contagious, fatal, lethal medical disease which has no cure or vaccine. *Demand* they propose and pass legislation which protects the *entire public,* not just the AIDS-infected or the AIDS-free people. Remind them that it is the healthy AIDS-free people who work and pay taxes that keep this great country going, and *it is these people who must be protected at all costs and at all times.*

(11) If you are pregnant, ask your physician to test you for AIDS every three months of your pregnancy. If you test HIV positive, obtain your obstetrical care in facilities and by physicians that specialize in the AIDS disease. By do-

ing this, both you and your baby will have the best chance of a favorable outcome.

If a person is already HIV positive, what should or can that person do?

Comment: In short – *stay alive!* Stay alive until a cure for AIDS is found. All people with the AIDS disease should get treatment and counselling as soon as possible. There is treatment for HIV-infected people, which helps them live longer and more comfortably. Counselling is a must. Aids-infected people must learn how to protect themselves from opportunistic diseases and they must learn how not to infect others with the HIV, which they carry in their bodily fluids. Most importantly, AIDS-infected people must be made to realize *they are not just like other people.* They must understand they have a disease which is slowly destroying their immune system; therefore, *their chances of becoming infected by other infectious organisms are steadily increasing.* Because of this fact, AIDS-infected people should stay away from crowds of people (especially in enclosed areas such as theaters and schools) and from people with other infections (such as upper respiratory infections, skin infections, wound infections, etc.). Also, I recommend that anybody infected by the HIV be treated by health care workers and in health care facilities which *specialize in the treatment of the AIDS disease*. This is not a disease which can or should be treated by anybody. It is a very complicated disease, one with many problems (the drugs for AIDS are few and toxic, all the body organ systems are involved, the immune system and/or the brain are steadily being destroyed, opportunistic disease can and do occur, etc., etc.).

In summary, anybody infected by the HIV must try to stay alive until a cure is found. To increase their chances of doing so, AIDS-infected people should get *specialized treatment and counselling* as early as possible. Lastly, these people should never give up hope because *a cure for AIDS is possible and probable*. The real questions is *WHEN?*

What is a lentivirus?

Comment: A lentivirus (the name is derived from the Latin word *lentus* which means "slow") is a virus which has a long incubation period before symptoms of the infection it causes occurs or develops. The lentivirus family has five different species – the human form (AIDS), the horse form (causes a fatal infectious anemia), the sheep form (causes a rare fatal pneumonia or a fatal brain disease), the cattle or bovine form (causes a fatal leukemia) and the goat form (causes a fatal encephalitis-arthritis). These viruses cause serious infections that are contagious and usually fatal in the species they are in.

I have often heard the AIDS virus (HIV) is a retrovirus. What is a retrovirus?

Comment: "Retro" stands for an enzyme (reverse transcriptase, to be specific) and retrovirus means this enzyme is found in the virus. There are different retroviruses, AIDS being one of them. A retrovirus has the ability, once it has entered a host or victim's cell, to take over the host cell's mechanism responsible for the production if its DNA (genetic or chromosomal material). With the aid of the invading virus' reverse transcriptase enzyme, the host cell is forced to make DNA from the retrovirus' genetic material (RNA), which is then incorporated into the chromosomes of the infected host. This changes or mutates the host's genetic code forever.

Once the HIV has infected a person, it forces the cells of that person (after it has changed the genetic code of that person's cells) to make more virus which can then go on to infect other cells of the same infected person. In summary, the genetically HIV changed cells of the infected person have become "HIV factories." These "HIV factories" then make more HIV to infect more host cells which in turn become "HIV factories" themselves and make more HIV to infect more host cells. This vicious, destructive circle continues until the infected person finally dies.

I know the above is complicated and sounds confusing, but the important thing to remember is a retrovirus attacks its victim's most vulnerable spot – its genetic material or chromosomes. Simply put, this disease is like the "sweet bug" (a fictitious species) which invades a candy making factory and then proceeds to eat all the candy in the factory and then forces the factory to make more "sweet bugs" instead of candy. These new "sweet bugs" then invade other candy factories to repeat the process ad nauseum, thus continuing the survival of the "sweet bug" species. This process continues until all the candy factories are destroyed. The end result of course, is the disappearance of all candy factories. This is why a retrovirus infection is almost (?) 100% fatal and so difficult to find a cure for.

If what you say is true and substantiated, that AIDS is a lethal contagious disease which threatens man's very existence, why are people being told differently by the authorities?

Comment: The answer to this question is as mysterious as the AIDS disease itself. Also many other equally baffling questions need answering as well. Why the deafening silence (about the AIDS threat) by the medical hierarchy? Why is organized medicine content to follow than lead the government in the war against the AIDS virus? Why is the government more concerned about the wants and needs, the legal and human rights and the medical care of the AIDS-infected people over those of the many more AIDS-free people? Why does the established media eagerly report all AIDS news, whether it is substantiated or not? Why does the U.S. public health service minimize the seriousness of the AIDS disease (which has no cure/vaccine) and maximize the seriousness of many other diseases (which do have cures/vaccines)? Why do our legislators *propose and pass laws that should not be passed and not propose and pass laws that should be passed* (to control the spread of AIDS)? Why aren't accurate statistics about the number of AIDS cases (in America and the world) revealed? Why aren't the real costs of the AIDS plague revealed? Why aren't the many social-economic-political problems of AIDS revealed and addressed? Why this and why that, etc.etc.? *My answer is – I DON'T KNOW!!!* I wish I did know, but I don't. If I knew, I would tell you. Until these and other such questions are answered and addressed, the AIDS virus will continue to infect and kill at an ever increasing rate. Once the critical mass of the disease is reached (when the virulency of the AIDS virus increases enough that it is able to claim many more victims in months instead of years), the AIDS plague will enter the exponential stage and then proceed to decimate the human race, much worse than the Black Death did. There is no room for error and no time for political-special interest group games with this killer virus. A cure must be found *now,* because there is little "sooner" and no "later" time left.

I'm the director of the local AIDS Chapter, and sir, let me tell you, you don't know what you are talking about? Are you a real medical doctor? How can you tell people such nonsense? Mr "Radio talk show host", how can you have such an AIDS-uniformed guest on your show? You, Mr. "Radio talk show host," are doing a disservice to your listeners by having this doctor as your guest, etc., etc.

Comment: I have been on radio talk shows all over the country – trying to educate and inform people about the AIDS virus and the disease it causes, and trying to help people protect themselves from the HIV infection. In so doing, I have talked to many concerned and interested people, both radio talk show hosts and their listeners calling in. *However,* there are always some doubting callers, like the ones making the above hostile statements and asking the above pointed questions. Their intent is not to seek AIDS information or to help people, but to discredit (in this case, me) anybody that disagrees with them. They don't want the public to hear the other side of the AIDS coin, the side the established media refuses to report (that AIDS is a lethal, fatal, contagious medical disease which threatens everybody). When doing these programs, I expect to have some callers who doubt or question what I am saying and to even attack me personally. Occasionally, I am not disappointed. However, what I have learned (but did not realize or expect) was that so called "AIDS experts" are monitoring the airways at all times. If anybody (like me) is on the airways with AIDS information, which is not expounded by the established media, they call in and try to discredit both the information and the bearer of the information. Why? *Because these people do not want the public to hear or think anything about AIDS but what they want them to hear or think.* I have found these so called "AIDS experts" (who call in) AIDS-uninformed and bigoted, with nothing to offer people but old mainstream AIDS nonsense; thus defending myself and discrediting them has been no problem at all. In fact, when these harassing "AIDS experts" call to discredit or embarrass me, I have found the information I give during the radio talk show has more "punch" and credibility with the listeners. What angers me is the thought that there are so many "AIDS experts" out there, who are unfortunately giving AIDS advice (solicited or not) which I believe is false and dangerous. Because of such "AIDS experts" (well meaning or not), I feel many people have and will become unnecessarily AIDS-infected and AIDS-dead. Anyway, I will continue to warn people about the AIDS plague and try to help them help themselves from the killer virus (HIV). I must admit here, I occasionally do get discouraged and feel bad, when attacked by such people. However, I then remind myself of two things which always keep me going.

(1) I am helping people, at least I hope I am helping people.
(2) The reassuring old saying that "sticks and stones may break my bones, but names will never hurt me."

Do you think physicians and dentists should have to be tested for AIDS? If they test positive for the AIDS virus (HIV), should they continue practicing medicine?

Comment: These questions are often asked and raise a host of possible answers, as well as other similar questions and issues. Simply answered, I think *all people should have to be AIDS-tested yearly,* not just physicians or dentists or any other segment of the population. Anybody who tests HIV positive has one of the three stages of AIDS and should be considered ill and contagious. Thereafter, such people should be treated and counselled (how not to expose/infect themselves with opportunistic diseases and how to avoid infecting others with the AIDS virus). The important fact that people do not consider (when they recommend all physicians and dentists get AIDS tested) is that if they are infected, *they most likely got infected by one of their patients.* This is the main reason doctors and dentists are considered one of the high risk groups of people to get AIDS – because *they can and do get AIDS-infected by their own patients or in their own work place.* If this a truism, and it is, then I think it is just as important (if not more so) to test all patients who go to a physician, dentist or health care facility (like a hospital). Since both groups can and do infect the other or even each other (patients infecting other patients, physicians infecting other physicians etc.), then it is equally important to AIDS test both groups. Also, if both of these groups (patients/health care workers and physicians/dentists) must be AIDS-tested, then everybody else should be AIDS-tested too, otherwise it is discrimination at its worst. In short, either or neither should be AIDS-tested to be fair. *What is good for the goose is good for the gander!* Wouldn't it be terrible for a pregnant woman to go to a hospital to have a baby and leave the hospital with either the baby or herself (or even both) AIDS-infected! Talk about a disaster!

I blame organized medicine for the above confusion and shortsightedness. Not only are our medical organizations not adequately protecting the public from the HIV (lack of proper AIDS education of the public, lack of leadership in the war against AIDS etc.), they aren't even AIDS-protecting their own members – especially those that have direct contact with patients, like myself. The AMA's present recommendations are for *all* physicians to voluntarily get aids-tested and if they test HIV positive, to voluntarily tell their patients they have AIDS and to voluntarily cease doing any invasive procedures on any patients. Here, the AMA completely ignores the safety and legal rights of *all physicians, including its own paying members!* Today, the AMA's *paying membership* doesn't even include one half of America's physicians and I doubt if it ever will have the majority, not with such irresponsible and one sided recommendations as these. "With friends like these, who needs enemies?" In America, there is no one organization that represents and speaks for all physicians – *not even the majority.* The term "organized medicine" is a misnomer and deceiving, but we unfortunately use it anyway, for lack of a better term. As a result, in my opinion, the practice of private medicine and the high quality of medical care in America is now being systematically destroyed, because we physicians (as a whole) have no effective organization to protect either. Politicians and self-serving special interest groups use the fragmentation and disorganization of the medical profession to harass, discredit, dictate and control it. It is this same "Achilles' heel" of medicine, which is helping the HIV spread, infect and kill.

Lastly, I think health care workers who are HIV positive should not directly (hands on) care for HIV negative patients. However, they should be allowed to practice their profession in areas where there is no direct contact with HIV-free patients (like in hospital administration) and in facilities which care for AIDS patients only. As time goes on and the plague worsens, such facilities will not only exist, but be mandatory and multiply in number. These are but some of the important questions, issues, and problems that must sooner or later be addressed, answered and corrected. *For the sake of us all, let us make it sooner than later!*

How dangerous do you think the AIDS virus really is?

Comment: As I said many times, the AIDS virus is a killer virus, without a known cure or vaccine and which is threatening the human race. It can infect anybody, anytime, anyplace, – man, woman, child, baby or fetus. If I could fantasize and see thru the "eyes" of an AIDS virus, what do you think I would see? I think I would see planet earth full of complacent reproducing human beings, who I could attack, infect, and feed off of. What a magnificent feeding ground! Best of all, there is nothing to stop me – *no cure, no vaccine, no nothing!* Better still, my ability to attack/infect/kill is *very underestimated by my victims*. Yes, the HIV is truly the worst predator man has ever faced! Equally true, is that man is the easiest victim a predator, like the HIV, could ever wish for.

Why do you think health care workers are so uninformed and/or dysinformed about AIDS?

Comment: For many reasons. Out of sight, out of mind and "ignorance is bliss" are two of the main reasons. Also the "fear of AIDS" is another. The more one knows about the AIDS disease, the more one realizes it is literally and figuratively a death sentence, if one is unfortunate to have it. Realizing this, many health care workers are afraid to talk or think or learn anything about this killer HIV. This is why I call this condition or state of mind "the fear of AIDS." Another reason is that health care workers also *know* AIDS is a "career killer." No way is a health care worker allowed to presently work with patients, if they are infected by a recognized contagious infectious disease, no matter what the disease is. *AIDS is such a disease and worse yet, it has no cure or vaccine! Health care workers know this!* They also know it is only matter of time until AIDS testing will be mandatory and until AIDS-infected health care workers will not *(by law)* be allowed to practice their profession. Therefore, if an HIV infection happens to them, and they certainly know it can, their livelihoods (as well as their lives) are ruined – a tragic personal and family disaster. Another reason is the government and organized medicine are not properly educating or informing health care workers about the dangers of the AIDS virus. In fact, they are minimizing the HIV dangers! If they did tell the whole truth, they know many health care workers will quit the medical profession. After all, how many health care workers are stupid enough to keep working, if they knew an AIDS- infection is a "career killer" and means certain death? Well, there are many health care workers (like me) who do know the truth and who are still working for one reason or another; but let me assure you, there are many other health care workers who are not working and many more who will not work once they know the truth. Also, common knowledge of the ominous characteristics and dangers of the HIV and the disease it causes will certainly decrease the already decreasing pool of young people entering the medical profession. This would certainly exacerbate the already growing health care worker shortage. These are but just some of the reasons which I can think of why most of our health care workers are so uninformed, misinformed, and/or dysinformed about AIDS.

Why aren't more AIDS tests done?

Comment: *Good question!* The main reason is that the American government, states and legal system have all made it too difficult for people to get AIDS tested. They have shackled the physician with legal restraints, obstacles and threats – breach of confidentiality and discrimination suits, ridiculous rules and regulations (must have written consent of the patient to order the HIV test, must use a "code" instead of the patient's name for the HIV test, the test result must remain in a sealed envelope labeled "confidential" etc.), cannot transfer a patient diagnosed as having AIDS (unless the patients and receiving entity *agree in writing*), cannot refuse to treat an AIDS patient (even if the physician doesn't feel qualified) etc. As a result, most physicians are now reluctant to mention AIDS testing, let alone order an AIDS test. Another reason is the majority of people have been lulled into a state of "AIDS complacency" by misinformation, dysinformation, and even no information. Unfortunately, AIDS complacency is when people don't consider AIDS is a threat to them; therefore these people don't think AIDS testing is necessary. The "fear of AIDS" is another big reason very little AIDS testing is done today. Most people don't want to know if they are AIDS-infected; because they know if they are, it means they are going to die prematurely, means they are going to lose their jobs and livelihood, and means a drastic change in their lifestyles forever. Contributing to the above obstacles are even more obstacles the *individual states* put up, which discourage AIDS testing even more. Such obstacles as mandatory counselling before the AIDS test is done, confusing and complicating instructions, limiting the number of testing sites, recommending only "high risk" people get tested, etc., all contribute to the low number of AIDS tests being done around the country. Add to this, the fact that *each state has different rules, regulations and laws about AIDS testing* certainly doesn't help the situation. Lastly, is the cost of the AIDS test. It differs from place to place and from state to state. Here in California, for example the test costs five dollars if done at Planned Parenthood, free of charge (if done "anonymously") and twenty-five dollars (if done "confidentially") at the local Department of

Health, and forty to forty-eight dollars if done at a private clinical laboratory or hospital. By the way, "anonymously" means very few questions are asked of the person getting the AIDS test and "confidentially" means more questions are asked – *ridiculous!* The test results are given only to the person being tested – no one else. AIDS tested people can give their test results to their physician or anybody else – *only if they choose to do so! No one else can get these results, unless the tested person agrees in writing.* So, if a person tests positive for the AIDS disease, he/she does not have to tell anybody. *This is ludicrous.* Bottom line of all this, is the little AIDS testing done in America today is a joke. I see no hope in controlling or containing, let alone eradicating, the AIDS plague today – not with this kind of absurd AIDS testing. If I had to bet how many Americans have been HIV tested, I would bet only about two percent (2+%) of America's 250 million people have been tested so far. Worse yet, I'll bet a far lesser percentage of people have been repeatedly HIV tested. There is no way such sparse testing can realistically tell us how serious the AIDS plague really is in America. Presently, we have no idea who has and who doesn't have AIDS, nor how extensive or how serious the AIDS plague is. How and why can/should anybody fight a problem they don't know they (or anybody else) have? The Centers for Disease Control (CDC) has estimated there are about 1.5 million people infected by the AIDS virus in America. The problem here, is they have been saying this since 1986. According to them, no one has become AIDS infected since 1986. Why is the CDC not telling the American people the truth? Another good question! The sooner we get rid of such obstacles to effective AIDS testing the better. We, as a nation, must find out how many of our people are AIDS infected as soon as possible. We must know how serious the AIDS plague is; and if it is as serious as I believe it is, our country must go into "overdrive" and address it head on. The time for nonsense and foolishness is past. It is time for serious fighting against the AIDS virus. *The clock is ticking!*

How long does it take an HIV test to turn positive from negative (thus diagnosing AIDS), once a person is infected by

the AIDS virus?

Comment: The blood banks across the country state a person tests positive (from the time of infection) for AIDS in over ninety percent (90%) of the time in three months and over ninety-five percent (95%) of the time in six months. However, they do admit a small percentage (exact amount is never disclosed) of the AIDS-infected people don't test positive for up to three years. *A few AIDS experts believe up to 20% of the AIDS-infected people don't test positive for AIDS for sixteen to thirty-four mouths (and some even beyond) after being infected by the HIV (The Alarming Reality,* by William T. O'Connor, M. D.).This being the case, it is no small wonder why many people do not want a blood transfusion and why most physicians today recommend autologous blood (one's own blood, given previously for their own use) or blood donated by close friends/relatives for blood transfusion. The important point to remember here is that anybody can test negative for the AIDS-virus, *and still be AIDS-infected.* This time period (the time an AIDS infection begins to the time the AIDS test converts from negative to positive, thus showing the person is AIDS infected) is called the "AIDS window." It is this "AIDS window" which is the problem, because it varies from person to person.Therefore, I believe it most important to test everybody every year, if we are ever to find out how severe the AIDS plague is and if we are making any progress in controlling it. Lastly, please remember a negative AIDS test is comforting, but it is not a 100% guarantee that you are AIDS free or you won't get AIDS infected in the future. The lesson of this last point is, *always keep your guard up against the lurking AIDS virus!*

Is the virus that causes AIDS man made?

Comment: Some people think it is, but most think it is not. Certainly no one is going to take credit for making the AIDS virus, not when it is now out of control and infecting/killing millions of people worldwide. Add to this the fact that no cure or vaccine for AIDS is available or even foreseeable, a person would have to be crazy to admit/take any credit or responsibility for the HIV. There are many theories around explaining how the AIDS virus came to be, but none are proven – at least according to the established media. Let us explore some of these theories:

(a) The HIV was released from the melting glaciers from a hibernated state. *Certainly possible!*
(b) The HIV fell to the earth from the heavens on some meteorite. *Certainly possible!*
(c) The HIV came from the depths of the ocean on some fish or plant. *Certainly possible!*
(d) An HIV infected green monkey in Central Africa bit a native and infected him with the HIV. He in turn infected his wife and girlfriend, who in turn infected others, etc. until now, we have over 75 million Africans infected. *Ridiculous and not possible!* Since the HIV does not infect animals or plants, and since the plague broke out in many places throughout the world at the same time (Africa, Haiti, Brazil), this theory makes no sense, epidemiologically speaking. I can just see the Little Green Monkey flying around the world on his (her?) jet airplane, biting people. It is beyond me how any AIDS expert can seriously support such a ridiculous theory, *but many do*. My question to them is, why?
(e) The HIV was made in the biological warfare center in Fort Dietrich, Maryland in the 1960's and early 1970's. It was made by crossing the bovine leukemia virus (causes a lethal, fatal leukemia in cattle) with the sheep visna virus (causes a lethal, fatal "brain rot" disease in sheep) on a human tissue plate. The end product was the AIDS virus(HIV), which infects *only man* and is contagious and 100% fatal. In testing it, it got loose and out of control and now threatens all the peoples on the planet Earth. True? *Possible and probable.* Of course I have greatly condensed this theory, but for more information on this theory and other such theories. I recommend contacting **America West Publishers** (P.O. Box 986, Tehachapi, CA 93581).

These are but some of the many theories of the possible origin of the AIDS virus. As time goes on, I am sure more theories will surface – maybe even one you, the reader, might come with. Realistically, however, I doubt if we will ever know the HIV origin – at least from the establishment and its media.

Do you think the origin of the AIDS virus is important?

Comment: When talking about AIDS, an African AIDS researcher once said "It is not important to know how the lion got into the house, what is important to know is how to get him out of the house!" Well I think this is only a half truth. If we knew how the lion entered the house, it might help us get him out and certainly should help us prevent any other lions from entering the house again. The point here is it would be very helpful to know how the AIDS virus (HIV) came to be. If we knew its origin, it certainly might help us find a cure and even a vaccine against the HIV.

Is there a cure for AIDS?

Comment: This is the $64,000.00 question. According to the established media, there is no cure for the AIDS disease and no cure is expected in the near future. This certainly is bad news for us all. However, according to some people, a cure is on the near horizon and/or already here. Who is right and who is wrong? Let me try, as best as I can, to shed some light on what various people think about an AIDS cure. The following are some of the most current opinions or theories on this question:

(1) There is no cure for the AIDS disease and there will never be one. If this is true, then we are all doomed and in time, mankind will cease to exist.

(2) There is no cure for the AIDS disease and none is expected in the near future, *but* an AIDS cure is possible and probable. Now this opinion is that of the established media and most people and it certainly does offer some hope for a cure.

(3) An AIDS cure is possible by removing the AIDS-infected blood from an AIDS-infected person, heating it enough to kill the AIDS virus (HIV) only and then transfusing the heated blood back into the same AIDS-infected person. Does

this work? According to some pretty knowledgeable people, this cure has been thoroughly evaluated and thereafter considered valueless. Still, I'm sure some people still believe this technique is or might eventually be effective.

(4) Electrophoresis/electrobiosis – Some AIDS researchers believe this method of treatment might eventually be the answer to the "containment" of the AIDS disease until a permanent cure is found. In fact, it might also eventually lead to an AIDS cure itself. Presently, this method is thought to only prolong the life of an AIDS-infected person. It entails removing the blood from the AIDS-infected person, treating it with ultraviolet light (thus killing the HIV in the blood) and then transfusing the treated blood back into the same AIDS-infected person. This method of AIDS treatment must yet be perfected, but it is feasible, simple, effective, and inexpensive – the technology is available. For further information, contact William Campbell Douglass, M.D., P.O. Box 1568, Clayton GA 30525.

(5) Pulsating electromagnetic irradiation – Some people around the world are convinced this method of treatment will ultimately be the answer for the cure of the AIDS disease. Simply put, the entire body of an AIDS-infected person is subjected to a barrage of radio waves/high frequency sound waves. These radio waves are specifically targeted or aimed and programmed to destroy all forms of the HIV in the infected person's body. Prior to this barrage, all the types of HIV viruses in the AIDS-infected person to be treated are identified. Once the HIV types are identified, the exact frequency of the radio wave necessary to destroy all the HIV types are programmed into the electromagnetic machine/device and the person's whole body is then treated. Since the HIV has a crystalline formation, it can be shattered by specific radio waves – much like a crystal wine goblet can be shattered by high frequency sound waves. This form of treatment destroys (shatters) the crystalline-like HIV and leaves the infected host cell intact. Once rid of the HIV, the infected host cell recovers back to its previous healthy state.

This theory ("biological transmutation of cells from the sick to the normal state") was discovered and promoted by two geniuses (Royal R. Rife and Nicholas Telsa) years ago. This method of possible AIDS treatment is complex and in need of more research, but headway is being made. To assist in the research is the new mind boggling Kurt Olbrich Ergonom 400 light-source microscope, which I believe will prove invaluable. The following excerpt from *The Conscious Connection* (Healing Therapies, page 34-35, August September 1990) describes the abilities of this microscope beautifully:

"This Ergonom 400 microscope (which does not kill cells by bombarding them with electrons in a vacuum as does the electron microscope) is also able to magnify specimens to 25,000 diameters in comparison with the normal light-source microscope capacity of only 1,800 diameters."

"Cells now may be seen LIVE at a higher magnification and resolution, showing such discoveries as the changes of a single micro-organism life cycle encompassing bacterial, fungoid and viral stages. Germs had previously been thought to remain in one stage: a virus remains a virus, a bacterium remains a bacterium, etc. However, videos made through the ergonom 400 shows germs changing from one form to another and back again through a process called pleomophism."

In any event, "pulsating electromagnetic irradiation" is an interesting and exciting concept for the ultimate cure of not only AIDS, but of other disease such as cancer. If you, the reader, want more information, please contact **America West Publishers** P.O. Box 986, Tehachapi, CA 93581.

(6) The electronic treatment of AIDS – Bio-electric medicine: There is a small but growing number of scientists who believe the electron treatment of various degenerative diseases, including cancer and AIDS, is the answer to a permanent cure. The theory here is to pump billions of electrons into the HIV infected human body which then energize the cells of the body and at the same time heat up the HIV to the

point where it bursts and disintegrates. "In summary, the free electrons restore the system, restore the cellular energy and destroy the AIDS viruses by causing them to heat up, expand and rupture their membranes. The heating action does not occur to the cells in the body, so only the viruses are destroyed." – *The McAlvaney Intelligence Advisor,* September 1990. One researcher, Evans A. Rapsomanikis (senior research scientist, Lockheed Corporation) has developed an electronic system (Bio-Sonic System II or BIS-II) with which he has had encouraging results treating AIDS patients – improvement in both the physical and mental conditions. Again, much more research is needed before this method of treatment for AIDS is perfected, let alone offered. However, bio-electric medicine may prove to be the first answer to an AIDS cure – it shows great promise.

(7) Conspiracy cure – What in the world is this? Well, some people believe that a small group of influential, well-off, international people believe the planet Earth can only support about 500 million human beings. Almost from man's beginnings, this is the number of people thought to have been sustained by Mother Earth – until the 18th Century. Since then, man's numbers on this planet increased exponentially, until now there are about six and one half billion people alive. This number of living people is more than have ever died – this fact is a good one for Ripley's "Believe it or not" isn't it? Anyway, these "conspirators" or "insiders" believe six billion people must be eliminated, one way or another, or it will mean the end of Earth as well as the entire human species. To insure the survival of both *(with them in control or charge of course), they developed the AIDS virus (HIV) and the AIDS cure.* They then unleashed this killer virus upon the peoples of the world without revealing the cure. When only about 500 million people remain on the Earth, then and only then, will the "insiders" reveal the AIDS cure. At that time, they hope to have complete control of the Earth and the people remaining on it. Far fetched? Ridiculous? Maybe and maybe not, I don't know. However, if you want more information on this theory,

contact **America West Publishers**, P.O. Box 986 Tehachapi CA 93581.

(8) High doses of vitamins – The theory here is if an AIDS infected person ingests daily high doses of various vitamins, his/her damaged immune system will eventually strengthen enough to suppress and/or eradicate the HIV infection. So far, however, this has not proven to be the case. I only wish the AIDS cure is this simple, but I am afraid it isn't.

(9) Vaccines – There is no available vaccine to cure or prevent the HIV infection. The vaccines being researched today are only to slow down the AIDS disease and prolong the lives of already AIDS-infected people. Thus far, all of them have proven unsuccessful for both AIDS prevention and AIDS cures. Because the HIV has $9,000^4$ (this is 9 x 9 x 9 x 9 followed by 12 zeros) different forms it can mutate or change to and because the HIV is so unstable (mutates almost at will), I don't believe a vaccine for the prevention of AIDS is possible. I hope I'm wrong.

Well, there you have it. As you can see, there is no known cure for AIDS – at least, not an AIDS cure which is recognized by the medical establishment and the public. The race for an AIDS cure, before the demise of mankind, is on. *We must win it, because we have no choice!* If an AIDS cure is truly known but not revealed for one reason or another (like some people believe), I can only hope the responsible parties abandon their own selfish, self-serving goals and reveal it for the good of all the peoples of the world.

What does a real plague do to a country?

Comment: If we want to know what a plague can do to a country, all we have to do is look back into history to find what we can expect. Plagues have always been bad news for countries – killing many people, causing many social and political changes and causing many economics calamities. During the three main plagues of the Black Death 200 to 400 years ago, the known world at that time was left in shambles. I believe AIDS will dwarf the killing and chaos of all three of those plagues combined, once it goes into overdrive. To say AIDS will change many things would be the understatement of the year. The effects of AIDS will be enormous, adverse and global, and will be felt well into the 21st Century.

Do you think the US government will ever classify or recognize AIDS as a plague?

Comment: Yes. In the near future, I believe the U.S. Government will officially declare AIDS as a plague and as the nation's #1 problem. It will finally recognize AIDS as the contagious, fatal, lethal, medical disease it is and not as a political or venereal disease which it is not. The government's main priorities will be to protect the AIDS-free public from the AIDS virus and to allocate huge sums of money for AIDS research, prevention and treatment.

Since 1981, the government has already spent over $4.7 billion on AIDS research and prevention. Last year, it spent $1.6 billion and this year, over $1.7 billion is requested. This amount is more than for any single disease, including cancer. In fact, it is far more than heart disease, hypertension, stroke and diabetes combined – afflictions that kill 35 times as many Americans as AIDS. As high as these figures now appear, they are but a "drop in the bucket" for what lies ahead. As more and more people (millions) become AIDS-infected and AIDS-sick, the more costs will soar to unbelievable heights. Hundreds of billions, to even trillions, of dollars will be needed for AIDS prevention and health care – assuming we continue to provide "state of the art" medical care for the AIDS-infected people.

Because of these high costs, the government will have to change its approach to AIDS medical care. It has to, because *it cannot afford not to*. It will have to take draconian steps, some of which may seem/be inhumane or even illegal, to control these costs and to contain the AIDS plague. Mandatory AIDS testing, rationing of health care, somehow minimizing the mixing of AIDS-infected and AIDS-free people, etc., are some of the changes I foresee, whether I or you approve of them or not.

What does all this mean for the American people? A drastic

change in lifestyles, *higher medical bills and higher taxes!* Each year the plague continues and worsens, the higher the medical costs wil be. Yes, our government will finally have to admit the seriousness of the AIDS plague, *the hard way* – when the "wrath of AIDS is all around us.

What do you foresee AIDS will do to America, socio-economically?

Comment: AIDS will have a dramatic effect on the American way of life. As the plague worsens and the "Fear of AIDS" increases, more and more people will leave the cities to live in small towns or in the country. They will marry sooner, have larger families, make more of their own clothes, grow more of their own food, and educate and entertain themselves at home. They will do most of their socializing with each other and with their neighbors. All this, they will do for one main reason – to lessen their chances of exposure and contact with the AIDS virus.

This being a truism, the following are some of the things I believe we can expect:

(1) **Cities.** As more and more people leave the cities for the country, there will be more buildings empty and more businesses disappearing. The prices of city residential and commercial real estate will plummet, because of less demand. Less people also means less taxes for the cities, which in turn means less money for city employees and city services (fire, police, garbage). The cities' infrastructures will deteriorate, even more than they are now, for lack of tax dollars. The bottom line of all this is that city life in the near future will not be very pleasant – more crime, more "fear of AIDS," less city services, rising unemployment, etc.

(2) **Towns and country.** Because people will be moving to these areas, the demand for rural land will rise dramatically. This in turn, will cause a huge demand for, people services – fire and police protection, food, fuel, etc. The worse the plague, the more the "Fear of AIDS" the more the people will relocate to the country. Yes, AIDS will greatly influence

life in the country – you can bet on it.

(3) **Business.** By this time, I am sure you have guessed what we should expect here. Businesses of *all types* will suffer in cities, but increase and benefit in small towns. Businesses that deal with large crowds of people will be adversely affected, more so in cities than in small towns – restaurants, theaters, coliseums, motels, hotels, operas, gambling casinos, airlines, etc. The point here is that people will want to stay out of an AIDS environment, that is in places where the AIDS virus is most likely to be found or with people who are most likely to be harboring the AIDS virus. In general, however, the AIDS plague will be bad news for business.

(4) **Religion.** Throughout history, man (when in trouble) has always turned to his Creator for help. This time, Man is in real trouble – a disease with no cure or vaccine is threatening his very existence. So as expected and like clockwork, man is starting to look at his Creator for some kind of help against AIDS. Already, more and more people (both AIDS-free and AIDS-infected, religious or not) are turning to religion for hope and comfort. This being another truism, I expect people will increasingly donate more money and time to religious causes than ever before. Why? *To help their religious leaders help them, that's why!*

(5) **Education.** More people will educate their young at home. As more people educate their children and themselves at home, the less schools will be needed, particularly public schools. This translates into less schools, less teachers, less aides, etc. Mail order educational courses (VCR and tape deck educational material, television, home workbooks, computer courses and special tutors) will all be increasingly utilized for home education.

(6) **Entertainment.** With time, more and more entertainment will be at the home level. Why? Again, because of the "Fear of AIDS." Many entities of "crowd" entertainment will suffer financially – theaters, operas, ball games, gambling casinos, etc. Investments in home entertainment (such

as television, games, radio, pool, and other types of home entertainment) will benefit handsomely.
- (7) **Food and clothing.** As more and more people grow their own food and make their own clothes, there will be less and less need for grocery and clothing stores. Mail order purchases of all sorts will explode. The larger shopping centers, as we know them, will have tremendous difficulty, because of high vacancy rates and the decreasing number of people supporting them.
- (8) **Health care.** People will do more and more of their own doctoring at home. They won't go to a physician, dentist, or health facility unless they really have to. Also, I believe we will see more health care providers making old fashioned house calls again – physicians, druggists, nurses, etc.

Until the AIDS plague is contained and finally eradicated, I believe we can expect to see many socio-economic changes, only some of which I have described above. Changes are always difficult, but when they are forced upon us (by government, famine, war or pestilence), they are even more difficult and usually unpleasant.

Do you think the AIDS plague will affect the economy?

Comment: Yes, and I'm afraid adversely. I believe our country is now in a recession (and maybe even in the early stages of an economic depression) and the AIDS plague will make it deeper and longer. To top it off, the recession will make the AIDS plague worse because there will be less money available to fight it. In short, *each will make the other worse.* As the plague worsens, more people will become AIDS infected/dead and thus unable to work. This means less taxes for the government to collect, which in turn means less money to fight the plague with. If one carefully analyses the information in the media, this "circle of misery" is already a reality. The solution is easy – a healthy economy and a cure for AIDS, a solution which I am sorry to say is not even on the horizon at this writing.

How will the AIDS Plague affect America's health care and health care costs?

Comment: In one word – unbelievably! Today, it costs about $200,000/year to medically treat one person dying of AIDS (third stage of AIDS). It costs $8,000 – $10,000/year to treat an AIDS patient (any stage) with AZT (a drug to prolong the life of an AIDS-infected person). Imagine what the costs would be treat 1 million AIDS-infected people with AZT *($10 billion/yr)* or 1 million people dying with AIDS *($200 billion /yr)*. How about treating 10 million AIDS-infected people with AZT *($100 billion/yr)* or 10 million AIDS-dying people *($2 trillion/yr)*. As high as these numbers are, they are nothing compared to what they will be when many millions (20+, 50+, 100+, ?) of America's 250 million people are AIDS-infected and dying. Who will pay these astronomical medical bills? The AIDS patient or his family? the government? You or me? I doubt it! I wish I had the answer, but I don't. All I know is we have an AIDS economical nightmare just in front of us, and sooner or later, somebody must face it – you can count on that!

As the AIDS plague worsens, so will the "fear of AIDS"; and because of this fear, more and more health care workers (physicians, nurses, laboratory technicians, etc.) will leave the medical profession – they already are! This, and the fact that less people will enter the health care profession, will result in a worsening shortage of health care workers to care for all sick people, let alone the AIDS-infected people. I foresee the government encouraging heath care workers to stay on the job with various incentives. All this will certainly increase the costs of medical care. Also, I think, both the life and health insurance industries will be decimated, once the AIDS plague accelerates its pace of infecting and killing. Anybody expecting any financial help, from these institutions for future AIDS healthcare, will be sadly disappointed.

In the near future, hospitals and hospices specializing in AIDS only will spring up, primarily for two reasons. One is to separate the contagious AIDS-infected patients from patient with other illnesses and the other, is to offer these unfortunate people more specialized health care. Again, all this will certainly increase health care costs.

Yes, the future of health care in the AIDS plague looks depressing and bleak. All we can do is the best we can do – *and we will do it!* I only hope the government and the medical profession finally admit what AIDS really is – a lethal, 100% fatal, medical, contagious disease – and start immediate effective treatment/research/prevention programs to control/eradicate it. Right now, I fear they are both underestimating the seriousness of the AIDS threat. As a result, I fear many more people will become unnecessarily AIDs-infected and AIDS dead. Their continued refusal to admit the obvious will also help increase the health care costs to even more unbelievable heights, a trait which delayed medical care is notorious for.

In any event, America's present form of health care is doomed and will soon change. The horrendous AIDS health care costs of the near future insures this change. What kind of health care will result is anybody's guess, but my bet is *"not very good!"*

What does all the "doom and gloom" talk of AIDS mean?

Comment: It means *hard times* ahead for all of us – like it or not, justified or not, fair or unfair, deserved or not. All we can do at this time is learn all we can about the AIDS virus and the disease it causes, learn how to best protect ourselves from the AIDS infection, see and foresee the problems AIDS is/will/might cause (so we can protect ourselves when they do occur) and *pray for an AIDS cure*. We have nothing to gain by ignoring, denying or minimizing the AIDS plague; but we have everything to lose – not only our lives, but our country as well.

Why are most physicians content to sit back and let government and special interest groups run the "War on AIDS"?

Comment: I don't really know, I can only surmise. I think physician ego, greed, AIDS-complacency, stubbornness, laziness, selfishness, fear, AIDS-ignorance, AIDS-uninformed, shortsightedness, and a few other not so nice adjectives all play some part in most physicians' reluctance to see the AIDS danger and speak out against it. A few of us are speaking out, warning America of the coming AIDS disaster, but at a heavy price. Just like Dr. Smart, the physician in the short story ("The Secret") in the front of this book, most of our colleagues are calling us alarmists, extremists, "casandras," etc. However, as time passes, we are convincing more and more of our colleagues that we are correct – the AIDS plague is rapidly becoming America's greatest problem and danger. Physicians, in general are good people and they certainly mean well, but please remember, physicians are human too – at least, I'd like to think so. Like all people, they won't admit there is a problem until there really is a problem – in this case, AIDS-sick and AIDS-dead people all around them. When physicians as a group finally see and admit AIDS is the problem I believe it is, you will see them take the lead in the "War on AIDS" – whether government, special interest groups, or anybody else likes it or not. We American physicians may occasionally be bad businessmen/women or arrogant or conceited or money hungry or whatever nasty thing we are often called, but one thing I know most of us are – *the providers of the highest quality medical care in the world.* It is this truism of my profession which tips the scales towards man's advantage in his war against the AIDS virus. It is this truism that should give hope to all HIV-infected people today. It is this truism, I believe, which will ultimately save America!

What are the hospitals doing to protect their health care workers and patients from the AIDS virus?

Comment: Most American hospitals are doing little, if anything, to HIV protect their health care workers. Worse yet, they aren't doing much to HIV protect their patients or their visitors. Unfortunately, hospitals don't insist on AIDS testing *any* patients or health care workers, let alone all of them. They don't even separate HIV-infected patients from patients with other illnesses, which would be considered sacrilege if done with any other lethal contagious disease. In fact, they don't even inform their health care workers which patients in the hospital have a diagnosis of AIDS (unless they are directly involved in the AIDS patient's care) so they can better protect themselves. In short, American hospitals do what they want when they want about AIDS. Why? The main reason is because there is no national AIDS policy to HIV protect people, *which everyone in the country must follow,* including hospitals. However, even though no such AIDS policy exists, responsible hospitals should be practicing stringent AIDS precautionary measures *voluntarily,* because *all hospitals should know this is good medicine.* Since they are not, why not? The answer should be obvious. *It is because not all people, that make hospitals function, are at equal risk for the HIV infection!* The hospital people with most HIV risk have the least say, the health care workers who give "hands on patient care" (physicians, nurses, technicians, housekeepers etc.). The hospital people with no "hands on patient care" have the least HIV risk, but they have the most to say about what is and what is not done in the hospital (administration, Board of directors, stockholders, bond holders, etc.). So you see, the "hands off" hospital people don't think the HIV danger is as great or as serious as the "hands on" people do, because *they aren't worried about getting HIV-infected;* therefore, the priorities for the hospital AIDS protective measures are and remain near the bottom of most hospital priority lists. If the "hands off" people were made to care for patients also, you would see AIDS protective measures at the top of hospital priority lists real fast – *you can bet on that!* I suggest the "hands off" people recognize, respect and address the AIDS fears of the "hands on" people, because if they don't, the hospital work force will melt away before their very eyes. Anyway, if hospitals implemented effective AIDS protective measures, the higher costs would greatly cut into hospital profits, thus adversely affecting the higher salaries, bonuses, and dividends of hospital administration and supporters. AIDS information, AIDS education, AIDS protective gear, "AIDS only" rooms and wards, AIDS precaution literature and posters etc. *All* cost money – *big money.* Don't get me wrong, we need hospitals. We need them badly, but we don't need them to help the AIDS virus (HIV) infect and kill us. Hospitals, along with the medical profession, must take the initiative and do what is right and responsible to protect the susceptible public from the HIV, no matter what the cost or the inconvenience. I urge you to visit your local hospital and make sure it has adequate AIDS policies to protect people in the Hospital (health care workers, patients and visitors) from the AIDS virus. If not, *demand* the hospital administration institute such HIV policies immediately, for the best interests of your community. If your demands are ignored, I suggest you support another hospital, one which is more "AIDS conscious." There is no time to only hope such protective AIDS policies are implemented voluntarily, it is time for public pressure to force all hospitals to comply. I don't mean to criticize hospitals unjustly and I certainly don't enjoy doing it, but in this case I feel I must. Like government, special interest groups and the medical profession, hospitals must recognize we have an AIDS plague on our hands and all must take immediate steps to protect the American people – *NOW!*

The above questions are but some of the many questions I have been asked, but they are what I believe to be the more important ones. My comments reflect basically what I believe and what I think about AIDS. They are intended to help people understand the HIV and the AIDS disease and to help people help themselves, which has been the purpose of me writing this book. In any event, my radio experience has certainly confirmed my conclusions – the majority of America's people are AIDS-uninformed and AIDS-complacent or AIDS-concerned and AIDS-scared. However, as the AIDS plague worsens and becomes more obvious, this will certainly change. Then, and only then, will America admit she has a problem, *a big problem – AIDS!* When this happens, I expect many changes in America's government and society, many of which will be very unpleasant indeed.

CHAPTER XI

THE FINAL CHAPTER: AUTHOR'S CRITICS ANSWERED

Wherefore I perceive that there is nothing better, than that a man should rejoice in his own works; for that is his proportion: for who shall bring him to see what shall be after him?
                                                          Ecclesiastes 3:22

    Many questions and doubts have probably arisen in readers' minds as they have read this book and digested its contents. Some of them may have been answered as they read on and some not. Many readers either believe or at least entertain much of what I have written. However, because of the controversial subject matter, I am aware that many readers doubt some of my opinions and comments.
    Consequently, the best way to answer many of these questions and to relieve the tension of some of the author's critics is to make this closing chapter an interrogatory, which can also serve as a summary of the book's principal points.

Critic: You have repeatedly stressed that our nation's leaders are treating AIDS as a political and not a medical disease, and that you seriously object to this. What gives you the right and what qualifications do you have to take such a position?

Author: I am a board-certified obstetrician/gynecologist and have been in solo private practice for more than twenty-five years. Every week I see more than a hundred patients, all of whom have some sort of medical problem and come for medical care. They depend on me to treat them professionally and competently, in the best manner I can.

I feel I have a moral, ethical, and legal obligation to do this, because this is how I was trained. Recently, however, the government, medical insurance companies, and medical bureaucrats have stepped in between the physician and his patient, thus breaking down their relationship. As a result, I feel the health care system is breaking down from high costs and almost unbearable legal regulations, liability, and roadblocks. All of this often interferes with the amount, type, and quality of care physicians can provide for their patients.

AIDS is a mystery to everybody – to you, to me, *and* to the so-called AIDS experts. Being a practicing physician, I can tell you AIDS is a contagious medical disease. There is no cure or vaccine for it; therefore, it kills almost all of its victims.

Knowing this, our politicians and medicrats still want us to value the "human rights" of the few dying AIDS-infected people over the lives of the millions of AIDS-free people. Of course, I care about the AIDS-infected patients, but no more than all other patients. All patients should get the best medical care we can give them, but without political or legal interferences.

As a nation, we must first protect our AIDS-free people – at all costs – if we want to give our country a chance to survive. The AIDS virus knows nothing about "human rights," it knows only how to kill humans. It must be attacked medically, not politically. This is why I say AIDS is a medical disease, not a political disease, and must be recognized and attacked as such.

Critic: Doctor, don't you think your "doom and gloom" scenario for AIDS is a bit exaggerated? How can you, and I suppose a few like you, be so dogmatic?

Author: No, I do not think I'm exaggerating one bit. In fact, I fear the situation is far worse than I have stated. Time, I believe, will unfortunately prove me correct. What amazes me more than anything is the complacency of the people and leaders about the entire AIDS problem, yet they seem to fear so many other, lesser life-threatening things.

Almost every day the established media tells us that this or that can cause cancer, brain damage, death, birth defects, and premature births, or cause us to be poisoned, hurt or maimed. The American people almost appear to enjoy always being frightened or in some sort of danger, and the media gives us more and more of this type of irresponsible information.

This being the case, what happened to AIDS? If anything should satisfy people's thirst for danger and the media's delight in frightening people with horrific health news, it's AIDS. Where's the media now? Why isn't it reporting the *real* AIDS threat?

I believe it's because the AIDS issue is too frightening, too life threatening, too real, *too political* and *too bad for good business*. Also, the media and the leaders are afraid of causing the people to panic if they are told the truth. I believe, however, that if people are given the truth about AIDS, instead of pabulum, they would "dig in" and face the AIDS threat head on. That's our nature and this nature is what helped make our country such a great nation. I repeat, I don't think I'm exaggerating!

Critic: The government is spending millions of dollars on AIDS research and researchers are working around the clock, trying to develop a vaccine against the AIDS virus. But you say a vaccine is impossible. Don't you think you could be wrong?

Author: I said the development of an AIDS vaccine is improbable, not impossible. The AIDS virus is mutating too rapidly for the development of an effective vaccine. Since there are so many trillions of different genetic combinations of the AIDS virus, I feel it is almost impossible for one vaccine to protect us from all of them.

However, this rapid mutating ability of the AIDS virus may be a blessing in disguise, because it could mutate into a predominantly benign form. In a fascinating movie called "The Andromeda Strain," an extremely contagious and lethal virus was rapidly killing all forms of animal life, including humans, in a small American town. Nothing could or did stop the virus' destruction – except itself. It mutated into a harmless benign strain. There is no reason to believe the AIDS virus could not do the same – at least, let us hope so.

Critic: Doctor, you stated that organized medicine's leaders are being irresponsible about the AIDS problem. Don't you think this is an irresponsible statement on your part?

Author: No. Because of organized medicine's silence and lack of leadership, physicians on the front lines have had to fight AIDS with their hands literally tied. They are forced to ignore their training as physicians and treat AIDS as a disease which has legal, civil, and moral rights. They cannot freely test patients for AIDS; they cannot freely tell people that they are or have been in contact with AIDS-infected patients; and they cannot even tell other physicians that they are treating AIDS patients.

When performing surgery on an AIDS-infected patient,

for example, physicians often cannot tell the rest of the surgical team that the patient has AIDS. I believe these health workers have a right to be able to choose whether or not they want to expose themselves to the AIDS virus.

The situation has become so bad that the protection of an AIDS-infected patient's human and civil rights comes before those of anybody else's. Patients come into the hospital and are indiscriminately mixed, whether they are high- or low-risk AIDS candidates or are AIDS-infected or not. The diagnosis of AIDS of a patient must be kept in strict confidence; hospital workers don't even know how many AIDS patients are being treated in the hospital at any one time. Because of this "special" treatment, physicians and other health care workers are forced to work in an environment of fear and danger – fear of both contracting the AIDS infection and of the discriminatory laws protecting the AIDS-infected people.

All this worsening insanity is presently enforced by law. The final result is predictable – a worsening shortage of physicians and nurses, a shortage of other health care workers and a raging AIDS plague, with all its horrors.

Organized medicine should not be supporting this ridiculous situation. Our medical leaders appear to have forgotten their responsibility to the public and have abandoned the rights and safety of their fellow physicians who work on the front lines. Their silence and lack of responsible leadership have placed the entire health profession and general public at great risk to the AIDS danger.

Critic: You have repeatedly stated that the rights of the AIDS-free people should come before those of the AIDS-infected people. Don't you feel you're discriminating against the AIDS-infected people by stating this?

Author: I believe civil and human rights of people are secondary to people's lives. We must realize that our nation, let alone the world, is in the early stages of a deadly AIDS plague. I feel that the issue of "discrimination" is unimportant when addressing this disease.

The real issue is who should be protected at all costs – the few dying AIDS-infected or the many AIDS-free people? Which of these two groups will live to work, reproduce, run the country, care for the sick and needy, and find an AIDS cure? *To say it is the AIDS-free group is not discrimination, it is reality.*

The very survival of our country depends on our recognizing the AIDS threat and taking rapid appropriate action. People need to be assured they will not be exposed to the AIDS virus, without their knowledge, just to satisfy some ridiculous law. People have good reason to fear the AIDS virus and a right to choose whether or not they want to expose themselves to it. They have a right to go to their doctor or dentist without worrying that they will unknowingly be mixed with AIDS-infected patients.

Health professionals who don't feel qualified or are unwilling to care for AIDS-infected people should not be intimidated or forced by law to do so. Physicians must be allowed to treat AIDS like the contagious and lethal disease it is. To do otherwise is national suicide.

Critic: You have repeatedly stated that the "fear of AIDS" is what concerns many physicians, as well as other health care workers. What do you mean by this statement?

Author: I mean far more than the fear of contacting the AIDS disease:

(a) The physicians' fear of accidently AIDS-infecting their

patients, friends, or families.
(b) The physicians' fear of the end of their medical careers if they become AIDS-infected.
(c) The physicians' fear of the adverse effect on their medical practices if people learn they treat AIDS-infected people.
(d) The physicians' fear of being shunned or boycotted by their AIDS-fearing colleagues, if they treat AIDS patients and/or are HIV infected.
(e) The physicians' own fear of contracting the AIDS disease and dying.

These are but a few of the fears physicians have. As the AIDS plague worsens, more fears will surely arise.

Critic: You said many physicians are retiring early and applications to medical schools have fallen off, a big reason being the "fear of AIDS." Have you taken any polls to confirm your statements?

Author: No, I have not taken any such poll, but the proof I have to support my statements is the "fear of AIDS" I see every day in the eyes, comments, and actions of physicians and other health care workers. Of course, there are many other reasons why physicians are leaving the practice of medicine and why the number of medical applicants to medical schools is dropping. Physicians today are being continually harassed by charges of fraud, incompetence, malpractice, and making too much money – all of which is beginning to make the practice of medicine as a whole a very stressful and unsatisfying profession. Add the "fear of AIDS" to the above (as well as the interference by government, medical bureaucrats, and insurance companies into the physician/patient relationship) and the result is a methodical decrease in the number and quality of physicians in America. Such a development will surely only aggravate the AIDS problem.

> As a point of interest, I am a member of the American Medical Association, California Medical Association, Santa Clara County Medical Society, American College of Obstetrics and Gynecology, American College of Surgeons, and the American College of Abdominal Surgeons and I have never been polled on anything concerning AIDS by these organizations.

Critic: Don't you think periodic mandatory HIV testing for everybody, as you recommend, is too expensive?

Author: Simply answered – NO! The AIDS virus is a contagious, deadly organism which will cause the plague of plagues – AIDS (if measures are not taken immediately to curtail it). This plague is now in its infancy and is found worldwide.

At this time, our only real weapon to combat this disease is to prevent its spread. No matter what the cost or inconvenience, we must all be tested for the AIDS virus and determine who is and is not AIDS-infected. I don't have all the answers on how to treat those who are AIDS-infected, nobody has; but I can say this, the AIDS-uninfected people must be protected from contracting the virus.

We are not dealing with a recoverable disease, like a cold or flu; we are dealing with a fatal disease. Anybody who does not take becoming AIDS-infected seriously is either "AIDS-ignorant" or a fool. I repeat, forget the cost and any other obstacle – test all people for the AIDS virus and take all precautions to help contain the spread of the AIDS plague. The sooner this is done, the more human lives will be saved and the better for the nation.

Critic: You stated that the AIDS virus can kill in two ways, indirectly by destroying the body's immune system and directly by destroying the body's central nervous system (CNS). How come we never see much evidence of the latter?

Author: The lack of information of CNS AIDS also concerns me very much. Most people don't even know CNS AIDS (AIDS dementia) exists, let alone know much about it. We know it is occurring, but we don't know to what extent.

We do know the AIDS virus often attacks and destroys the CNS, causing AIDS dementia and finally death, but we don't have any accurate statistics. Everyone seems to be concentrating on the immune system type of AIDS disease, completely ignoring the CNS AIDS dementia type.

This type of AIDS infection concerns me a great deal, because such an AIDS-infected person may be more dangerous to people from his progressive loss of brain cells and brain function, than from his being an AIDS-virus carrier. As an example, a CNS AIDS-infected person (who outwardly appears normal) could very well be an airplane pilot, a surgeon, or a bus driver. Unintentionally and accidently, such a person with brain damage could hurt and/or kill people because of his/her inability to perform his/her duties properly.

Early CNS AIDS-infected people have no outward physical signs and symptoms of a degenerating brain, which makes it very difficult to recognize them unless we have mandatory AIDS testing for everybody. **Imagine how terrible it could be, if one of our leaders (or worse yet, one of our enemy leaders) has AIDS dementia and his finger is on the red button, which fires off nuclear missiles.**

Critic: If the AIDS virus, and the disease it causes, is such a threat to the survival of mankind, then why aren't more people concerned?

Author: Throughout history, man's human nature and behavior is a constant and thus, man is destined to repeat his mistakes of the past. This being a truism, I expect the people of America to react as people have done in past plagues. They will remain unconcerned and complacent about AIDS until millions of people are visibly AIDS-sick, AIDS-dying, and AIDS-dead. Then, and only then, will all people know they are dealing with a worldwide plague – one that will most likely prove to be the plague of plagues.

Critic: Throughout this book, you have quoted statistic after statistic. How do the readers know they are accurate and of what real value are they?

Author: First, I want to emphasize that only a small percentage of our people are tested for AIDS ond only the AIDS-sick (third stage) patients are counted and reported as the number of AIDS cases in the United States. The known HIV-infected people of the first stage (asymptomatic) and the second stage (ARC), as well as the people with CNS-AIDS (AIDS Dementia), are not counted or included in the number of AIDS cases reported to the people by the government. Also, many AIDS infected people are not diagnosed and many diagnosed AIDS infected people are not reported. This deception, I feel, is deplorable and masks the true severity of the AIDS disease. A formula I use for a rough "guesstimate" **of the total number (all three stages) of living HIV-infected people in the United States is:**

(a) Multiply each reported AIDS-dead person by ten to get the probable number of AIDS-sick people (third

stage) alive.
(b) Multiply each AIDS-sick person by 100 to get the probable number of alive HIV-infected people in the first and second stages.
(c) Multiply each AIDS-dead person by 1000 to get the probable number of all alive HIV-infected (first, second, and third stage) people. **All these people have AIDS.**

Realizing the figures obtained by this formula are very rough, they do give you some idea of the number of AIDS-infected people that are probably alive. **Scary, isn't it!**

Second, the statistics available on AIDS are incomplete and many are questionable, but all show similar trends of the AIDS problems. These trends are most important:

(1) The number of American people being infected by the AIDS virus is increasing.
(2) The number of American people who become AIDS-sick is increasing.
(3) The number of American people who die of AIDS is increasing.
(4) The medical costs to care for American AIDS patients is increasing.
(5) The number of problems the AIDS virus and disease cause the people, society, economy, and government of America is increasing.
(6) The number of people worldwide, who become AIDS infected and eventually die of AIDS, is increasing.
(7) The horrors, misery and fear AIDS causes mankind is increasing.

While the scattered available statistics may not always be accurate, the trends they reflect are. These alarming trends show what the AIDS virus is doing and what we should expect it will do in the future. We need to use this information in our efforts to control the future course of the AIDS plague.

Critic: Since you are a practicing obstetrician/gynecologist in a high risk environment for the AIDS infection and since you are so concerned about the AIDS problem, why are you still practicing medicine?

Author: I still practice medicine because it is my profession and my livelihood. I enjoy this work and try to do it well; but with the increasing interference by government and special interest groups, it is rapidly becoming less satisfying and more difficult to do properly, especially in light of the increasing AIDS problem.

Each physician and health care worker has to personally decide if and how they will work with the AIDS problem. As the AIDS plague worsens, the decision as to whether to treat or not treat AIDS-infected patients will become more and more difficult for all health care providers to make. As time goes on, the "fear of AIDS" will grow and spread throughout the medical community, further complicating the already complicated AIDS medical care problems.

Critic: You believe AIDS can be transmitted by means other than sex, from the cough or sneeze of an AIDS-infected person or the bite of an AIDS-contaminated insect. Since you are definitely in the minority on this point, don't you feel you could be wrong?

Author: Of course I could be wrong, but unfortunately I don't believe I am. The most important points concerning the transmission of the AIDS virus from person to person are:

(1) The AIDS virus is found in all the bodily fluids of an AIDS-infected human being.

(2) Blood (composed of blood cells and liquid), serum (the liquid portion of the blood), saliva, sputum, breast milk, semen and vaginal secretions are the bodily fluids where the AIDS virus is most likely to be found.

(3) The AIDS virus must reach the blood of an AIDS-free person, from where it can then invade the cells in the blood or in the central nervous system.

(4) There are many ways or modes for the AIDS virus to reach the blood of an AIDS-free person, but these ways vary tremendously in rate of success.

(5) The rate of success (for the AIDS virus to reach the blood and then infect an AIDS-free person) varies from "most likely" (**very efficient**), "likely" (**moderately efficient**) and "unlikely" (**inefficient**).

(6) Examples of these modes are:

    (a) **"Very efficient"** – The use of AIDS-contaminated needles; the use of AIDS-contaminated blood for transfusions; perverse sex practices, which help the AIDS virus reach the blood; AIDS-infected women who have babies; AIDS-infected mothers, who breast feed their babies.

    (b) **"Moderately efficient"** – Oral sex and French (deep) kissing; oral salivary contact between small children; needle-stick injuries with AIDS-contaminated needles; chance contact of sores or abrasions with AIDS-contaminated blood, serum, saliva or sputum.

    (c) **"Inefficient"** – Social kissing, inhalation of respiratory aerosols caused by coughing or sneezing; bites by blood-sucking insects.

(7) The AIDS virus is virulent and durable – it can stay alive and viable for 7-14 days in a dry state and longer in a liquid state. It can mutate often and there is no medicine to cure, or vaccine to prevent, the disease it causes.

With these points in mind, I believe that the AIDS virus can spread by many modes of transmission, including oral sex, kissing, and the aerosol of a sneeze or cough.

Why do we believe the bite of a mosquito can cause malaria, or the bite of a flea can cause the Black Plague, but not AIDS? We know the AIDS virus is much smaller than either of the other two infectious viruses and can be carried by a mosquito or flea in much larger numbers. Why do we not believe saliva from a kiss or the aerosol of a cough or sneeze can transmit the AIDS virus, when we know the AIDS virus can be found in the saliva or sputum of an AIDS-infected person? Why do we believe it impossible to get the AIDS disease from AIDS-contaminated clothes, plates, glasses, etc., when we know the AIDS virus can be activated from a dry state?

The evidence to support my position of multiple modes of AIDS transmission is beginning to surface. When enough evidence surfaces to convince most people I am correct, the AIDS problem will become the nation's most important issue, as well as nightmare.

Critic: Don't you think the massive AIDS education efforts by the government and organized medicine have been successful in helping the people understand the AIDS disease and its problems?

Author: I don't think the people are being AIDS educated properly. The true extent and severity of the AIDS disease is not being reported and is minimized; thus the American people are lulled into a sense of complacency and lack of concern for the AIDS virus. The AIDS education, if you can call it that, most physicians are presently getting is very superficial and more of a political/ethical/moral nature than of a medical/scientific nature. The end result is that we as a nation are unprepared to face the AIDS plague and our physicians are unable to treat the AIDS disease properly.

When the AIDS disease really surfaces and people by the millions become AIDS-sick or AIDS-dead, people will be horrified. The social, economic, political and medical problems the AIDS disease will cause will overwhelm the nation, including the very people who are supposedly educating us – the government and organized medicine. Our leaders must stop minimizing the severity of the AIDS disease and start telling us the truth. They must fully inform and educate the people about the severity, danger and extent of the AIDS virus and how to protect themselves from it.

Critic: Don't you think your statement that all pregnant women should be tested for AIDS is unnecessary and not cost effective?

Author: The HIV or AIDS test is expensive now; but if the test is mandatory for all pregnant women, its cost would quickly become very reasonable. The AIDS test should be mandatory for all pregnant women, because any such woman who tests positive is diagnosed as having the AIDS disease and is condered as having a high risk pregnancy. An HIV-infected pregnant woman can transmit the AIDS infection to her baby in more than 50% of the time; therefore, she should receive her obstetrical care in a facility which specializes in such high risk pregnancies. Here, this pregnant woman can receive the most appropriate care for the most favorable outcome for her and her baby. Also, she can be well counseled on how not to infect other people with the AIDS virus and herself with an opportunistic disease.

Critic: Should an AIDS-infected mother breast feed her baby? If not, why?

Author: A recent study by Dr. Stephanie Blanche of Necker Hospital, Paris (reported in the New England Journal of Medicine and the CDC AIDS Weekly August 14, 1989, Page 7) showed that AIDS-free babies who are breast fed by their AIDS-infected mothers are much more likely to become AIDS infected than if not breast fed. The AIDS virus in the cells of the colostrum and the free AIDS virons in both the colostrum and breast milk can infect the baby through the lining of the baby's mouth and/or stomach. This is a frightening observation because it shows the AIDS virus can infect humans when in the mouth or stomach. Knowing this, I ask you these few questions:

(1) Would condoms protect these babies from the AIDS virus?
(2) Can this same AIDS-contaminated breast milk infect adults, if they drink it?
(3) Can a person get AIDS-infected by eating AIDS-contaminated food or off AIDS-contaminated eating utensils?
(4) Can a person get AIDS-infected by drinking AIDS-contaminated liquids, like water, tea or milk?
(5) Can a person get AIDS-infected by inhaling the aerosol of a cough or sneeze from an AIDS-infected person?

The main point of the above questions is that the AIDS virus can find its way from a person's mouth, stomach, or intestinal tract to his/her blood stream, where it can/might then infect that person. If this mode of transmission becomes a common one, man is in deep trouble. In summary, I don't think an AIDS-infected mother should breast feed her AIDS-free baby. If she does, the baby's chances for becoming infected are extremely high.

Critic: You haven't mentioned any drug for the treatment of the

AIDS disease. Is there any such effective drug?

Author: There is no drug available to cure the AIDS disease at this time. There are some drugs for AIDS being used, but the most effective, recognized drug is AZT (Zidovudine), and it is only partially effective against the AIDS disease. This drug does not cure AIDS, it only retards its rate of growth; thus the AZT-treated AIDS victim can live longer.

There is a good side and a bad side of AZT. The good side is it can extend the life of an HIV-infected person. Hopefully, the AIDS patients on AZT therapy can thus stay alive until a cure is found. The bad side of this drug is as follows:

(1) AZT therapy is expensive. It costs $8,000 to $10,000 a year for a person to take this drug effectively.
(2) AZT is not effective for all HIV-infected people. Some are helped by it and some are not.
(3) AZT has side effects, some of which are severe or dangerous enough for a person to discontinue using the drug.
(4) Since an HIV-infected person in all three stages of the AIDS disease is contagious and infectious, the longer such a person lives, the more people this person can possibly infect.
(5) The economics of AZT therapy are frightening. Let us assume there are 1,000,000 (one million) HIV-infected people being treated a year with AZT.

   (a) The cost to treat these people will be $10 billion/year (1 million people x $10,000/year). The more people taking AZT, the higher the cost. Today, it is estimated by some people that up to 5 million people in America are HIV infected (all three stages). This means the cost of AZT therapy for all these people will be $50 billion/year (5 million people x $10,000/year).

(b) Continuing this exercise in mathematics, an AIDS-sick patient (where death is prolonged one year by AZT therapy) will cost somebody $210,000/year ($10,000/year for the AZT drug and $200,000/year for medical care of an AIDS patient in the third stage). This cost will continue each year the patient lives.

(c) If we estimate there are 10,000 AIDS-sick (third stage) people out of our example of one million, the medical costs would be 10,000 x $210,000 or $2.1 billion/year. Therefore, as more AIDS-sick people are kept alive, the higher the medical costs will be.

In summary, AZT appears to be a drug which does help HIV-infected people. But the questions we must all ask ourselves are:

(1) Is the prolongation of the AIDS disease worth this cost?
(2) Who will pay this cost?
(3) Can the HIV-infected people or their families afford this cost?
(4) Should this nation assume this cost?
(5) Can the nation afford this cost?

Several things are certain: medical costs for HIV-infected people are necessary, but if these medical costs are not controlled, our present medical system will soon be destroyed and our country, bankrupt.

Critic: Are you really serious about proposing mandatory HIV testing for all people getting married?

Author: *Absolutely.* Not only is it illogical, it is insane to require people to be tested for syphilis and German measles and not AIDS. The AIDS virus is infecting people by the millions, while the other two organisms combined are not. Since there is no cure, infection with AIDS is a death sentence. Infection by the other two disease is treatable and not lethal. If one or both people are unknowingly HIV-infected at the time they marry, their marriage is doomed from the very beginning.

If either or both parties test positive for AIDS, they should be well counseled as to what this means for them personally, for any pregnancies they may have, and for their friends and relatives. Also, the HIV-infected party should be appropriately counseled on how not to HIV infect AIDS-free people and treated. Lastly, anybody having any contact with the HIV-positive person should be found, informed, HIV tested, and counselled, as well. These are but a few of the reasons I believe people getting married should be tested for the AIDS virus.

Critic: Most people believe testing everybody for the AIDS disease is unnecessary, expensive and "overkill," but you advocate just the opposite, especially in the health care field. Don't you think, "just maybe," you are wrong?

Author: To make a long answer short – *NO! I think all people should be routinely tested for AIDS – including all patients and health care workers*. There are now many potential victims for the HIV in the health care environment – the patients in the hospital, the visitors in the hospital, all health care workers and patients going to a physician's or dentist's office. Since we are not routinely HIV testing everybody, we don't know who is and who is not AIDS-infected; thus all these people (patients, visitors and health care workers alike) can and do infect each other – one way or another. To mandatory AIDS test one group and not the others makes no rational sense, plus such a policy violates the legal and civil rights of those being forcibly AIDS tested. If a person walked into a health care facility and bubonic plague or smallpox was suspected, he/she would immediately be quarantined and appropriate testing for the diagnosis would be done as soon as possible. Once the diagnosis was confirmed, the patient would be treated under strict quarantine conditions. No one I can think of would say this violates this patient's human, legal or civil rights or anything else – *it is just accepted good medicine!* Why is AIDS different? Because AIDS in America is treated as a political disease, a disease with civil rights and not as the lethal, contagious, killer disease it is – *RIDICULOUS!* In summary, AIDS should be treated like any other lethal, contagious, infectious medical disease. America's population must be protected from the HIV and people with AIDS must be diagnosed and treated/counselled as soon as possible – *AMEN!*

Critic: Why do repeat yourself, especially the "doom and gloom" talk, so often in your book?

Author: It is a learning technique that really gets a point across and helps people remember/learn things. I have used this technique throughout my education and I know it is effective. So, I have purposely repeated much of the book's more important information and points to help the reader better understand and learn about the HIV and AIDS disease – a subject which is very complex and important, *to say the least*.

Critic: Doctor, you have repeatedly stated that the rights of the AIDS-infected people are inappropriately protected above those of the AIDS-free people by the government and special interest groups. Do you believe it is the moral and ethical duty of a physician to treat society in general, and the AIDS-infected people in particular?

Author: In America, every citizen has inalienable individual rights. This is a principal which assures us all life, liberty and the pursuit of happiness and has given us unmatched freedom and prosperity. Our society is composed of individuals, all of whom have these rights; therefore, no one has a duty to serve anybody unless he/she wants to. All of us must respect each other's inalienable rights, as guaranteed by the United States Constitution, or we will surely lose both our freedom and country.

So to answer your question – No! I do not think a doctor (or any other health care provider) has any duty to serve "society" or his "community," or to treat any patient (including an AIDS-infected patient) unless he/she voluntarily chooses to do so. To force any health care provider by any means to treat any patient against his/her wishes is a form of involuntary servitude and violates his/her personal rights. This principal also applies to all patients, not just AIDS-infected patients. When AIDS-free patients are treated by health care providers, their rights must be honored, just as equally as those of the AIDS-infected patients. The AIDS-free patients have the right to choose if they want to be treated or not treated by AIDS-infected health care providers or to be mixed or not mixed with AIDS-infected patients.

In fact, all people have the same right to know when they are being placed in a high risk AIDS environment, where the risk of HIV infection is increased. Presently, this is not the case. Our government and various special interest groups are unfortunately protecting and enforcing the inalienable rights of the AIDS-infected people over those of the AIDS-free people. This misguided, insane policy will surely insure the spread of the AIDS plague and exacerbate and multiply all the problems the AIDS virus is causing and will cause in America.

Critic: Why are you the only physician who is such an alarmist about the HIV and the AIDS disease?

Author: I am not the only physician who is trying to warn the public and the medical profession about the coming AIDS disaster. A few people like William Haseltine M.D., Robert Strecker M.D., William O'Conner M.D., Gene Antonio ("The AIDS Cover Up"), and George Green (American West Publishers) are also out there warning everybody who will listen. Unfortunately, the majority of people and the established media aren't listening – *not yet!* Soon, very soon, they will not only listen, *they will see!* People will then see the "Wrath of the HIV," which for many of them will be too late.

Critic: Why are you one of the few physicians, who is recommending everybody be AIDS tested regularly?

Author: I have given my reasons repeatedly throughout the book why and how often everybody should be tested for the HIV infection, but I cannot answer why most physicians aren't recommending such HIV testing also. Why America's Infectious Disease physicians aren't screaming and demanding everybody be regularly HIV tested (with all the available evidence that AIDS is a *lethal, fatal, infectious, contagious, medical disease*) baffles me. Also, why aren't the medical leaders in the obstetrical field demanding regular HIV testing for all pregnant women? Are these physicians AIDS uninformed or fearful of the consequences or playing politics or catering to special interest groups or just plain irresponsible? You choose the answer, but let me help you a little – I doubt if they are AIDS uninformed.

Critic: In closing, Doctor, what final suggestion or advice do you have for the readers to consider?

Author: My final comment is that we, as a nation, must find out how serious the AIDS plague really is – NOW! Once we truly know the extent of the disease, appropriate and prompt action must be taken.

Organized medicine needs to assume its abrogated role as the leader in this war with the AIDS virus. Throughout history, the medical profession has led the fight against diseases and plagues, but not in the case of AIDS. So far, America's medical profession has allowed government, business groups, special interest groups, etc. to interfere with its duty to protect the health and safety of the nation's people from the AIDS virus.

If AIDS is far worse than we now know or suspect, we must proceed with much more aggressive methods of containing and managing it. Many of these methods may be unpleasant, and some even appear inhuman, but they must be done if the AIDS plague is to be fought successfully.

As a start, I recommend we begin by anonymously AIDS testing all people (babies, adults, males, and females of all races) who die from anything – including suicides, accidents, old age, disease, and murder. *This, I believe, will give us a much better perspective of the extent of the AIDS plague today.* Once accomplished, we should expand the AIDS testing to everybody alive, as soon as feasible. If the disease is much more prevalent (as I suspect), *we must stop rationalizing and begin aggressive, appropriate action against the AIDS virus!*

"HAPPINESS USA REVISITED" 1995

We have piped unto you, and ye have not danced;
we have called unto you, and ye have not answered;
we have mourned unto you, and ye have not wept.
Luke 7:32

After Jill Well died of AIDS, the Well's "secret" became common knowledge. Even though Dr. I. M. Smart was correct in honoring Jack and Jill's "secret," both ethically and legally, the town held him responsible for the AIDS infection of so many other innocent people. Within months his reputation as a good obstetrician was slipping, as was his medical service. His friends disappeared, his colleagues avoided him and his patient load melted away. Professionally, he was ruined. "Why and how did this happen – especially to me? Maybe if I tell everybody what the 'secret' has taught me about AIDS, I can save many lives. Maybe I can even save my deteriorating medical practice. Yes, that's what I'll do. I know they will listen and understand – after all, this is a wonderful place, full of understanding loving people!" thought Dr. Smart.

For the next six months, Dr. Smart proceeded to warn everybody who would listen about the dangers of the AIDS virus. He told them he was originally complacent and uninformed about the AIDS disease. As a result, he failed to diagnose Jill's AIDS earlier and thereafter take proper precautions. Also, his failure subjected many unsuspecting people around Jill to the AIDS virus. He urged all people to get tested for AIDS, to respect the AIDS virus, to consider anybody who is AIDS-infected as contagious and sick at **all** times, to **always** use precautions from the AIDS virus, to expose all other "secrets," to encourage the town leaders to pass laws which protect the AIDS-free pubic, to always remember AIDS has no cure or vaccine, to always remember AIDS is literally a death sentence and much, much more. He warned the people, time and time again, that if they didn't heed the dangers of the AIDS virus, the disease it causes (AIDS) would surely destroy both them and their town. Dr. Smart used every means he knew of to inform, educate and warn the town's people about AIDS – the radio, the newspaper, flyers, person to person, television, etc.

As time passed, more and more people began to call Dr. Smart a lunatic, an alarmist, a madman – every derogatory name they could think of. His nickname became "Cassandra Smart M.D." Instead of heeding his warnings and learning from his disastrous experience with AIDS, the people of Happiness USA laughed at him and continued their daily routines, without any concern or thought about AIDS. AIDS is a problem for the people of Africa or Haiti or Brazil – for everybody but them, they rationalized. After all, they weren't homosexual, drug addicts or any other such high risk group, which the HIV attacks and infects. The verbal attacks and abuses continued, not only against Dr. Smart, but against his family as well. His wife and two children were increasingly harassed, ridiculed and berated – in the grocery store, in school, in church, etc. It was one thing to see his practice ruined but quite another to watch his family slowly destroyed. No way would he allow that. Enough was enough! Humiliated, discredited and frustrated, Dr. Smart finally left town with his family. Why? Because Dr. Smart had to protect his family and had to make a livelihood, which he could no longer do in Happiness USA. Also, he had decided to specialize in the treatment and prevention of AIDS. He was convinced that someday soon, such AIDS specialists/experts would be needed, and they would be the only hope the nation would have to lead it out of the AIDS plague – **maybe!**

Five years passed and Dr. Smart's predictions and warnings blossomed – the AIDS plague was raging in Happiness USA. Over sixty percent of the people were thought to be AIDS-infected and thousands were already AIDS-dead. The AIDS Plague and the fear of AIDS virus (HIV) had literally paralyzed the city. At first, the mayor (Mr. N. O. Leader) appealed to his fellow politicians, as well as to the business and medical communities, for any help or suggestions. When this failed, he then **pleaded** for their help to stop the plague – but to no avail. Nobody knew how, or even where to begin. The town was dying, right before their eyes. Finally, the President (M. A. Fathead, M.D.) of the local medical society had an idea. He remembered his old friend Dr. Smart. He knew he had specialized in AIDS prevention and treatment after he left Happiness USA, and was now one of the leading AIDS experts in the country. "Why not ask Dr. Smart back to Happiness USA to help save it from the AIDS plague? After all, he owes it to the people, who once supported him for so many years before he left." thought Dr. Fathead. Thinking this a great idea, Dr. Fathead consulted with Mayor N. O. Leader. Both agreed the idea was brilliant and to fully cooperate with Dr. Smart, if they could convince him to return. So, Dr. Fathead promptly telephoned Dr. Smart and asked him for his help. Of course Dr. Fathead first apologized for the dismal way the people treated Dr. Smart the last year he was in Happiness USA, and then proceeded to plead with him for his help. Even though he was literally run out of town, Dr. Smart put his personal feelings aside and agreed to return to help control the AIDS plague. He felt it was his duty as a human being and as a physician to help, that is if he could.

As Dr. Smart drove into the little town of Happiness USA, he couldn't help but recall the many reasons he left his private practice in 1990 and went back into medical training, to become a well known specialized AIDS expert. Such memories as Jack and Jill's terrible "secret" (which resulted in the AIDS infection and death of so many innocent people), the AIDS-complacency of the people, the eagerness of attorneys to profit from AIDS litigation and the ever mounting cases of AIDS all flashed thru his mind. Now, he thought, he was willing, ready and qualified to address the AIDS plague. But how does he start and from which direction does he begin?

Throughout the next day, Dr. Smart drove all over town and talked to many people. What he saw and what he heard horrified him. The situation was much worse than he had imagined.

• The AIDS plague was obviously raging and out of control.

> Over 60% of the people were obviously AIDS-infected and many people had already died from AIDS. The cemeteries were literally overflowing with "customers".
> - Unbelievable numbers of houses and shops were empty or boarded up. "For Sale" and "for lease" signs were everywhere.
> - Shopping centers were sparsely occupied and some were even abandoned, their parking lots being used by children as playgrounds.
> - Empty lots throughout the town were overgrown with weeds and littered with garbage.
> - Business activity was virtually at a standstill, because of the people's obvious "fear of AIDS". Theaters, hotels, restaurants, and other such public gathering places were either closed or on the verge of closing. In short, where the AIDS virus was "thought" to be, the people avoided.
> - The town's public hospital was closed, because of the lack of funds. The other private hospital was chuck full of patients – **mainly AIDS patients**. Also, there was an apparent shortage of physicians, nurses and other health care providers.
> - The town's infrastructure was in need of drastic repair:
>   - Streets were full of potholes.
>   - Sidewalks were falling apart.
>   - Sewers were plugged.
>   - many street lights were broken or burned out.
>   - City buildings were dirty and badly in need of paint and repair.
>   - Garbage and litter were everywhere.
>   - Policemen were few and far between.
> - Many complaints of poor or lacking city services (police, garbage, transportation, social services, etc.) were heard everywhere.
> - The "Fear of AIDS" was noticeable everywhere (on people's faces, in the newspapers on the radio, etc.). The wrath of AIDS seemed to have engulfed the town.
> - The town's government was obviously collapsing. The lack of funds resulted in huge cutbacks (employees, city services, city

business, salaries, etc.) which created and exposed the town to many other dangers and problems (poor police/fire protection, deteriorating social services, etc.).
- The public schools were half full and in terrible condition.
- To say the town's economy was depressed, would be a gross understatement.
- Crime was commonplace and worsening with time. The streets at night were essentially barren. Anyone on the streets at night was asking for trouble and usually got it.

Dr. smart knew the AIDS plague would be bad when he arrived, but not this bad. He concluded the AIDS complacency of the people, the disastrous AIDS policies of the town government (which still considered AIDS a political disease instead of a lethal, contagious, medical disease), the lack of the medical community's duty and responsibility to protect the public from the AIDS virus (HIV) and the counter productive actions of various self-serving special interest groups all helped expose the town to the "wrath of the HIV".

Several days after his arrival, Dr. Fathead and Mayor Leader met Dr. Smart in the mayor's office at city hall. Both thanked Dr. Smart for coming and proceeded to tell him of the sorry state the town was obviously in. They asked him to take all the time he needed to assess the situation and thereafter, recommend what the town and people could do to control the AIDS plague, to treat the AIDS-infected people and to get the town back on its feet. Dr. Smart said he already had seen and heard some of the problems but would like to take two or three more days to thoroughly evaluate the seriousness of the plague. Then he said he would make his recommendations. Mayor Leader said "Take all the time you need and please remember, money is no problem. If you need any assistance, just ask. We are at your command." After a delicious lunch, the only pleasant part of the meeting, everybody left with some degree of hope for success.

For the next few days, Dr. Smart continued to interview more people and literally drive up and down every street in town. The principal of the only high school told Dr. Smart the school was half empty because of both the lack of funds and the "Fear of

AIDS." He said that many parents would not allow their children to come to school for fear of them getting AIDS-infected and this was the main reason for the lack of students. This same "Fear of AIDS" was heard again and again throughout the community. As stated before, the town's only open hospital was overflowing with patients, 80% of which were AIDS-infected. This resulted in a terrible shortage of hospital beds for people with other illnesses. The health care workers, most of whom were AIDS-infected, were not well AIDS-informed or AIDS-educated and were in short supply. Dr. Smart heard many people complain that the mounting needs of the AIDS-infected people were causing many problems and shortages throughout the town – hospital beds, health care funds, funds for town services, housing, etc. Wherever Dr. Smart went, he found no separation, quarantine or isolation of AIDS-infected from AIDS-free people. In fact, no one knew who was AIDS-tested and who was not, or who was HIV-infected and who was not. The little AIDS testing done was voluntary and all test results were strictly confidential. In fact, it was strictly against the law to tell anybody who was HIV-infected without the written consent of the HIV-infected person. To do otherwise was a civil offense, punishable by heavy fines and even incarceration (jail). Physicians told Dr.smart their hands were literally tied by legal restraints (breech of confidentiality and discriminatory suits, fines, penalties, etc.), when dealing with the AIDS disease. They too could not AIDS test anybody unless they had their patients written permission and they too could not tell anybody (the local department of public health or even other health care workers) which of their patients had AIDS. Shades of the "Secret" – **nothing had changed in the past five years.** The physicians were being politically and legally forced to literally treat AIDS as a venereal disease with "civil rights" instead of the contagious, 100% lethal, medical disease it is. The law protected the AIDS-infected people at the expense of the health of the rest of the public. **An insane situation!** In summary, Dr. Smart saw chaos, confusion, death, fear, depression, deception, anger and despair every where he went. "What a blooming mess! This is a nightmare of nightmares!" he thought.

After his investigation of the town and its people, Dr. Smart *formulated his thoughts on what to do and say., Finally, he again met with Dr. Fathead and Mayor Leader and asked to address the town, both on radio and television. He wanted to tell everybody what he had to say at the same time. Dr. Fathead and the mayor were at first surprised by this strange request, but agreed to abide by his wishes. The next few days, Dr. Smart's presentation was widely promoted. The people were told Dr. Smart was going to tell them how to stop the AIDS plague dead in its tracks. The people were elated and their hopes went higher and higher with each passing minute. Finally, they thought, someone was going to save them from this killer AIDS virus. Thank God for Dr. Smart, we knew he would save us!*

One week after Dr. Smart arrived, he addressed the town on live T.V. and radio. He spoke at 8 pm, hoping everybody could then hear him. As he looked at his notes, he slowly began:

"As you may recall, five years ago, I lost a patient to the AIDS disease, here in Happiness USA. Because of that experience, I was convinced we were facing a lethal disease – a disease which could reach plague proportions and which could literally destroy Happiness USA and even our nation, as we know it. I then proceeded to warn you time and time again about this potential AIDS threat. My reward was for me and my family to eventually be run out town – discredited, humiliated, alone and penniless. That, however, was in the past and now unimportant."

"Now, Happiness USA is in the grips of the AIDS plague of which I warned you about and now, you ask me to return to help you. Since I am a conscientious physician and since many of you were once my cherished patients, I came. And so, for the past seven days I have evaluated your dilemma. In short, your town is now besieged by the killer AIDS virus and is literally in shambles."

"Not only have thousands of people died from AIDS, but thousands of people are now AIDS-infected and dying, and others, who are AIDS-free, are leaving Happiness USA. To make matters worse, very few new people are moving into your town because of the AIDS plague. As more and more of you leave or die, more vacancies are created in both the residential and commercial sectors, and more businesses either close or go bankrupt. Since there are less

people and less businesses to pay taxes, the town collects less tax money to keep its government properly running. This in turn is resulting in the deterioration of the towns infrastructure (streets, sidewalks, etc.) and services (police, fire, garbage, etc.). Also, with less police to enforce the law, crime is now increasing, adding to your plight. As the plague continues to worsen, the "fear of AIDS" will also continue to increase. So, because of more AIDS fear and more crime, more people will leave Happiness USA. This vicious cycle will unfortunately continue until the town is literally empty of people, unless the AIDS plague is contained. I estimate over 80% of you, not 60%, are already HIV-infected and in one of the three stages of AIDS. Since there is no separation of AIDS-free from AIDS-infected people, since no precautions against the AIDS virus are being practiced or encouraged and since there is very little AIDS testing being done, no one really knows who is or who is not HIV-infected or how severe the AIDS plague is. As things now stand, the remaining 20% AIDS-free people will probably not be AIDS-free for very long. What do you expect when:

- *There is no mandatory AIDS testing for everybody. Worse yet, there is even no testing of people serving the public (physicians, dentists, nurses, bus drivers, cooks, airplane pilots, etc.) or people getting married or women having babies or people going to hospitals or high risk people (for the HIV infection). Why?*
- *I see very few precautions against the AIDS virus being practiced by any of you. There are virtually no such precautions in your restaurants, theaters, shops and other such public gathering places.* **Not even in your hospital!** *Why? Are you purposely on a course of self-destruction?*
- *There is no treatment or counselling of known AIDS patients or available facilities that specialize in the AIDS disease. This is not a disease which anybody can treat. It is too complicated and too lethal!*
- *You people out there who are AIDS-infected... don't you realize you are sick?* **Super Sick!** *You are not "just like anybody else!" Your immune systems are slowly and methodically being destroyed by the AIDS virus; thus you are increasingly at risk to*

contract other diseases, that your damaged immune systems cannot protect you from. These diseases can and will kill you. Civil rights, human rights, discrimination, breech of confidentiality, etc. are important issues in a healthy society, but their importance is secondary when that society is being besieged and destroyed by a deadly disease like AIDS. You must protect yourselves at all times from these secondary so called "opportunistic diseases," which can and will shorten your already shortened lives. **Your goal is to stay alive until a cure for AIDS is hopefully found and, just as important, to not infect others with the AIDS virus.** *Why is this so difficult for you to understand?*

- *AIDS-free and AIDS-infected people intermingle as if there is no problem or danger. The problem and danger is that each can infect the other with a killer disease – the former infecting the latter with an opportunistic disease and the latter infecting the former with the AIDS virus. Why can't or don't any of you want to believe this?*
- *There is no isolation, quarantine, or separation of any kind of AIDS-infected people from the rest of the public.* **Not in restaurants, not in theaters, not in schools, not in hospitals, not anywhere!** *Why?*
- *Most of you still consider the AIDS disease as a political or venereal disease, which it is not. You don't believe, or don't want to believe, AIDS is a lethal, fatal, contagious medical disease of all people. Why? How much proof do you need?*
- *Most of you still think the AIDS virus has some kind of civil rights. This is absurd! The AIDS virus can infect and kill anybody, anyplace, and anytime –* **you and your town are living proof of this!**
- *Few of you seem to know there is no cure or vaccine for AIDS. Also, too many of you believe an AIDS cure or vaccine is just around the corner –* **wrong, it is not!**
- *Too many of you treat the AIDS disease as a disease of other people, until you (or one of your family) are AIDS-infected. Then, you become concerned and finally realize what it really is – a death sentence!*

- *Your local government is in shambles and unable to govern the town properly. Have you wondered why? For two reasons. One is for lack of funds from taxes, but this is understandable and correctable. The second, however, is more serious and not understandable – the self-serving politicians in your government. The majority of them put their own interests (their salaries, their pensions, their reputations, their obsessions to stay in office, etc.) over those of the people they are supposed to govern and protect. Since their personal interests are more important than the health and welfare of the public, bad laws are proposed and passed and good laws are not even proposed, when addressing the AIDS plague. To do so, they believe, would jeopardize their political careers. How? Because they know effective laws to protect the people from the HIV and control the AIDS plague would alienate many of their supporters. I guess they never looked any further than the end of their noses to see there would be no elections and nobody to govern if the plague emptied the town of people and made it a ghost town. Unfortunately, this type of behavior (from the local to the federal level) is commonplace for many of our politicians across our nation.
- *Your medical community is not adequately prepared to deal with the AIDS plague, because it is AIDS-uninformed and AIDS-uneducated. Your only hospital is short of beds and terribly understaffed. It has no policies for the management of his disease. AIDS-infected and AIDS-free patients are mixed haphazardly, there are no AIDS educational programs for the health care workers, there is very little AIDS-testing being done, there is very little AIDS-protective equipment available for the health care providers, etc. The majority of the physicians are uninformed, misinformed or dysinformed about the AIDS disease. In fact, the entire hospital staff is as uninformed about AIDS as is the rest of the community. Maybe even worse! Why? Throughout the hospital, both patients and health care workers are terrified of being infected by the HIV. Since no AIDS precautions are practiced, I can see why. This "fear of AIDS" greatly interferes with the care of the sick, whether it

is AIDS or some other disease. Who is to be blamed for all this – **all of you, but especially my fellow physicians!** They should have prepared themselves long ago to manage this disease and led the war on AIDS, not follow it. Instead, they did nothing and now the AIDS plague is out of control, in and out of your hospital. Some of you might wonder, why didn't at least one physician in the community speak up and warn everybody about the AIDS danger. I again remind you, one once did and you ran him out of town. **Remember?**
- With all this pestilence, death, crime and fear around, you still have not taken any reasonable precautions on your own to protect yourselves from the AIDS virus. Why?

Now, when most of you are AIDS-infected and your town is decimated, you ask an AIDS expert (like me) to help you. You and your town have again proven that mankind does not admit he has a problem **until he really does have a problem!** Finally, however, you have admitted you have a problem, but not until most of you are dying or have died."

"I am sure you are now eagerly awaiting to hear the magic solution to your AIDS problem. Well, I am sorry to tell you that **there is no magic solution!** The AIDS plague has spread too far and has infected too many of you for any chance of such a solution for Happiness USA. God has given all of you a body and a brain to use wisely; but most of you have allowed, and even helped, the AIDS virus to infect both. I don't know why, but you have."

"Five years ago, I warned you what would happen if you failed to heed the dangers of the vicious AIDS virus and failed to take any necessary precautions to protect yourselves against it. You chose to ignore my warnings. Now, I do not have to say I told you so, **but I will!** Now, I do not have to say your town is dying, **but it is!** Now, I should say I am going to help you, **but I can't!** I want to, but I can't. Why? Because it is simply a matter of priorities. Happiness USA and its people are to far down the path of AIDS. You have waited too long to ask for help. What I am trying to say is there too little time and too little money left for the government or anybody else to save you. There are too many other towns and too many other people which/who still have a chance to survive, because there, the AIDS plague has not yet surfaced. **It is these people who I can and must help!** As I said, it basically comes down to a matter of priorities and Happiness USA, I hate to say, is at the bottom of the list. So in parting – goodbye, good luck, and may God help you."

As Dr. Smart drove out of Happiness USA, he looked back, shook his head and thought, "Why? Oh, why didn't they listen? Throughout the world, mankind is fighting a war for survival against the AIDS virus. Here in Happiness USA, there is no war because a war takes two opposing parties to fight. The attacking AIDS virus is feeding, not fighting, on the AIDS-complacent human fodder of Happiness USA. It's beyond me why this pathetic situation has been allowed to develop and to continue. All this misery and death was and is so unnecessary – what a nightmare! I really hope God does help them, because now I'm afraid, **nobody but God can help them!**"

Author's Comment: Unrealistic? Unbelievable? Exaggerated? I think not! One only has to research history to see what plagues can do to people and to countries. Again I repeat, man never learns from history – it is man's human nature and behavior to repeat his mistakes of the past. This, unfortunately, is man's greatest weakness – a weakness which may ultimately destroy him. Our present handling of the AIDS virus is proving we have not changed. We as a nation will not admit we have a problem until we really have a problem – in this case, people AIDS-sick and AIDS-dead all around us. Our "problem," I think, will unfortunately surface somewhere between 1993 and 1995. Then and only then will America admit she has a serious AIDS plague on her soil. Then and only then will the sleeping giant (America) awake and begin the real "war on AIDS." Happiness USA eventually realized it had an AIDS plague, but too late! Let's hope the good old USA doesn't make the same mistake.

DEFINITIONS

AIDS
- Acquired Immune Deficiency Syndrome
- A disease caused by the HIV (Human Immunodeficiency Virus)
- A disease composed of three stages:
    First Stage – the asymptomatic stage
    Second Stage – AIDS Related Complex stage (ARC)
    Third Stage – The AIDS-sick stage

AIDS-infected
- Refers to the first and second stages of the AIDS disease.

AIDS-sick
- Refers to the third stage of the AIDS disease.

ARC
- AIDS Related Complex, the second stage of the AIDS disease.

AIDS Dementia
- An infection of man's central nervous system by the HIV.

AIDS-uninfected
- Not infected by the HIV; free of the AIDS disease.

AIDS-free
- Not infected by the HIV; free of the AIDS disease.

AIDS-ignorant
- A person who is adequately informed about the HIV and the AIDS disease, but refuses to believe it.

AIDS-vulnerable
- A person at risk for the AIDS disease.

AIDS-expert	• A person who is well-informed about the AIDS disease.
AIDS-high risk	• A person who has a good chance of getting the HIV infection. • A place where the HIV is most likely to be found.
AIDS Environment	• An area where the HIV or AIDS disease is most likely to be found.
AIDS-contaminated	• Something or someone contaminated by the AIDS virus (HIV).
AIDS-test	• A test to detect the AIDS virus (HIV); a diagnostic test for the AIDS disease.
AIDS-uninformed	• Refers to a person who is not informed about the AIDS virus or disease.
Antigen HIV test	• A test to detect the AIDS virus (HIV), the organism which causes the AIDS disease.
Full-blown AIDS	• The third stage of the AIDS disease.
HIV	• Human immunodeficiency virus, the virus which causes the AIDS disease.
HIV test	• A test to detect the HIV; a diagnostic test for the AIDS disease.
HIV carrier	• Refers to a person who is infected by the HIV and who is contagious.
HIV-infected	• Infected by the HIV.
HIV-uninfected	• Not infected by the HIV.

HIV-free	• Not infected by the HIV.
HIV-contaminated	• Something or someone contaminated by the AIDS virus (HIV).

FOOTNOTES

(1) Margaret Kennedy, *Interest and Inflation Free Money*, Permaculture Institute Publications, Steyerberg, Federal Republic of Germany, 1988, pages 10-13.

(2) Ibid.

(3) Jonas and Jonat Salk, *World Population and Human Values*, Harper Books, 1981.

(4) *The Timing Device*, Vol IV-17, April 22, 1988 and Gene Antonio, *The AIDS Cover-up*, page 110.

(5) *The Merck Manual of Diagnosis and Therapy*, Fifteenth Edition, pages 288-294.

(6) Gene Antonio, *The AIDS Cover-up*, pages 14-15.

(7) Gene Antonio, *The AIDS Cover-up*, page 20.

(8) Dr. William Campbell Douglas, *The Cutting Edge* monthly newsletter, November 1987.

(9) Irene Wielowski, "AIDS virus not new, researcher says," *The Washington Times*, October 2, 1987.

(10) "The AIDS Epidemic: A Bio-Warfare Conspiracy?" *Health Freedom News*, May 1988.

(11) Dr. William Campbell Douglas, " Who Murdered Africa?" *The Cutting Edge* monthly newsletter, November 1987.

(12) Ibid.

(13) "Women with AIDS – cases grow, but risks relatively confined," *American College of Obstetrics and Gynecology Newsletter,* July 1988, page 10.

(14) "Early HIV Infection Appears Unaltered in Pregnancy," *OB-GYN News,* Vol. 23, No. 15, page 25.

(15) Gene Antonio, *The AIDS Cover-up,* page 12.

(16) "Children and AIDS," *Science News,* Vol. 134, page 72.

AUTHOR'S MESSAGE TO THE READERS 1989

Now that you have read this book, you are AIDS-informed. Use this information wisely. Use it to protect yourself and loved ones. Share it with your friends, neighbors and the people of your community. Write your local, state, and federal elected officials and insist they recognize AIDS as a contagious disease, not a political or venereal disease. Insist they tell the American people the truth about AIDS and they take immediate effective steps to protect the AIDS-free public. Insist they protect the rights and health of all people, not just the AIDS-infected people. Lastly, and most important, remind them that it is the working healthy public that pays the taxes that pays their salaries and runs America.

Remember, don't assume anything about the AIDS virus. Question all AIDS-information and evaluate it carefully before you believe or follow it. By so doing, you will always be increasing your chances of Surviving the AIDS Plague and its terrible consequences.

AUTHOR'S MESSAGE TO THE READERS 1991

It has been 2 years since my last message to the readers and what progress have we made against the AIDS virus? *Little if any!* The majority of the American people, including the health care professionals, are still AIDS uninformed and AIDS complacent. Why? *Mainly because our government and various self-interest groups are still leading the war against AIDS, with the medical profession far behind.* Where are our medical leaders who should be leading, not following, this war? Why isn't America HIV testing all her people, especially couples getting married and women having babies? Why is America allowing other countries' AIDS patients to enter her territory and endanger her people? Why isn't America protecting her HIV-free people from the AIDS virus? Why is America procrastinating in calling AIDS what it really is – a lethal, contagious, infectious disease which is worse than all the Bubonic Plagues of the past combined? Are we Americans waiting for our country to be inundated by the AIDS virus before we get concerned and angry? Is it when millions of our people are HIV-infected, HIV-sick and HIV-dead when we will say *enough*? Is it only then when we will seriously fight the AIDS virus? Gosh, I sincerely hope not!

It is time for America's "silent majority" to speak up, before it is too late. It is time to undo the damage the vocal, irresponsible "silent minority" has done – which has helped the HIV spread, infect and kill. The time for niceties or urging is past, now is the time for DEMANDING! DEMAND our government officially recognize the AIDS plague and make the protection of HIV-free people from the killer HIV its number one priority. DEMAND our government quit catering to the AIDS special interest groups and to the wants and needs/legal rights/health care/civil rights/human rights/ etc. of AIDS infected people *at the expense of the health of the country and its HIV-free people.* DEMAND the medical profession quit playing possum and start leading the war on AIDS. DEMAND your hospitals protect its health care workers, patients and visitors from the HIV. DEMAND your personal physicians put the pressure on their medical societies and health care facilities to start urging immediate legislation at all levels of government to contain the AIDS plague.

In short, we must all stop treating AIDS as a political/venereal disease with civil rights, *NOW!* In any society, moral and ethical issues and behavior are important; but when a society is being inundated and destroyed by a contagious disease (like AIDS), *responsible action against that disease is the most important and essential response for its survival!* We must win this "war against AIDS" – *there is no compromise, no option and little time!!!*

ABOUT THE AUTHOR

TAKI NICK ANAGNOSTON, M.D., a USAF veteran, is a board certified Obstetrician-Gynecologist who received his medical training at Stanford and Cincinnati Schools of Medicine. He has been in private practice for over twenty-five years and currently, maintains an active, solo, obstetric-gynecology practice in California.

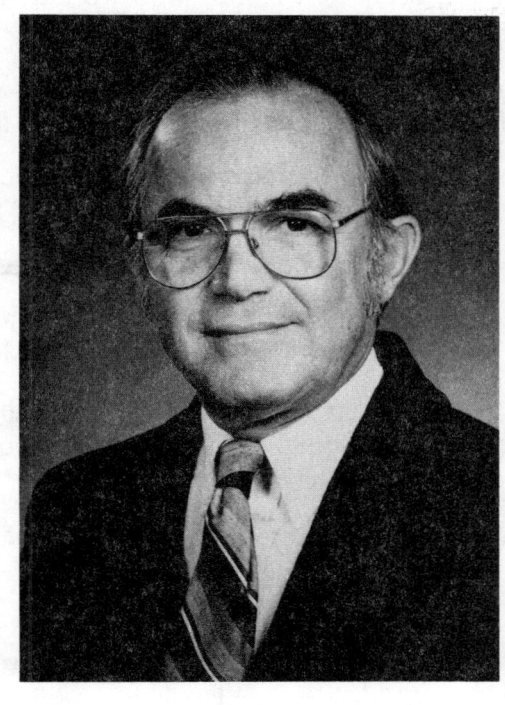

He is a member of the American College of Obstetricians and Gynecologists, the American College of Surgeons, the American Medical Association, the California Medical Association and the Union of American Physicians and Dentists. Because of his concern for the welfare of his fellow man and because of his strong belief that AIDS is man's greatest threat to his very survival, he has managed to write this book. Dr. Anagnoston is a busy clinician, not an author, but he felt obligated to at least try to warn his country and people about what he sees and foresees the lethal AIDS virus is and will do to the peoples of planet earth.

Dr. Anagnoston has compassion, sympathy and caring for HIV infected people; but he is just as concerned about our HIV free pregnant women and the babies they are carrying, our HIV free health care workers, our nation and its millions of HIV free people and, most importantly, the very survival of mankind itself. It is our HIV free people, who must be protected from the killer AIDS virus; because it is they who work and pay the taxes which keeps our nation alive, well, free and strong.

Because of these concerns, he has written "Surviving the Aids Plague." The goals of his book are six-fold:

1. To help inform and educate people about the HIV and the disease it causes, AIDS.

2. To help people protect themselves from the deadly HIV virus.

3. To encourage and help unfortunate HIV infected people to stay alive, until a cure for AIDS is hopefully found.

4. To help people see and foresee the problem AIDS is and will cause socially, financially, and politically – so they can better survive today and tomorrow.

5. To warn people, all peoples of the world, that the AIDS disease is global and can infect anybody, anytime and anyplace.

6. To give notice to all peoples that mankind is at war with the AIDS virus and that his very survival on this depends on whether he wins or loses this war – this is a truism that cannot be ignored!

Dr. Anagnoston urges all Americans to work together, along with the other people of the world, to find a cure for the killer AIDS disease. Meanwhile, he urges people to learn all they can about the deadly HIV and the AIDS disease, to know and follow the recommended precautions, which help avoid the HIV infection, and to question all AIDS information before they believe and/or follow it.

Lastly, anybody reading "Surviving the AIDS Plague" should have more insight of the problem AIDS is and will cause and thus have a better chance of surviving the "plague of plagues" – AIDS.

AIDS

THE LAST GREAT PLAGUE
by Sananda, Hatonn, Ashtar, Nikola Tesla & Walter Russell

This book TRUTHFULLY ASSESSES the AIDS crisis. You will learn the shocking truth about the World Health Organization's (WHO) DIRECT involvement in the spread of AIDS world-wide as well as the U.S. Public Health Service's DIRECT involvement with the spread of AIDS in the U.S. You will learn how the experimentation of animal retroviruses in humans, namely Bovine (cow) Leukemia virus and Visna virus (Brain rot of sheep) were combined to create the deadly AIDS virus and so why the African Green Monkey Theory is totally dispelled. You will learn WHY condoms offer NO protection from AIDS and WHY the vaccine option will not work since recombinant retroviruses replicate at least 9000 to the 4th power which means every AIDS virus diagnosed to date is <u>different</u> with each individual! Other questions answered herein are WHY would anyone perpetrate such evil upon humanity? And **who** is responsible for this horrible disease? What OTHER viruses are THEY dumping on mankind?

This disturbing report may leave you in shock. Where is the HOPE? There IS hope with knowledge of TRUTH and UNITY, mankind can stop the spread of AIDS. AIDS will NOT die out naturally, so we are being given clues for cures of this disease and OTHER diseases as well. From the work of Dr. Royal R. Rife we learn about electromagnetics and SEM waves, since viruses are crystalline structures they are therefore affected by sound vibrations and light. Walter Russell speaks about the "secret" of light, about electricity, octaves and atomic structures. You will learn about the works of Bruce Cathie, John Crane and Nikola Tesla. Remember, there is assistance coming from God and our Heavenly Hosts. It is up to mankind to take the necessary steps with the tools and "clues" provided. Will YOU join us?

The following quote by Dr. Michael Urban, Ph. D.:

"AIDS is the most electrifying, terrifying, exaggerated, hyped, misunderstood and misrepresented disease of modern time."

CHAOS IN AMERICA
by Dr. John L. King
$11.95 . . . Trade Paper . . . ISBN:0-922356-24-6

John L. King, author of *How to Profit from the Next Great Depression,"* was accused of being too gloomy and negative about the future of our economy. If anything, his research convinced him that HE HAD UNDERESTIMATED THE CRISIS WE FACE! Some examples about what YOU should be preparing for:

- As our banking system collapses, your bank will close its doors—permanently! The government will not be able to bail the system out! Depositors could be paid off with pennies on the dollar—despite government "insurance."
- This will create a devastating credit collapse and deflation!
- The value of your home—and of real estate across the country—will be devastated, perhaps worth as little as ten cents on the dollar within a couple of years!
- The stock market will crash to levels not seen since the Great Depression. In inflation-adjusted terms, the Dow will end up where it was in 1933, when it fell as low as 41!
- Short-term interest rates will climb as high as 40%!
- At least temporarily, gold and silver prices will soar—gold to $2000 an ounce and silver to more than $100 an ounce!

And that is just the beginning! The simple truth is: We are facing an economic crisis of unimaginable proportions—a period of swift and steep economic decline that will completely alter the world we live in. *Chaos in America* also teaches about both history and economics. Learn how to survive and prosper despite the Chaos. Dr. King will share 3 investments where your money will be safe; where to live during depression; what to do about real estate; what goods to stockpile, starting now; what to do about energy shortages and self-defense and much more!

SPIRAL TO ECONOMIC DISASTER
LIFEBOAT MEASURES - IF YOU ACT NOW
by Gyeorgos Ceres Hatonn

Waking-up to some economic realities. Exposing the "grey-men" and the secret government, their manipulations from a historical perspective, the degree of their diabolical capabilities, and the perfection of their plan on the unsuspecting "masses". Depression imminent. Get ready, it is coming down fast. New currency and some solutions for not getting caught in the new money and debit card system. Get your hands on cash (under 50s) and stash it (not in a bank). Financial strategies across the board. The solution of Incorporation (for everyone). The Nevada secret. Prophecies of these times previously given. Sananda and Aton state 'how it will be'.

RAPE OF THE CONSTITUTION; DEATH OF FREEDOM RRPP-VOL. II
by Gyeorgos Ceres Hatonn

As you journey through this passage, this may well be the most important single Journal you will ever read. It is of physical importance and impacts your soul growth tremendously, that which you do in this cycle of experience. This book is not pleasant--it was not written for entertainment; you are on the edge of the abyss in your nation and the "anti-Christ", of which you have waited, is upon you. Rarely are things as you expect or at first perceive for it is the way of the enemy of Godness.

You ask and again ask, "What can I do?" Herein we tell you that which you can do. The time for letting "someone else" do of your work is finished--you will stand forth and participate in the journey of God or you will be passed by. Your Constitutional rights as written by the Founding Fathers are being replaced by the New Constitution which is already in operation without your realization of same.

You have a right and obligation to know that which is in store for you at the hands of the conspirators for The New World Order, and further obligation as a citizen, to act. You have been people of the lie far too long, my friends, and it has all but cost you every vestige of freedom. What you do now can change your world. Do nothing, and you had better increase your prayer time, for it is serious indeed. The projected prophecies are at your door and it is time you recognize your enemy!